T0259499

Cardiovascular Diseases

Editor

ROBERT D. SHEELER

PRIMARY CARE:
CLINICS IN OFFICE PRACTICE

www.primarycare.theclinics.com

Consulting Editor
JOEL J. HEIDELBAUGH

March 2013 • Volume 40 • Number 1

ELSEVIER

1600 John F. Kennedy Boulevard • Suite 1800 • Philadelphia, Pennsylvania, 19103-2899

http://www.theclinics.com

PRIMARY CARE: CLINICS IN OFFICE PRACTICE Volume 40, Number 1
March 2013 ISSN 0095-4543, ISBN-13: 978-1-4557-7144-8

Editor: Yonah Korngold

Primary Care: Clinics in Office Practice (ISSN: 0095–4543) is published quarterly by Elsevier Inc., 360 Park Avenue South, New York, NY 10010-1710. Months of issue are March, June, September, and December. Periodicals postage paid at New York, NY and additional mailing offices. Subscription prices are $216.00 per year (US individuals), $353.00 (US institutions), $108.00 (US students), $264.00 (Canadian individuals), $415.00 (Canadian institutions), $169.00 (Canadian students), $329.00 (international individuals), $415.00 (international institutions), and $169.00 (international students). Foreign air speed delivery is included in all *Clinics* subscription prices. All prices are subject to change without notice. POSTMASTER: Send address changes to *Primary Care: Clinics in Office Practice*, Elsevier Periodicals Customer Service, 11830 Westline Industrial Drive, St. Louis, MO 63146. Customer Service Health Sciences Division, Subscription Customer Service, 3251 Riverport Lane, Maryland Heights, MO 63043. **Customer Service: 1-800-654-2452 (U.S. and Canada); 314-447-8871 (outside U.S. and Canada). Fax: 314-447-8029. E-mail: journalscustomerservice-usa@elsevier.com (for print support); journalsonlinesupport-usa@elsevier.com (for online support).**

Reprints. For copies of 100 or more, of articles in this publication, please contact the Commercial Reprints Department, Elsevier Inc., 360 Park Avenue South, New York, NY 10010-1710. Tel. (212) 633-3812; Fax: (212) 482-1935; E-mail: reprints@elsevier.com.

Primary Care: Clinics in Office Practice is covered in *MEDLINE/PubMed (Index Medicus)* and *EMBASE/ Excerpta Medica, Current Contents/Clinical Medicine,* and *ISI/BIOMED.*

Printed and bound by CPI Group (UK) Ltd, Croydon, CR0 4YY

Transferred to digital print 2012

Contributors

CONSULTING EDITOR

JOEL J. HEIDELBAUGH, MD, FAAFP, FACG
Clinical Associate Professor, Departments of Family Medicine and Urology, Clerkship
Director, Department of Family Medicine, University of Michigan Medical School,
Ann Arbor, Michigan; Ypsilanti Health Center, Ypsilanti, Michigan

EDITOR

ROBERT D. SHEELER, MD
Consultant, Department of Family Medicine, Mayo Medical School, Rochester, Minnesota

AUTHORS

AKOCHI O. AGUNWAMBA, MD
Department of Family Medicine, Mayo Clinic, Rochester, Minnesota

JACK ANSELL, MD
Chairman, Department of Medicine, Lenox Hill Hospital, New York, New York

SANDRA L. ARGENIO, MD
Department of Family Medicine, Mayo Clinic, Jacksonville, Florida

DAVID S. BACH, MD
Professor, Department of Internal Medicine, Park W. Willis III Collegiate Professor of
Cardiovascular Medicine, University of Michigan, Ann Arbor, Michigan

BARRY E. BLESKE, PharmD
Associate Professor, Department of Clinical and Social Administrative Services, College of
Pharmacy, University of Michigan, Ann Arbor, Michigan

BRUCE BURNETT, MD, FACP
Medical Director, Thrombosis and Anticoagulation Services, Park Nicollet Clinic, St Louis
Park, Minnesota

WILLIAM E. CHAVEY, MD, MS
Associate Professor, Departments of Family Medicine and Emergency Medicine,
University of Michigan Medical School, Ann Arbor, Michigan

EDMUND P. COYNE, MD, FACC
Consultant Cardiologist, Cardiovascular Medicine, PC, Davenport, Iowa

CHRISTOPHER DITTUS, DO, MPH
Chief Medical Resident, Department of Medicine, Lenox Hill Hospital, New York,
New York

TRAVIS M. DUMONT, MD
Endovascular Surgical Neuroradiology Fellow, Department of Neurosurgery, Gates Vascular Institute, Kaleida Health, School of Medicine and Biomedical Sciences, University at Buffalo, State University of New York, Buffalo, New York

GRANT T. FANKHAUSER, MD
Department of Vascular Surgery, Mayo Clinic, Scottsdale, Arizona

MOHAMMAD TARIQ FAREED, MD, FAAFP
Department of Family Medicine, Mayo Clinic, Rochester, Minnesota

RAMIL GOEL, MD
Department of Cardiovascular Disease, Mayo Clinic, Scottsdale, Arizona

MICHELE A. HANSON, MD, FAAFP
Assistant Professor, Department of Family Medicine, Mayo Clinic, Rochester, Minnesota

TERESA R. HANSON
Creighton University School of Medicine, Omaha, Nebraska

ADAM S. HELMS, MD
Clinical Lecturer, Department of Internal Medicine, University of Michigan Health System, Ann Arbor, Michigan

ROBERT V. HOGIKYAN, MD, MPH
Associate Professor, Department of Internal Medicine, Division of Geriatrics and Palliative Medicine, University of Michigan, Ann Arbor, Michigan

TAREQ KASS-HOUT, MD
Stroke Neurology Fellow, Department of Neurology, Emory University, Atlanta, Georgia

YEONG KWOK, MD
Assistant Professor, Department of Internal Medicine, Division of General Medicine, University of Michigan, Ann arbor, Michigan

ELAD I. LEVY, MD, FACS, FAHA
Professor, Departments of Neurosurgery and Radiology, Gates Vascular Institute, Kaleida Health, Toshiba Stroke Research Center, School of Medicine and Biomedical Sciences, University at Buffalo, State University of New York, Buffalo, New York

MAXIM MOKIN, MD, PhD
Endovascular Surgical Neuroradiology Fellow, Department of Neurosurgery, Gates Vascular Institute, Kaleida Health, School of Medicine and Biomedical Sciences, University at Buffalo, State University of New York, Buffalo, New York

MARTINA MOOKADAM, MD
Department of Family Medicine, Mayo Clinic, Scottsdale, Arizona

ROBERT H. NELSON, MD
Assistant Professor of Medicine, Division of Endocrinology; Assistant Professor of Family Medicine, Mayo College of Medicine, Mayo Clinic, Rochester, Minnesota

JOHN M. NICKLAS, MD, FACC, FAHA
Associate Professor, Department of Internal Medicine, Division of Cardiovascular Medicine, University of Michigan, Ann Arbor, Michigan

RAFAT F. PADARIA, MD, FACC
Consultant Cardiologist, Cardiovascular Medicine, PC, Davenport, Iowa

NICOLAS W. SHAMMAS, MD, EJD, MS, FACC, FSCAI
Founder and Research Director, Midwest Cardiovascular Research Foundation; Adjunct Clinical Associate Professor of Medicine, University of Iowa; Consultant Cardiologist, Cardiovascular Medicine, PC, Davenport, Iowa

FADI ELIAS SHAMOUN, MD, FACC
Department of Carviovascular Medicine, Mayo Clinic, Scottsdale, Arizona

JOSE A. SILVA, MD
Department of Cardiology, John Ochsner Heart and Vascular Institute, Ochsner Clinic Foundation, New Orleans, Louisiana

KOMANDOOR SRIVATHSAN, MD
Department of Cardiovascular Disease, Mayo Clinic, Scottsdale, Arizona

LAURA A. TUTTLE, MA
Clinical Research Specialist, Department of Family Medicine, University of North Carolina at Chapel Hill, Chapel Hill, North Carolina

RICHARD VAN HARRISON, PhD
Professor, Department of Medical Education, University of Michigan, Ann Arbor, Michigan

ANTHONY J. VIERA, MD, MPH
Associate Professor, Department of Family Medicine, University of North Carolina at Chapel Hill, Chapel Hill, North Carolina

CHRISTOPHER J. WHITE, MD
Professor of Medicine and System Chairman of Cardiology, Department of Cardiology, John Ochsner Heart and Vascular Institute, Ochsner Clinic Foundation, New Orleans, Louisiana

KATHERINE H. WINTER, MD, MPH
Family Medicine Resident, Department of Family Medicine, University of North Carolina at Chapel Hill, Chapel Hill, North Carolina

Contents

> Coronary artery disease (CAD) is the leading cause of death worldwide. There are several presenting clinical syndromes, including sudden cardiac death. Risk factor analysis can help the primary care provider identify patients who may need more extensive evaluation or treatment. Treatment may be medical or surgical and depends on the individual patient's comorbidities and preferences. In the future, growth of new blood vessels or cardiac cells may aid in the treatment of CAD.

> Heart failure (HF) often presents as dyspnea either with exertion and/or recumbency. Patients also experience dependent swelling and fatigue. Measurement of the left ventricular ejection fraction (LVEF) identifies HF patients who may respond to pharmacologic therapy and/or electrophysiologic device implantation. Angiotension converting enzyme inhibitors, beta blockers, and aldosterone inhibitors can significantly lower the mortality and morbidity of HF in patients with an LVEF less than 35%. Cardiac defibrillators and biventricular pacemakers can also improve outcomes in selected patients with a decreased LVEF. The authors provide a guide for therapeutic decisions based on the inclusion criteria of the major clinical trials.

> Cardiac arrhythmias comprise of a heterogenous group of disorders which manifest in a wide range of clinical presentations. They can be associated with underlying cardiac disease and portend a grave prognosis, with some arrhythmias being rapidly fatal. Other arrhythmias, however are relatively benign and can be asymptomatic or may be a mere inconvenience for the patient. All primary care physicians can expect to encounter some forms of arrhythmias during the course of their practice. This review article provides a brief overview of the commonly seen tachyarrhythmias for the general practitioner and provides relevant updates on the recent developments in our understanding of their mechanisms and management.

bowel disease is difficult to determine, acute mesenteric ischemia (AMI) has been reported to cause in 1 in 1000 hospital admissions, whereas chronic mesenteric ischemia (CMI) is estimated to affect 1 in 100,000 individuals. Mesenteric ischemia generally manifests in its chronic form as postprandial abdominal pain resulting in significant weight loss, and in its acute form as an abrupt development of abdominal pain, lower gastrointestinal bleeding, and subsequent intestinal necrosis. This article discusses the cause, clinical manifestations, diagnosis, and management of AMI and CMI.

The medical management of patients with an abdominal aortic aneurysm (AAA) includes modification of risk factors, smoking cessation, cardiovascular risk treatment, and hypertensive therapy. No specific therapy has been shown to alter disease outcome. Many AAA and thoracic aortic aneurysms are amenable to endovascular treatment. Endovascular repair offers the benefit of shorter hospital stays and lower perioperative morbidity and mortality. Most patients with peripheral arterial disease (PAD) are asymptomatic or have atypical symptoms; only a few present with classic intermittent claudication or critical limb ischemia. Smoking and diabetes mellitus are the most important risk factors for developing PAD.

Hypertension is the most common modifiable risk factor for cardiovascular disease. Antihypertensive treatment substantially reduces the risk of heart failure, stroke, and myocardial infarction. Current guidelines recommend screening all adults for high blood pressure (BP). Lifestyle modifications to help control high BP include weight loss, exercise, moderation of alcohol intake, and a diet low in sodium and saturated fats and high in fruits and vegetables. Out-of-office BP monitoring should be used to confirm suspected white coat effect, especially in patients with apparent resistant hypertension.

Elevated levels of blood lipids are well-documented risk factors for cardiovascular disease. Current classification schemes and treatment levels for hyperlipidemia are based on the National Cholesterol Education Panel's Adult Treatment Program-3 (ATP-III) guidelines. Extensive research over the past decade has raised the question whether or not ATP-III guidelines are sufficiently aggressive. New guidelines from ATP-IV are expected to be released in the near future, but in the meantime physicians are faced with uncertainty about how low to target low-density lipoprotein cholesterol, whether to pharmacologically treat high-density lipoprotein cholesterol and triglyceride levels, and how best to achieve target goals.

PRIMARY CARE:
CLINICS IN OFFICE PRACTICE

Foreword

"Life Ticks Away Faster Every Day"

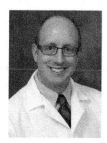

Joel J. Heidelbaugh, MD, FAAFP, FACG
Consulting Editor

As the promise of dramatic health care reform approaches a practical reality, we are thrust into a deeper responsibility of minimizing morbidity and mortality from the greatest killer of both men and women in the United States: cardiovascular diseases. The role of the primary care clinician in the diagnosis and management of these conditions will continue to have greater importance and influence, as we will be increasingly held accountable by insurance payors for financial incentives, and disincentives for poor outcomes.

This volume of *Primary Care: Clinics in Office Practice* provides a diverse array of articles on topics related to cardiovascular diseases. They provide the harrowing statistics on the prevalence of hypertension, hyperlipidemia, acute coronary syndrome, and other common diseases that primary care clinicians encounter. Impressively, the authors provide subtle details on the diagnosis of atypical presentations of common cardiovascular disorders. Significant attention is given to pharmacotherapy of cardiovascular conditions, including options for anticoagulation. Moreover, a look toward the promise of novel genetic markers and new laboratory tests provide additional knowledge for inquisitive clinicians.

Although our lives and those of our patients may seem to tick away faster every day, the optimism of decreasing the burden of cardiovascular diseases depends on our ability to integrate new knowledge of pharmacotherapy and innovative testing and techniques in daily practice. Dr Robert Sheeler and his colleagues deserve tremendous adulation and respect for their efforts in compiling a timely, evidence-based, and invaluable resource for primary care clinicians to aid in improving the cardiovascular health of our patients. In this rapidly evolving field of medicine, this collection is both unique in breadth and important in scope regarding preventive medicine and advancing technology.

Prim Care Clin Office Pract 40 (2013) xiii–xiv
http://dx.doi.org/10.1016/j.pop.2012.12.002
0095-4543/13/$ – see front matter © 2013 Published by Elsevier Inc.

primarycare.theclinics.com

I encourage clinicians at all levels and across all specialties to review this volume with the same enthusiasm and passion that initially led them to improving the life and longevity of their patients.

Joel J. Heidelbaugh, MD, FAAFP, FACG
Departments of Family Medicine and Urology
University of Michigan Medical School
Ann Arbor, MI 48109, USA

Ypsilanti Health Center
200 Arnet Suite 200
Ypsilanti, MI 48198, USA

E-mail address:
jheidel@umich.edu

Preface

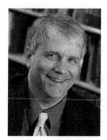

Robert D. Sheeler, MD
Editor

Cardiovascular medicine is one of the most highly evolved clinical fields in the practice of medicine based on a strong commitment in the field to the analysis of outcomes of large, well-designed clinical trials. At the same time, the field continues to advance along many fronts from basic science at the cellular level to the interpretation and application of technical procedural studies. The degree to which the specialty will question even its basic assumptions and dogma to advance the science has been exemplary. The real beneficiaries of this are the millions of patients worldwide who live longer and healthier lives from both the aversion of cardiovascular disease and the treatment of its myriad manifestations.

In primary care we have the benefit of a rapidly evolving pharmacologic armamentarium to both preserve the health of blood vessels and the heart and treat diseases. Atherosclerotic diseases of multiple vascular beds are becoming all too common because of our sedentary office-based and couch-based lifestyles. The manifestations of the typical presentations of common diseases are well known to the practitioners and too much of the public at large. However, atypical presentations and presentations in complex areas such as the abdomen where symptoms may be masked or mistaken for other disease states remain a substantial diagnostic challenge to the clinician and a hazard to the patient.

To get superb outcomes, physicians at the front line of medical practice in primary care practice need to have a solid map of the territory they are helping their patients to navigate. This can be difficult when a field as broad as cardiovascular medicine continues to evolve rapidly along many fronts simultaneously. This can be accomplished in part by strong referral and consulting relationships where primary care doctors have continuous access to the knowledge and expertise of local specialists and co-manage a variety of cases together. This provides the specialist the needed practice base and the primary care doctor both access to the most up-to-date care for his or her patients and fosters continuous learning. To gain the most benefit from such a consulting relationship, the primary care provider needs to have an up-to-date working knowledge of the field to ask the right questions and to educate their patients about the risks, benefits, and choices. A current volume such as this issue can provide a detailed yet highly efficient overview of the state of the art.

Prim Care Clin Office Pract 40 (2013) xv–xvi
http://dx.doi.org/10.1016/j.pop.2012.12.003
0095-4543/13/$ – see front matter © 2013 Published by Elsevier Inc.

As the biotechnology revolution continues, the degree to which targeted therapy will be available at the cellular pharmacologic level will increase rapidly. This will return more therapy to primary providers when it is the pill rather than the procedure that reaches the most precise target. To gain the benefits for their patients and their practices, primary care providers will need to stay current on both the standards of care and the rapid transformation of the practice of today to the practice of tomorrow. They are at a unique vantage to help their patients bridge this technology gap by providing a human face that encourages relationship-centered patient-driven care, which fosters allowing patients to make prudent choices.

I was incredibly fortunate to have a number of leading specialists in a wide variety of cardiovascular disciplines agree to write articles for this issue. Their work spans many aspects of the field and provides leading-edge information combined with distilled wisdom in the practice of cardiovascular medicine. I was truly impressed by their commitment to provide information that was concise, up to the minute, and pragmatic in such a clear manner. This issue relies on their substantial accumulated knowledge as well as the latest research and should be of great value to those in primary care who take the time to read and study this material. It is so well written that it should also be of value to cardiologists and other specialists as an overview of the latest materials in the field.

Robert D. Sheeler, MD
Department of Family Medicine
Mayo Medical School
200 First Street SW
Rochester, MN 55905, USA

E-mail address:
sheeler.robert@mayo.edu

Coronary Artery Disease

Michele A. Hanson, MD[a],*, Mohammad Tariq Fareed, MD[a],
Sandra L. Argenio, MD[b], Akochi O. Agunwamba, MD[a],
Teresa R. Hanson[c]

KEYWORDS

- Angina • Aspirin • Ischemia • Troponin

KEY POINTS

- Coronary artery disease (CAD) is the leading cause of death worldwide.
- Diagnosis of acute myocardial infarction (MI) is made when there is typical rise and fall in levels of biomarkers of myocardial necrosis, troponin and creatine kinase-MB (CK-MB), plus at least one or more of the following:
  - Symptoms of myocardial ischemia
  - Ischemic electrocardiographic (ECG) changes (ST segment ↑/↓)
  - Development of pathologic Q waves (ECG)
  - Imaging evidence of new loss of viable myocardium or new regional wall motion abnormalities (RWMA)[3]
- Risk factor analysis can help the primary care provider identify patients who may need more extensive evaluation or treatment.
- Treatment may be medical or surgical and depends on the individual patient's comorbidities and preferences.
- In the future, growth of new blood vessels or cardiac cells may aid in the treatment of CAD.

CAD is the leading cause of death worldwide. Approximately every 25 seconds, an American will have a coronary event, and approximately every 1 minute someone will die of one.[1] CAD refers to the pathologic process of atherosclerosis affecting the coronary arteries. CAD includes a spectrum of diagnoses including angina pectoris, MI, silent myocardial ischemia, and sudden cardiac death.

EPIDEMIOLOGY

- CAD is responsible for approximately one-third of all deaths in individuals older than 35 years.

---

[a] Department of Family Medicine, Mayo Clinic, 200 First Street Southwest, Rochester, MN 55905, USA; [b] Department of Family Medicine, Mayo Clinic, 4500 San Pablo Road, Jacksonville, FL 32224, USA; [c] Creighton University School of Medicine, 2500 California Plaza, Omaha, NE 68178, USA
* Corresponding author.
E-mail address: hanson.michele@mayo.edu

Prim Care Clin Office Pract 40 (2013) 1–16
http://dx.doi.org/10.1016/j.pop.2012.12.001
0095-4543/13/$ – see front matter © 2013 Elsevier Inc. All rights reserved.

- Nearly half of all middle-aged men and one-third of all middle-aged women in the United States develop some manifestations of CAD.
- In the Framingham Heart Study, the lifetime risk of CAD was studied in 7733 subjects aged 40 to 94 years who were initially free of CAD. The lifetime risk for individuals aged 40 years was 49% for men and 32% for women. At the age of 70 years, the lifetime risk was 35% in men and 25% in women.
- Incidence increases with age with women lagging behind men by 10 years.

CLINICAL PRESENTATIONS
Angina Pectoris

Some patients have stable angina. Low-risk angina typically remains stable for at least 60 days. This fact means that there is no significant change in frequency, duration, precipitating causes, or ease of relief.[2] There should also be no evidence of recent myocardial damage.

High risk or unstable angina (UA) has the following features:

- New occurrence of angina
- Worsening of chronic stable angina pattern with increased frequency or duration of symptoms as well as new triggers and incomplete relief with symptom management
- Evidence of recent myocardial damage
- Symptoms of peripheral vascular disease

Patients with UA should be referred to cardiology for further evaluation.

Acute Coronary Syndrome

The classical symptoms include chest pain and diaphoresis; however, upper abdominal pain, back pain, throat/jaw pain, and arm pain may also occur. There may also be gastrointestinal (GI) symptoms such as nausea, fullness, pressure, or gas. Patients may also complain of shortness of breath or dizziness. Prompt recognition is critical. Emergency room evaluation is often necessary with cardiology consultation if there is evidence of myocardial damage or dysfunction.

Diagnosis of acute MI is made when there is a typical rise and fall in the levels of biomarkers of myocardial necrosis, troponin and CK-MB, plus at least one or more of the following:

- Symptoms of myocardial ischemia
- Ischemic ECG changes (ST segment ↑/↓)
- Development of pathologic Q waves (ECG)
- Imaging evidence of new loss of viable myocardium or new RWMA[3]

Fig. 1 shows the typical pattern of biomarkers in acute MI.

As seen in the figure, with reperfusion therapy for acute MI, with either thrombolysis or angioplasty, coronary perfusion is restored and the marker levels peak higher and earlier with more rapid washout declines when compared with the nonreperfused state.[4]

Cardiac biomarkers may be elevated without acute coronary syndrome. Levels of CK-MB may be elevated with skeletal myopathy/trauma, cardiac trauma, myocarditis, severe hypothyroidism, seizures, cardioversion/defibrillation, or renal failure. Troponin T levels are elevated with many of the preceding states as well as in heart failure, pulmonary embolism, demand ischemia, coronary angioplasty, or myocardial infiltration.

The differential of acute chest pain includes acute coronary syndrome, aortic dissection, pulmonary embolism, pericarditis, GI problems such as gastroesophageal

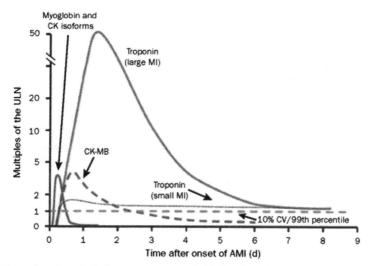

Fig. 1. Biomarkers trends during acute myocardial infarction. AMI, acute myocardial infarction; CV, cardiovascular; ULN, upper limits of normal. (*From* Kumar A, Cannon CP. Acute coronary syndromes: diagnosis and management, part I. Mayo Clin Proc 2009;84:917–38; with permission.)

reflux disease, peptic ulcer disease , or biliary problems and finally musculoskeletal causes.

The ECG changes are essential in the diagnosis, localization, risk stratification, and management of acute coronary syndromes. Acute infarctions are now subdivided into ST-elevation MI (STEMI) and non–ST-elevation MI (NSTEMI). STEMI indicates a transmural infarct in evolution, whereas NSTEMI is usually subendocardial. Pathologic Q waves usually develop after STEMI, but they may also occur after NSTEMI. UA is often associated with ischemic T-wave inversion and some ST-segment depression during acute symptoms, but levels of biomarkers do not increase significantly (**Fig. 2**).

Fig. 3 shows the examples of ECG findings in both ST-elevation and non–ST elevation acute MI.

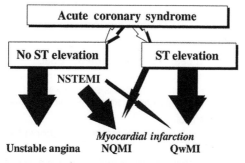

Fig. 2. Types of acute coronary syndromes. NQMI, Non Q-wave myocardial infarction; QwMI, Q-wave myocardial infarction. (*Adapted from* Antman EM, Braunwald E. Acute myocardial infarction. In: Braunwald EB, editor. Heart disease: a textbook of cardiovascular medicine. Philadelphia: WB Saunders; 1997; with permission.)

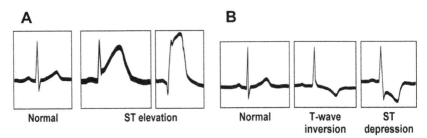

Fig. 3. ECG examples of cardiac ischemia (*A*) STEMI. (*B*) NSTEMI. (*Courtesy of* William Freeman, MD, Rochester, MN.)

Silent Myocardial Ischemia

Some patients have no known event but are found to have ECG evidence of previous myocardial damage. It has been estimated that between 2% and 4% of healthy asymptomatic middle-aged men have significant CAD. If they have 2 or more major coronary risk factors, the prevalence may approach 10%.[5] Silent ischemia is more likely to occur in persons with diabetics, older adults, and those with prior MI or revascularization procedures. This condition is more likely to occur in patients with diabetes mellitus. Additional evaluation of the current cardiac status of such persons may be necessary to optimize their ongoing care.

Sudden Cardiac Death

In some patients, the first manifestation of CAD is sudden cardiac death. Ideally, recognizing those at risk for CAD would help identify such individuals and decrease the incidence of this ominous presentation.

The presentation of CAD in women can be somewhat confusing. Even though cardiovascular disease is the leading cause of death in women, many women—and sometimes even their health care providers—do not consider heart disease when they develop symptoms. Also, women are more likely to have less-typical symptoms such as shortness of breath, vomiting, or jaw pain. Women are also likely to delay seeking treatment.[6]

RISK FACTORS

There are some nonmodifiable risk factors for CAD such as male sex and family history of CAD. However, there are several risk factors that can be managed through lifestyle and medication management such as

- Tobacco use—smoking cessation should be the goal.
- Hyperlipidemia—identification and treatment can improve outcome. Treatment should include lifestyle recommendations as well as medication if indicated.
- Hypertension—again, there should be an emphasis on lifestyle with medications to achieve optimum control.
- Diabetes mellitus—this is a major risk factor and is considered to be a coronary heart disease equivalent.
- Obesity—this needs lifestyle management, with a smaller role for medical and possible surgical intervention
- Sedentary lifestyle—the American College of Cardiology endorses a minimum of 30 to 60 minutes of aerobic activity most days of the week.

There are some additional historical factors that may need to be considered such as history of hormone replacement therapy. There are some emerging risk factors that are being identified and may be useful to evaluate in some patients. Typical items present in a novel cardiac profile include evaluation of lipoprotein (a), highly sensitive C-reactive protein, fibrinogen, and homocysteine. If patients have any of these risk factors, they may want to consider more aggressive therapy such as the earlier addition of medication to lifestyle management of hyperlipidemia.

DIAGNOSIS OF CAD

The gold standard test for diagnosing CAD has been cardiac catheterization with angiogram. This is obviously an invasive test that is not used first line. There are several tests that can help the primary care provider determine whether or not the patient with symptoms suggesting CAD does indeed have CAD.

ECG

ECG is the most commonly performed cardiac test. This test shows the rhythm and rate of the heart at that point in time. In the acute situation, the ECG may show changes that suggest ischemia such as ST elevation. There may also be evidence of old MI with Q waves present. If the heart is not under any stress, patients may have normal result of ECG even if they have CAD.

Stress Tests

The treadmill exercise stress test (TMET) or exercise stress test can be done to evaluate the heart during exercise. ECG and blood pressure (BP) monitoring are done while a patient exercises. Evidence of CAD may only be present in situations when the heart is being challenged. A patient may develop angina during the test, or there may be changes in ECG or BP suggesting cardiac ischemia.

Patients may develop exertional hypotension or hypertension. The decrease in BP during exertion to values lower than the resting systolic pressure is called exertional hypotension. The finding often indicates severe heart failure or multivessel CAD.[7] Other causes of hypotension include fixed cardiac output, which occurs with stenotic valvular disease and hypertrophic cardiomyopathy, volume depletion, and certain drugs such as vasodilators. The test should be stopped if hypotension occurs.

Exertional hypertension may also occur. This condition is defined as a peak systolic pressure greater than 210 mm Hg in men and greater than 190 mm Hg in women. A normotensive patient with a hypertensive response is more likely to develop hypertension.[8] Exertional hypertension is not typically as worrisome as exertional hypotension during TMET.

Sometimes a patient is physically unable to exercise because of orthopedic or medical issues. In these cases, the heart may be chemically stimulated with a medication to mimic the effects that would be obtained if the patient were able to exercise. Dobutamine is a medication that is often used for chemical stress tests.

A stress echocardiogram is another option for assessing the potential of cardiac dysfunction during exercise testing. If any area of myocardium is compromised during exercise, the echo may show reduced or absent muscle wall activity.

Myocardial Perfusion Imaging

Thallium and sestamibi scans are tests that can show how well blood is flowing to various portions of the heart. These tests are typically done with a stress test. The radioactive substance is injected through a vein, and a special camera takes images.

Normal myocardium takes up more thallium/sestamibi than myocardium being supplied by a blocked or partially blocked coronary artery. Ideally, these tests are done with a patient actively exercising. However, if the patient is unable to exercise, pharmacologic agents can be used such as dipyridamole, dobutamine, or adenosine (Adenoscan). Adenosine is preferred because of a very short half-life, rapid reversal, and more predictable vasodilation.[9]

Multiple-Gated Acquisition Scan

The multiple-gated acquisition (MUGA) scan is basically a radionuclide angiogram. A radioactive substance, technetium 99, is attached to patients' red blood cells. These blood cells are then injected into the patients' bloodstream. A gamma camera is then used to take images of the beating heart. This technique is useful in obtaining an accurate left ventricular ejection fraction (LVEF). The MUGA scan can also identify areas of the heart that may have been previously damaged.

Coronary Artery Calcium Scans

In CAD, the atheromatous plaques often contain calcium. A cardiac CT scan can be done and the calcium level can be measured. The assumption, then, is that if there is a significant amount of calcium on the scan, there is a higher probability of having CAD. The scoring is based on the Agatson score.[10]

- 0: no identifiable disease
- 1 to 99: mild disease
- 100 to 399: moderate disease
- 400+: severe disease

The coronary calcium scan is most useful in patients in the intermediate risk category for CAD. If patients have been working on aggressive lifestyle management with diet and exercise and have a high score on a coronary calcium scan, they may be more apt to begin medication management with statin therapy to improve their long-term risk of symptomatic CAD.

Cardiac Magnetic Resonance Imaging

Magnetic resonance imaging (MRI) has been a useful modality for examination of the brain, spine, and joints. However, this method has also become useful in diagnosing congenital heart disease, cardiac tumors, and aortic dissection. MRI is being studied in the evaluation of CAD. The challenge has been getting accurate pictures of a moving heart. As technology improves, MRI may become a way to noninvasively examine the coronary arteries, but at this time is not typically used for CAD evaluation.

Cardiac Catheterization and Angiography

The best way to determine if coronary arteries are affected by CAD is to image them directly with angiogram. A catheter is inserted into the blood vessels through the groin, arm, or neck. The catheter is then advanced to the heart. A dye is injected through the heart while a series of radiographs are obtained. This technique gives a moving picture of the heart and coronary arteries. Information can be obtained about the valves and coronary arteries. The LVEF can be estimated and wall motion abnormalities can be analyzed. The angiogram is a diagnostic procedure, but the catheter can be used in multiple therapies such as angioplasty, stenting, or valvuloplasty.

Table 1 reviews the various tests that are available for the evaluation of CAD and compares their advantages and disadvantages.

Table 1
Comparison of cardiac tests

Test	Sensitivity (%)	Specificity (%)	Advantages	Disadvantages
ECG	68	97	Inexpensive	—
Exercise stress test	Males: 68 Females: 31–33	Males: 77 Females: 52–76	Well validated, inexpensive, readily available	Less useful in women or those with atypical presentation
Myocardial perfusion imaging	90	70	High sensitivity	Expensive
Stress echo	76	88	Information of LV mass and valve function	Subjective interpretation
Coronary artery calcium CT	91	46	Adds prognostic value to intermediate risk group	Low specificity
Coronary CT angiography	94	82	Noninvasive	High cost, high radiation exposure, new modality, needs HR control
Cardiovascular MRI	72	97	No radiation or iodine contrast, no need for HR control	High cost, new and limited availability
Cardiac PET	92	85	High sensitivity	New and experimental
Coronary angiogram	—	—	Gold standard	Invasive and expensive

Abbreviations: CT, computed tomography; HR, heart rate; PET, positron emission tomography.
Data from Holman JR. Cardiac Testing. CME Bull 2011 Dec;10(2):1–6.

There are many options for evaluation of an individual's risk for CAD. Not all tests are as readily available at all medical centers, and the evaluation of an individual patient may depend on the availability and expertise at the evaluating center. The first and most important step in assessing a patient for CAD is taking a careful history and reviewing risk factors. Most cardiac testing is reserved for the patient in the intermediate-risk category, which needs more advanced testing to make the diagnosis of CAD.

GENERAL MEDICAL MANAGEMENT OF ACUTE CORONARY SYNDROME

In the absence of contraindications, certain medical therapy should be given immediately to all patients at the time of presentation with an acute coronary syndrome. These therapies include oxygen, aspirin, β-blockers, nitrates, and morphine. Continuous ECG monitoring is recommended to monitor for potentially malignant ventricular arrhythmias or heart block. Heart rate (HR), BP, and O_2 saturation are monitored closely looking for signs of left ventricular (LV) dysfunction or congestive heart failure. Ongoing assessment for symptoms of ischemic pain, dyspnea, and anxiety and measures to decrease these symptoms are performed to reduce myocardial oxygen demand.

Aspirin

Aspirin inhibits platelet aggregation. The recommended acute dose is 162 to 325 mg, chewed to maximize immediate absorption. If there is a documented allergy to aspirin, clopidogrel should be used.

β-Blockers

The most widely used agent is metoprolol given intravenously (IV) for short-term than in oral form. There are multiple pharmacologic effects from β-blockers (**Fig. 4**):
Contraindications to β-blocker therapy in acute MI include

- Cardiogenic shock
- Moderate to severe LV failure
- Second- or third-degree atrioventricular heart block
- Hypotension with systolic BP less than 100 mm Hg
- Sinus bradycardia with HR less than 69
- Severe reactive airway disease

Precautions should be taken in mild LV failure, severe peripheral arterial occlusive disease, and severe chronic obstructive pulmonary disease (nonreactive airway disease).

Nitrates

Nitrates cause smooth muscle relaxation and act in several ways to decrease ischemia. LV preload is reduced. Coronary vasodilatation occurs. Vasospasm is reversed. Nitroglycerin is given sublingually initially and is then often administered IV.

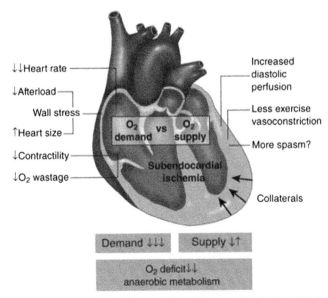

Fig. 4. β-blockade effects on ischemic heart. (*From* Morrow DA, Boden WE. Stable ischemic heart disease. In: Bonow RO, Mann DL, Zipes DP, et al, editors. Braunwald's heart disease - a text-book of cardiovascular medicine. 9th edition. Philadelphia: Elsevier; 2012; with permission. *Modified from* Opie LH. Drugs for the heart. 4th edition. Philadelphia: WB Saunders; 1995.)

Morphine

Morphine is the narcotic given for pain control during an acute MI. This drug is given IV and titrated to decrease pain and as a result decreases patient anxiety by diminishing oxygen demand on the cardiac muscle. Morphine also reduces preload by venodilatory effects.

Oxygen

All patients are given supplemental oxygen during initial evaluation for acute coronary syndrome.

SPECIFIC MANAGEMENT OF ACUTE CORONARY SYNDROMES
Acute MI Management: ST-Elevation MI

Landmark studies in 1980 documented the presence of occlusive intracoronary thrombus in nearly all patients with acute STEMI.[11] As a result of this finding, thrombolytic therapy emerged targeting the acute coronary thrombosis. Streptokinase and tissue plasminogen activators (t-PAs) are used to promote clot breakdown. Percutaneous coronary intervention (PCI) is the most rapid way to achieve reperfusion; however, most hospitals (80%) do not have 24/7 access to immediate PCI.

The algorithm in **Fig. 5** shows the plan of action in STEMI.

If one does not have PCI immediately available, thrombolytic therapy should be initiated. In the global utilization of streptokinase & tissue plasminogen activator for occluded coronary arteries (GUSTO) trial of 1993, t-PA agents were found to be superior to streptokinase.[12] However, all types of thrombolytic reperfusion have had a profound impact on mortality.

Minimizing the time from presentation to thrombolysis can save lives. About 65 lives can be saved for every 1000 patients treated within the first hour of STEMI. These 60 minutes are referred to as "the golden hour" (**Fig. 6**).[13]

In the absence of contraindication, thrombolytic therapy with a t-PA agent should be given to all patients with STEMI and to those with the following features:

- Symptom onset less than 12 hours before presentation
- Ischemic ST-segment elevation of 0.1 mV or more in 2 or more contiguous limb leads or 2 mV or more in 2 or more contiguous precordial leads

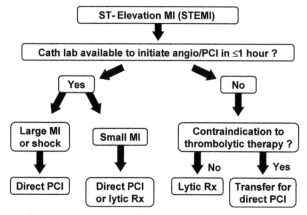

Fig. 5. Algorithm for management of STEMI. Cath lab, catheterization laboratory, Rx, therapy. (*Courtesy of* William Freeman, MD, Rochester, MN.)

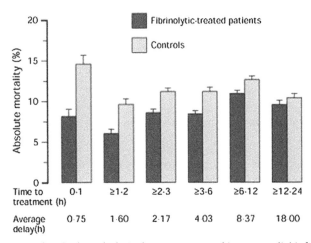

Fig. 6. Comparison of early thrombolytic therapy to control in myocardial infarction. (*From* Boersma E, Maas AC, Deckers JW, et al. Early thrombolytic treatment in acute myocardial infarction: reappraisal of the golden hour. Lancet 1996;348(9030):771–5.)

- Symptoms compatible with acute MI and new or presumably new left bundle branch block

Bleeding complications are the greatest risk with use of thrombolytics. Intracranial hemorrhage is the most serious bleeding complication. Risk factors for intracranial hemorrhage include

- Age greater than 75 years
- Systolic BP of 160 mm Hg or more
- Any prior stroke
- Body weight less than 80 kg (men) or less than 67 kg (women)

The current (2007) American College of Cardiology/American heart Association (ACA/AHA) guidelines for absolute and relative contraindications are as follows: Absolute contraindications for thrombolytic therapy include

- Any prior intracranial bleed
- Ischemic stroke within 3 months
- Active bleeding
- Known intracranial neoplasm (primary or metastatic)
- Head or facial trauma within 3 months
- Suspicion of aortic dissection

Relative contraindication for thrombolytic therapy

- History of prior ischemic stroke of more than 3 months
- Internal bleeding within 1 month
- Systolic BP greater than 180 mm Hg or diastolic BP greater than 100mm Hg
- Major surgery within 3 weeks
- Prolonged cardiopulmonary resuscitation (>10 minutes)
- Active peptic ulcer
- Pregnancy

Timely reperfusion therapy can save the myocardium and decrease mortality.

Other Acute Coronary Syndromes: Unstable Angina (UA) and Non–ST-Segment Elevation MI (NSTEMI)

A clinical risk score for UA and NSTEMI has been derived from the thrombolysis in myocardial infarction (TIMI) trials. Management is directed by the TIMI score.

In general, patients with intermediate to high risk UA or NSTEMI syndromes are evaluated directly with coronary angiography anticipating PCI while stabilizing with medical therapy. These patients have a TIMI score of 3 or more. Patients with low-risk UA and NSTEMI are first stabilized with medical therapy and then risk stratified with stress testing to assess the need for coronary angiography and possible PCI (**Fig. 7**).

MEDICAL MANAGEMENT OF CHRONIC CAD

The primary care provider has several categories of medication that can be used to optimize the care of a patient with CAD.

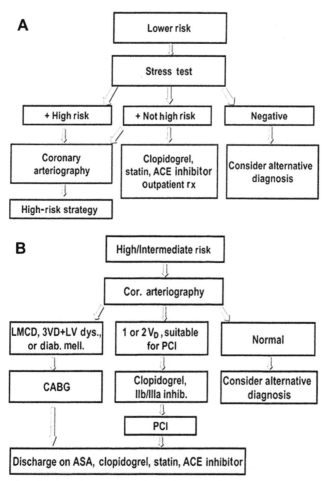

Fig. 7. (*A, B*) Management of UA/NSTEMI. ACE-I; CABG, coronary artery bypass grafting; Cor, coronary; diab. mell, diabetes mellitus; dys, dysfunction; LMCD, left main coronary disease; Rx, therapy; 1 or 2 V_D, 1 or 2 vessel disease; 3VD+ LV dys, 3 vessel disease plus left ventricle dysfunction. (*From* Baunwald E. Cerebrovascular thromboprophylaxis in mice by erythrocyte-coupled tissue-type plasminogen activator. Circulation 2008;118:1442–9; with permission.)

Aspirin

Evidence from basic science and clinical research, epidemiologic studies, and randomized clinical trials have provided strong support for use of aspirin in decreasing the risk of cardiovascular disease events in a wide range of patients. Daily aspirin is used as primary prevention of a first cardiovascular event in individuals at moderate to high risk. Aspirin is used in the treatment of an acute cardiac event as well as for secondary prevention after MI, stroke, transient ischemic attack, or coronary revascularization. The 2006 ACC/AHA guidelines on secondary prevention recommends daily doses of 75–162 mg for secondary prevention.

β-Blockers

The ACC/AHA recommends β-blockers as first-line therapy in the treatment of chronic stable angina, particularly effort-induced angina. Therapeutic goals of β-blocker therapy include

- Reduce frequency of angina
- Reduce severity of angina
- Improve exercise capacity without significant side effects

Cardiovascular effects of β-blockers involve a reduction in myocardial oxygen demand by decreasing HR and contractility. This reduction decreases the LV wall stress and thus decreases the oxygen demand.[14]

β-blockers are generally well tolerated. In patients with reactive airways, β-blockers may cause bronchoconstriction. Some patients may experience worsening of peripheral arterial disease or Raynaud phenomenon. Fatigue is a side effect that may be caused by reduction in cardiac output or by direct effects on the central nervous system. Depression has been mentioned but has not been proven in randomized trials. Men may experience erectile dysfunction.

Angiotensin-Converting Enzyme Inhibitors or Angiotensin Receptor Blockers

Angiotensin-converting enzyme (ACE) inhibitors are recommended for patients with MI, LVEF less than 40%, hypertension, diabetes, or chronic kidney disease. If a patient is intolerant to an ACE inhibitor, an angiotensin receptor blocker may be tried.

ACE inhibitors reduce LV afterload, which is particularly important in patients with large infarcts. ACE inhibitors also enhance coronary microcirculation by promoting endothelium-mediated vasodilation. These actions are helpful in preventing pathologic LV remodeling.

ACE inhibitors are typically started within 24 hours of the acute event after stabilization of hemodynamics. The greatest benefit has been found in patients with an STEMI and LVEF less than 40%. ACE inhibitor therapy has been shown to be additive to the use of aspirin and β-blockers and reduces the rate of recurrent MI, rehospitalization for heart failure, and death.

Nitrates

Nitroglycerin acts as a venodilator, coronary vasodilator, and modest arteriolar dilator. The primary anti-ischemic effect of nitrates is to decrease myocardial oxygen demand by producing more systemic vasodilations than coronary vasodilatation leading to reduction of LV systolic wall stress. In patients with exertional stable angina, nitrates improve exercise tolerance, time to onset of angina, and ST-segment depression during exercise testing. In combination with β-blockers or calcium channel blockers (CCBs), nitrates produce greater antianginal and anti-ischemic effects.

One problem with nitrate use is development of tolerance. Intermittent therapy with an adequate nitrate-free interval is recommended. Common side effects include headache, flushing, and hypotension. Some of the contraindications to nitrate use include hypertrophic cardiomyopathy, right ventricular infarction, severe aortic stenosis, and volume depletion.

There are several commonly used nitrate preparations. Sublingual nitroglycerin is the therapy of choice for acute anginal episodes, and it may be also used prophylactically for activities known to elicit angina. Proper patient education in use of nitroglycerin is essential. Patients need to be aware that nitroglycerin pills degrade with time and may need to be replaced even if they are not used. Isosorbide dinitrate or mononitrate can be used orally. Nitrates can also be administered by transdermal or IV routes.

Calcium Channel Blockers

CCBs are a heterogeneous group of compounds used in a variety of cardiovascular disorders such as stable angina, vasospastic angina, hypertension, hypertrophic cardiomyopathy, and supraventricular arrhythmias. Some of the commonly used CCBs include nifedipine, amlodipine, verapamil, and diltiazem. Nifedipine and amlodipine are in the dihydropyridine group. These medications block slow calcium channels in a dose-dependent manner and vasodilate coronary arteries, reduce coronary resistance, and increase coronary artery blood flow. Verapamil is a negative inotrope and chronotrope. It is effective in angina as it decreases myocardial oxygen demand. Diltiazem is potent coronary but mild arterial vasodilator; therefore it has fewer side effects related to peripheral vasodilatation.

Statin Therapy

Patients with known coronary disease are at high risk for cardiovascular events. Statin therapy has been shown to reduce events and all-cause mortality.[15] Intensive therapy with atorvastatin, 80 mg, daily reduces mortality in patients with acute coronary syndrome. The current recommendation is to start early in the hospital course rather than titrating up in the outpatient setting.[16,17] Starting of statin therapy is recommended regardless of prior lipid levels. The low-density lipoprotein target for those with established disease is less than 70 mg/dL.

PERCUTANEOUS CORONARY INTERVENTION (PCI)

Angioplasty is the technique of mechanically widening narrowed or obstructed arteries. Angioplasty has also been called percutaneous transluminal coronary angioplasty; however, the preferred term at present is percutaneous coronary intervention.

Balloon angioplasty is a procedure in which a balloon catheter is passed over a guide wire to the narrowed blood vessel locations. The balloon is then inflated to 75 to 500 times the normal BP. The balloon crushes the fatty deposits and opens up the blood vessel.

Stents

A stent may be placed during a PCI procedure. A stent is a metal mesh tube that acts as a scaffold and holds open the coronary artery. During a balloon angioplasty, the stent is expanded when the balloon expands; however, the balloon is collapsed and withdrawn, whereas the stent remains in the artery permanently. Over time, the artery heals around the stent.

There are a variety of stents available. Stents can be characterized by the material composition, size, and whether or not they are drug eluting. Most procedures at present use drug-eluting stents. Drug-eluting stents consist of a standard metallic stent, a polymer coating, and an antirestenotic drug such as sirolimus or paclitaxel. The drug is mixed with the polymer and is released over a period ranging from days up to a year. The drug decreases the local proliferative healing response. After PCI and stent placement, the patient is typically placed on antithrombotic therapy with aspirin and clopidogrel for 6 to 12 months.

Indications for PCI

Initially, angioplasty was used in the treatment of patients with stable angina with atherosclerotic lesions in a single vessel. Now there are multiple indications such as

- Acute STEMI
- Non–ST-elevation acute coronary syndrome
- Stable angina
- Anginal equivalent with known CAD (ie, dyspnea, dizziness, arrhythmia, and syncope)
- Asymptomatic or mildly symptomatic patient with objective evidence of moderate to large area of viable myocardium or moderate to severe ischemia on noninvasive testing

Complications of PCI

Complications related to the balloon angioplasty procedure can occur. Some of these include dissection or perforation of the blood vessel. Complications with the use of stents include failure of stent deployment, stent thrombosis, and stent infection.

PCI has been a major advancement in less-invasive reperfusion of compromised myocardium. The use of stents has helped maintain the dilation of the vessel by providing scaffolding. Drug-eluting stents have been found to decrease the rate of closure. The number of indications for PCI has increased as the equipment has evolved to deal with more complex lesions. Patients typically will be placed on antithrombotic therapy during the postprocedure time.

SURGICAL TREATMENT OPTIONS

Conventional Coronary Artery Bypass Grafting (CABG)

Coronary artery bypass grafting (CABG) is a surgical procedure that improves blood flow to the heart by bypassing the diseased portion of a blood vessel. Conventional CABG surgery is done by surgically opening the patient's chest with an incision over the sternum and dividing it to expose the heart. Typically, the vessel used to bypass the disease artery is taken from the patient. Originally, the saphenous vein was used, but now more typically the internal mammary arteries are used. Other arteries that may be used include the radial artery or the gastroepiploic artery. An arterial vessel is likely to remain unobstructed longer than a venous vessel.

Minimally Invasive Coronary Artery Bypass (MIDCAB)

Minimally invasive coronary artery bypass is a procedure that is done through a much smaller incision over the patient's heart. Because the procedure has a smaller incision and excludes the use of the heart-lung machine, there is typically less pain and a more rapid recovery. However, this technique is indicated as an option for only certain coronary vessels—the left anterior descending artery and the right coronary artery.

Indications for surgery

There are several clinical indications when surgery may by appropriate in CAD.

- Angina—if a patient continues to have angina despite medical treatment or has specific vessel disease with high risk of MI or death
- Extensive disease—patients with extensive CAD, including left main or multiple arteries, and patients with poor LVEF
- After MI—patients who have had an MI may undergo CABG if their vessels cannot be opened by angioplasty or by stent placement

Choice of appropriate intervention for CAD depends on the extent of disease, age, comorbidities, patient's preference, and evidence for potential benefit.

SURGICAL COMPLICATIONS

As with any surgical procedure, there are complications such as bleeding or infection. During CABG, a patient is placed on a bypass pump to allow the surgeon to operate on a nonbeating heart. A complication related to the use of the bypass machine is called postpump syndrome.[18] The postpump syndrome is characterized by leukocytosis, systemic inflammation, and multiorgan dysfunction thought to be triggered by surgical trauma, lung reperfusion, and blood contact with artificial bypass circuitry.

NEW HORIZONS—HIBERNATING MYOCARDIUM, STEM CELLS, AND GROWTH FACTORS

The term hibernating myocardium refers to a state when myocardial myocytes adapt by lowering their functional state to match the low energy supply.[19] The low energy results from persistent asymptomatic ischemia that produces LV dysfunction that can mimic nonischemic causes of heart failure. The heart tissue is still viable, so if blood flow can be improved, the hibernating myocardium can be reversed. Stem cells have been used to grow both new blood vessels and new cardiac cells.[20] A variety of growth factors are also being studied as a stimulant to angiogenesis.

SUMMARY

- CAD is the leading cause of death worldwide.
- There are several presenting clinical syndromes, including sudden cardiac death.
- Risk factor analysis can help the primary care provider identify patients who may need more extensive evaluation or treatment.
- Treatment may be medical or surgical and depends on the individual patient's comorbidities and preferences.
- In the future, growth of new blood vessels or cardiac cells may aid in the treatment of CAD.

REFERENCES

1. Roger VL, Go AS, Lloyd-Jones DM, et al. Executive summary: heart disease and stroke statistics—2012 update: a report from the American Heart Association. Circulation 2012;124:188–97.
2. Gibbons RJ, Abrams J, Chatterjee K, et al. ACC/AHA 2002 guideline update for the management of patients with chronic stable angina. Available at: www.acc/org/qualityandscience/clinical/statements.htm. Accessed August 24, 2006.

3. Thygesen K, Alpert JS, White HD, Joint ESC/ACCF/AHA/WHF Task Force for the Redefinition of Myocardial Infarction. Universal definition of myocardial infarction. J Am Coll Cardiol 2007;50:2173.

4. Wu AH, Apple FS, Gibler WB, et al. National Academy of Clinical Biochemistry Standards of Laboratory Practice: recommendations for the use of cardiac markers in coronary artery diseases. Clin Chem 1999;45:1104.

5. Silent Myocardial Ischemia. UpToDate.

6. Mosca L, Appel LJ, Benjamin EJ, et al, American Heart Association. Evidence-based guidelines for cardiovascular disease prevention in women. Circulation 2004;109:679.

7. Dubach P, Froelicher VF, Klein J, et al. Exercise-induced hypotension in a male population. Criteria, causes, and prognosis. Circulation 1988;78:1380.

8. Weiss SA, Blumenthal RS, Sharrett AR, et al. Exercise, blood pressure and future cardiovascular death in asymptomatic individuals. Circulation 2010;121:2109.

9. Lee TH, Boucher CA. Clinical practice. Noninvasive tests in patient with stable coronary artery disease [review]. N Engl J Med 2001;344(24):1840–5.

10. Agatston AS, Janowitz WR, Hildner FJ, et al. Quantification of coronary artery calcium using ultrafast computed tomography. J Am Coll Cardiol 1990;15(4): 827–32.

11. DeWood J, Spores J, Notske R, et al. Prevalence of total coronary occlusion during the early hours of transmural MI. N Engl J Med 1980;303:898–902.

12. GUSTO trial results. American Federation of Clinical Research. Clin Res 1993;41: 207–8.

13. Thrombolytic Therapy for acute MI. Lancet 1996;348:771.

14. Lopex-Sendon J, Swedberg K, McMurray J, et al. Expert consensus document on beta-adrenergic receptor blockers. Eur Heart J 2004;25:1341.

15. Randomised trial of cholesterol lowering in 4444 patients with coronary heart disease: the Scandinavian Simvastatin Survival Study (4S). Lancet 1994;344: 1383.

16. Cannon CP, Braunwald E, McCabe CH, et al. Intensive versus moderate lipid lowering with statins after acute coronary syndromes. N Engl J Med 2004;350: 1495.

17. Hillis DL, Smith PK, Anderson JL, et al. 2011 ACCF/AHA Guideline for Coronary Artery Bypass Graft Surgery: a report of the American College of Cardiology Foundation/American Heart Association Task Force on Practice Guidelines. Circulation 2011;124(23):e652–735.

18. Aranki S, Aroesty JM, Suri RM. Early noncardiac complications of coronary artery bypass graft surgery. UpToDate. Available at: http//www.uptodate.com/contents/early-noncardiac-complications-of-coronary-artery-bypass-graft-surgery?source=search results&selectedTitle1-150. Accessed August 14, 2012.

19. Slezak J, Tribulova N, Okruchlicovva L, et al. Hibernating myocardium: pathophysiology, diagnosis, and treatment. Can J Physiol Pharmacol 2009;87(4):252–65.

20. "Clinical research." Cardiac angiogenesis: four approaches to restoring cardiac function. Columbia University medical Center, Department of Surgery; 2012. Available at: http://www.columbiasurgery.org/pat/cardiac/angiogenesis.html. Accessed July 24, 2012.

Heart Failure
Clinical Problem and Management Issues

John M. Nicklas, MD[a],*, Barry E. Bleske, PharmD[b],
Richard Van Harrison, PhD[c], Robert V. Hogikyan, MD, MPH[d],
Yeong Kwok, MD[e], William E. Chavey, MD, MS[f]

KEYWORDS

- Heart failure • Cardiomyopathy • Angiotensin converting enzyme inhibitor
- Beta blocker • Aldosterone antagonist • Implantable cardiodefibrillator
- Biventricular pacemaker

KEY POINTS

- Heart failure (HF) often presents initially either as dyspnea with exertion and/or recumbency. Patients also commonly experience dependent swelling, rapid fatigue, cough, and early satiety. These symptoms are sometimes mistakenly attributed to other causes including pneumonia, asthma, and peptic ulcer disease.
- Patients with a presumed diagnosis of HF should have an assessment of *left ventricular ejection fraction* (LVEF). The assessment should be repeated when the clinical situation is changed and is not easily explainable through history or physical examination. LVEF should be measured or remeasured 6 months after surgical or percutaneous revascularization.
- Over the past 3 decades, large, prospective, randomized, placebo-controlled trials have demonstrated conclusively that angiotensin converting enzyme inhibitors, beta blockers, and aldosterone antagonists can significantly lower the mortality and morbidity of HF in patients with left ventricular systolic dysfunction (LVSD), specifically in patients with an LVEF less than 35%.
- In addition to pharmacologic therapy, clinical trials have also demonstrated conclusively that implantable cardiac defibrillators can significantly lower mortality in patients with symptomatic HF and LVSD and that biventricular pacemakers can significantly lower mortality and morbidity in selected patients with LVSD and prolonged QRS intervals.

[a] Department of Internal Medicine, Division of Cardiovascular Medicine, University of Michigan, CVC Room 2391, 1600 East Medical Center Drive, Ann Arbor, MI 48109-5853, USA; [b] Department of Clinical and Social Administrative Services, College of Pharmacy, University of Michigan, 428 Church Street, Ann Arbor, MI 48109-1065, USA; [c] Department of Medical Education, University of Michigan, G1103 Towsley Center, 1500 East Medical Center Drive SPC 5201, Ann Arbor, MI 48109-5201, USA; [d] Department of Internal Medicine, Division of Geriatrics and Palliative Medicine, University of Michigan, 2215 Fuller Road, 11G, Ann Arbor, MI 48105, USA; [e] Department of Internal Medicine, Division of General Medicine, University of Michigan, 4260 Plymouth Road, Ann Arbor, MI 48109, USA; [f] Departments of Family Medicine and Emergency Medicine, University of Michigan Medical School, 1500 East Medical Center Drive, L2003 Women's SPC 5239, Ann Arbor, MI 48109, USA
* Corresponding author.
E-mail address: jnicklas@med.umich.edu

Prim Care Clin Office Pract 40 (2013) 17–42
http://dx.doi.org/10.1016/j.pop.2012.11.010
0095-4543/13/$ – see front matter © 2013 Elsevier Inc. All rights reserved.

primarycare.theclinics.com

INCIDENCE

More than 5 million Americans currently have heart failure (HF). An additional 400,000 develop HF annually.[1] Each year, 990,000 patients are hospitalized with HF as the primary diagnosis. Overall, nearly 50% of HF patients die within 5 years of the onset of symptoms. The incidence of HF increases with age. HF is the most common cause of hospitalization in older adults. Because the American population is aging, the incidence of HF and associated morbidity and mortality will increase in the future.

ETIOLOGY AND NATURAL HISTORY

HF results from the inability of the heart to deliver adequate perfusion to meet the body's metabolic demands using normal cardiac filling pressures. Multiple cardiac abnormalities can cause HF. Left ventricular systolic dysfunction (LVSD) is a common cause of HF and can be identified by documenting a reduced left ventricular ejection fraction (LVEF) using widely available imaging tools. Over the past several decades, investigators have studied HF patients with LVSD intensively and have demonstrated that several pharmacologic interventions can reduce mortality and morbidity. To date, no other cause of HF has been as extensively studied, nor have effective interventions been conclusively identified. Therefore, this article primarily reviews HF secondary to LVSD.

The most common cause of LVSD is coronary artery disease producing an ischemic cardiomyopathy. Nonischemic cardiomyopathies may be familial or may be caused by a variety of insults including inflammation and toxins. The cause of nonischemic cardiomyopathy is frequently not identified and may resolve within 12 months of the onset of symptoms in approximately 30% of cases. Patients with HF secondary to LVSD, either ischemic or nonischemic, suffer frequent hospitalizations and are at increased risk of premature death. Dietary indiscretion in sodium intake and medication nonadherance can worsen symptoms. Progressive pump failure and malignant arrhythmias cause most deaths among HF patients, with the relative proportions of pump failure versus arrhythmic deaths varying based on symptomatic status, pharmacologic treatment, and device interventions.

As many as 50% of patients with HF have a preserved left ventricular ejection fraction (HF-PEF). Historically, these patients were thought to have diastolic dysfunction. Diastolic dysfunction may be identified on the basis of echocardiographic criteria, such as the ratio of early-to-late diastolic filling, short deceleration times, and isovolumic relaxation times. However, many patients with HF-PEF do not have echocardiographic evidence of diastolic dysfunction. Some patients may have concomitant systolic and diastolic HF. HF may be more simply conceived in terms of reduced (HF-REF) or preserved ejection fraction, HF-PEF, rather than in terms of systolic or diastolic dysfunction, respectively. Other causes of HF are less common.

SIGNS AND SYMPTOMS

HF is recognized as a syndrome of clinical symptoms and physical signs. HF often presents initially as dyspnea either with exertion or with recumbency. Patients also commonly experience dependent swelling, rapid fatigue, cough, and early satiety. These symptoms are sometimes mistakenly attributed to other causes including pneumonia, asthma, and peptic ulcer disease. Arrhythmias causing palpitations, dizziness, or aborted sudden death can be the initial manifestations of the disease. Elevated cardiac filling pressures can lead to physical signs of congestion including dependent edema, jugular venous distention, and pulmonary rales. Compensatory ventricular dilation producing an enlarged and laterally displaced cardiac apical impulse can be palpated in some patients.

HF CLASSIFICATIONS

HF limits exercise capacity. In general, patients with more severe functional limitations have poorer survival. The New York Heart Association (NYHA) classification of functional capacity, a system originally designed as a research tool, has been used to estimate prognosis in clinical practice and to selectively define study populations in clinical trials.

NYHA Class	NYHA Symptom Description
NYHA Class I	Asymptomatic
NYHA Class II	Mildly symptomatic
NYHA Class III	Moderately symptomatic
NYHA Class IV	Symptoms at rest

In 2001, the American College of Cardiology (ACC) and the American Heart Association (AHA) proposed a new stratification scheme.

ACC/AHA Class	Description
A	At risk
B	Asymptomatic
C	Symptomatic
D	Refractory

This article provides a guide for therapeutic decisions based on the inclusion criteria of the major clinical trials. **Table 1** shows the relationship between these classification schemes.

DIAGNOSTIC TESTING AND EVALUATION
Left Ventricular Ejection Fraction

Patients with a presumed diagnosis of HF should have an assessment of LVEF. The assessment should be repeated when the clinical situation has changed and is not easily explainable through history or physical examination. LVEF should be measured or remeasured six months after surgical or percutaneous revascularization.

Echocardiography is commonly used to assess LVEF. Other imaging modalities are also used including radionuclide ventriculography, contrast ventriculography, cardiac magnetic resonance imaging, cardiac computed tomography, and gated single-proton emission computed tomography (SPECT).[2]

Transthoracic echocardiography provides noninvasive diagnostic information readily and safely. It provides information on ventricular shape and function, wall thickness, and valvular function. It is commonly used, widely available, and inexpensive.

Although radionuclide ventriculography or gated SPECT imaging may also be used to assess LVEF and right ventricular ejection fraction, they do not allow assessment of valvular function or wall thickness. Gated SPECT may have better interobserver reliability than echocardiography in assessing LVEF.[3] However, the cost and radiation exposure support echocardiography as an appropriate initial evaluation.

Table 1
Treatment recommendations for heart failure patients with left ventricular systolic dysfunction

ACC/AHA	B	C		D
NYHA	I	II – III		IV
Symptoms[a]	Asymptomatic	Symptoms, Current or Prior		Recurrent or Ongoing Rest Dyspnea
		Never Hospitalized	History of Hospitalization	
Angiotensin converting enzyme inhibitor	Yes	Yes	Yes	Yes
Beta blocker	Yes[a]	Yes	Yes	Yes[b]
Aldosterone antagonist		Yes	Yes	Yes
Isosorbide dinitrate-hydralazine		Selected patients[c]	Selected patients[c]	Selected patients[c]
Diuretic		PRN congestion	PRN congestion	Yes
Angiotensin receptor blocker		PRN[d]	PRN[d]	PRN[d]
Digoxin		PRN[d]	PRN[d]	PRN[d]
Consider AICD/Bi-V pacemaker	Selected patients[e]	Yes	Yes	Yes
HF disease management			Yes	Yes
Referral to advanced HF program				Yes[f]

Shading: ▨ = Recommended, ▨ = Consider.

Abbreviation: AICD, automatic implantable cardioverter defibrillator.

[a] No explicit evidence of benefit exists for beta blockers among asymptomatic patients, although many patients in this class will have other indications for beta blockers such as coronary artery disease (CAD).

[b] Beta blockers may be continued safely for patients with rest dyspnea except in patients with signs of congestion or hemodynamic instability.

[c] The combination of isosorbide dinitrate and hydralazine benefited patients self-reported as African American. This combination may be added for patients who remain symptomatic despite therapy with angiotensin-converting enzyme inhibitors (ACEIs) and beta blockers and as tolerated without reducing the doses of ACEI or beta blocker to subtarget doses.

[d] These interventions may provide symptomatic benefit. If no benefit is perceived, the medications may be withdrawn. In the case of digoxin, however, withdrawal may lead to clinical deterioration and should be done with caution. Little evidence exists to support the safety of ACEI/aldosterone antagonists/angiotensin receptor blockers in the same patient. Beause all agents can increase potassium levels, avoiding this combination may be prudent.

[e] See **Fig. 2**. Indication only for asymptomatic patients with ischemic cardiomyopathy.

[f] Refer for shared medical decision making regarding left ventricular assist device or transplant.

Functional Testing

Exercise stress testing may have a role in the evaluation of some patients with HF. Exercise stress testing is useful in evaluating active and significant concomitant coronary artery disease and in assessing functional capacity.

Cardiopulmonary exercise testing can quantitate a patient's functional capacity. Testing may be indicated to document disability for insurance. Patients with poor ventilatory efficiency (VE/VCO2 slopes > 35) or very low peak oxygen consumptions

($Vo_2 < 14$) may be candidates for advanced HF interventions including ventricular assist devices and cardiac transplantation.[4,5]

Cardiac Catheterization

Coronary angiography and left heart cardiac catheterization are useful in the management of HF when the discovery of significant coronary artery disease or valvular heart disease would either impact medical treatment or provide the necessary information to proceed to surgery. Right heart catheterization may be useful in the development of a differential diagnosis and to guide therapy in patients for whom volume status is unclear.

Electrocardiography

Standard 12 lead electrocardiography (ECG) should be used to help determine whether ischemic heart disease is likely and to identify some arrhythmias. For example, atrial fibrillation may not be apparent on physical examination especially in patients who are ventricularly paced, but can be recognized on the ECG. Additionally, an ECG can be helpful to assess for left ventricular dyssynchrony. Left bundle branch block suggests dyssynchrony. Those with a QRS duration less than 120 msec may still have dyssynchrony that can be detected on an echocardiogram.

Ambulatory Rhythm Monitors

A major cause of death in HF is sudden death presumably due to ventricular arrhythmias. Ambulatory monitoring should be a part of the evaluation of any heart failure patient suspected of rhythm disturbances.

B-type Natriuretic Peptide

Measuring B-type natriuretic peptide (BNP) and its closely related N terminal fragment is useful in the diagnosis and prognosis of patients with HF. These biologically active proteins are present in cardiac myocytes and are released in response to a complex array of stimulants including stretching of myocytes. They are biologically active: augmenting urine volume and sodium excretion, inhibiting renin-angiotensin activation, and relaxing vascular smooth muscle. Their analogues may have useful clinical applications in the future.

An elevated BNP can establish the diagnosis of HF in patients who present with dyspnea. BNP does not differentiate the cause of HF. In acute care settings, high BNP levels correlate directly with the probability of HF and low BNP levels make HF unlikely. For example, a BNP of 50 pg/mL has a negative predictive value of 96%, whereas a BNP of 100 pg/mL has a positive predictive value of 79%, and a BNP of 150 pg/mL has a positive predictive value of 83%. At a BNP of 250 pg/mL, the relative risk of HF is 7.0 (**Fig. 1**).[6] BNP levels can be increased by renal insufficiency and to lesser extremes by age and female gender. Obesity tends to lower BNP levels.

Elevated BNP levels in patients with an established diagnosis of HF are also powerful indicators of prognosis. Relative risk of death increases by 35% for each 100 pg/mL increase in BNP. Persistently elevated levels in patients being treated for HF indicate a poorer prognosis. Trials of BNP or N-terminal proBNP (NT proBNP) guided outpatient management have shown mixed results. The largest study did not show a significant improvement in clinical endpoints when NT proBNP–guided management was compared with symptoms-guided management.[7] However, a benefit occurred in a prespecified subgroup analysis of patients younger than 75 years. The utility of BNP measurements in the emergency setting to guide decisions about admission or therapy has yielded mixed results.

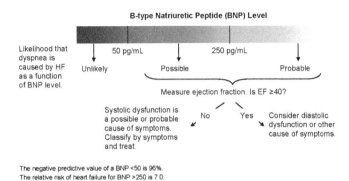

Fig. 1. Graphic representation of the relationship between B-type natriuretic peptide (BNP) level and likelihood of HF as a cause of dyspnea.

Potassium and Magnesium

Monitoring of potassium and magnesium serum concentrations is essential in most HF patients. Diuretics may significantly lower potassium and magnesium concentrations. Angiotensin-converting enzyme inhibitors (ACEI), angiotensin receptor blockers (ARB), aldosterone antagonists, and dietary factors (eg, bananas and salt substitutes) may significantly increase potassium concentrations, especially in the presence of renal impairment or when used in combination. In general, based on clinical perspective, potassium levels should be maintained between 4.0 and 5.0 mEq/L.[8] Circadian variation may lower potassium levels by up to 0.5 mEq/L during the early morning hours in a given patient.[9] Artifactually elevated potassium levels may occur because of hemolysis of the sample and hand clenching during phlebotomy.

If required, potassium supplementation should be administered; usual dose range is 10 to 80 mEq/d with a potassium chloride preparation.[10] Other salt forms include potassium phosphate and potassium bicarbonate. Microencapsulated formulations may have better patient appeal and gastrointestinal tolerance.

Magnesium levels should be maintained between 1.5 and 2.4 mEq/L. The usual dose range for magnesium supplementation for asymptomatic patients with minor alterations in serum concentrations is 1 to 4 tablets of a product such as magnesium oxide 400 mg (242 mg elemental magnesium content). Diarrhea can be a dose-limiting side effect. Hypokalemia is often easier to correct if hypomagnesemia is also corrected.

Sodium

Patients with HF may have low serum sodium levels. Often these low levels are the result of extracellular fluid excess leading to a dilutional hyponatremia. Fluid restriction and diuresis may correct the dilutional hyponatremia. In contrast, diuretic use in patients with free access to fluid can lead to total body sodium depletion.

LIFESTYLE MANAGEMENT
Patient Education

Patient education on several topics at the time of discharge from a hospitalization for HF is a Joint Commission core measure. Many heterogeneous studies have examined the role and the effectiveness of patient education in HF.[11–13] Most interventions successfully increased patient knowledge about HF and measures to control HF. However, more comprehensive disease management programs involving nurses or case managers who made repeated contacts with patients were more successful at improving clinical outcomes.

Exercise

Many clinical trials (some randomized) have examined the benefits of a variety of exercise training formulas in HF. A Cochrane review of available studies in 2010 concluded that although exercise in HF appeared to be safe, it had no significant impact on short-term or long-term all-cause mortality or overall hospital admission rates.[14] Likewise, in the HF-ACTION trial, 2331 participants safely exercised at 60% to 70% of heart rate reserve 3 to 5 times per week, but did not gain significant reductions in mortality or hospitalizations.[15]

Diet

No large prospective clinical trials of salt or fluid restriction exist for the treatment of HF. Common clinical practice is to recommend limiting sodium intake to 2000 mg daily and fluid intake to 2 L or less daily, especially in patients with hyponatremia. One prospective study suggested that fluid restriction might be more important than sodium restriction.[16]

CARDIAC SURGERY
Coronary Artery Bypass Grafting

Ischemic HF is potentially reversible. Revascularization of viable but dysfunctional myocardium that has been transiently ischemic (stunned) or chronically ischemic (hibernating) may improve systolic function and LVEF. A meta-analysis in 2002 of observational studies suggested that coronary artery bypass grafting (CABG) in patients with HF and viable myocardium improved survival.[17] However, in 2011, STICH, the only large prospective trial of CABG in patients with HF, demonstrated no improvement in all-cause mortality during 5 years of follow-up, though a nonsignificant trend favored CABG.[18] Significant crossover occurred between groups and led to an as-treated analysis that suggested a significant 30% reduction in all-cause mortality for patients undergoing CABG. Assessment of myocardial viability did not identify patients more likely to benefit from CABG.[19]

Surgical Left Ventricular Reconstruction

In patients with HF and LVSD, the left ventricle enlarges and changes from an ellipsoid to a less mechanically efficient spherical shape. A variety of surgical interventions including the Dor, surgical anterior ventricular endocardial restoration, and Batista procedures have attempted to remodel the left ventricle in patients with HF to reduce left ventricular size and restore mechanical efficiency. However, in HF patients undergoing CABG, left ventricular reconstruction did not improve mortality or symptoms.[20]

Mitral Valve Repair

Left ventricular enlargement and shape change distort the mitral valve apparatus, dilating the annulus and displacing the papillary muscles, frequently producing mitral regurgitation (MR). Surgical repair of the mitral valve can decrease the degree of MR, but repair does not improve survival.[21] Medical therapy and electrophysiologic pacing interventions, especially in patients with dyssynchrony, can also decrease the degree of MR.

Advanced Heart Failure Interventions

Left ventricular assist device (LVAD) implantation or cardiac transplantation is potentially indicated in patients with recurrent or ongoing rest dyspnea (see **Table 1**). An

LVAD may serve as a bridge to transplantation or as palliative destination therapy especially in older patients.

ELECTROPHYSIOLOGIC DEVICES
Automatic Implantable Cardiac Defibrillators

Prophylactic implantation of implantable cardiac defibrillators (ICDs) has been demonstrated in large trials to decrease mortality significantly in patients with HF and LVSD.[22-26] ICD placement should be considered in all HF patients who are symptomatic or have a history of ischemic cardiomyopathy with an ejection fraction less than or equal to 35%. Survival benefit from an ICD is only realized after one year, so patients should have an estimated life expectancy of more than 1 year. An ICD should not be implanted within 1 month following myocardial infarction or within 3 months following CABG.[27,28] Appropriate patients should be referred for ICD implantation regardless of gender. However, some data question whether women benefit from ICDs and whether they have more device implantation complications than men.[29-31] In the past, fewer ICDs have been placed in women, so data are limited.

Cardiac Resynchronization Therapy

Cardiac resynchronization therapy (CRT) with biventricular (Bi-V) pacing has been shown to decrease the composite of all-cause death or hospitalization by 19% in HF patients with NYHA III or IV symptoms, an LVEF less than or equal to 35%, and a QRS interval greater than or equal to 120 msec.[32] All-cause mortality alone was reduced by 24%. When an ICD was added to the Bi-V pacer, all-cause mortality was reduced by 36%. Also, when Bi-V pacing alone was restricted to HF patients with NYHA class III or IV symptoms, an LVEF less than or equal to 35%, and a QRS interval either greater than or equal to 150 msec or greater than or equal to 120 msec with echocardiographic evidence of cardiac dyssynchrony, the combined endpoint of mortality or cardiovascular hospitalization was reduced by 37%.[33] Bi-V pacing also improved symptoms and quality of life. Benefit occurred primarily in patients with left bundle branch block.

Bi-V pacing may also benefit less symptomatic HF patients (NYHA I and II) with an LVEF less than or equal to 40% and a QRS interval greater than or equal to 120 msec. In 2 clinical trials in this group of patients, time for first hospitalization or death was significantly delayed by 56% and 62%.[34,35] Again, benefit occurred primarily in HF patients with left bundle branch block. **Fig. 2** illustrates an algorithm for referring patients for device therapy.

PHARMACOLOGIC THERAPY

Over the past 3 decades, large, prospective, randomized, placebo-controlled trials have demonstrated conclusively that some medications can significantly lower the mortality and morbidity of HF in patients with LVSD, specifically in patients with an LVEF less than 35%. See **Table 1** for drug use by patient classification and **Table 2** for dosing and cost.

Angiotensin-converting Enzyme Inhibitors

Landmark randomized controlled trials including CONSENSUS and the SOLVD treatment and prevention trials demonstrated the effectiveness of ACEI in lowering morbidity and mortality in both asymptomatic and symptomatic patients with HF and LVSD.[36-38] The benefit from ACEI was inversely related to LVEF, greatest in the patients with the lowest LVEF.

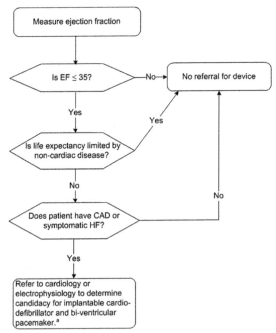

^aDevice therapy, i.e. implantable cardiodefibrillator or bi-ventricular pacemaker, can significantly improve mortality in appropriate patients. Determining appropriate clinical criteria can be complex and may require the assistance of a cardiologist or an electrophysiologist. The algorithm above gives guidance but is designed to be inclusive so that all eligible patients can at least be considered for a device.

Fig. 2. Algorithm for referring patients for implantation of either a cardiac defibrillator and/or a biventricular pacemaker.

ACEIs are often avoided in patients with HF because of perceived risk and contra-indications. Patient factors such as lower blood pressure, elevated serum creatinine level, and cough should not be considered absolute contraindications. When initiating treatment, careful monitoring is warranted if the systolic blood pressure is less than 100 mm Hg or the creatinine level is elevated. Some patients will not tolerate ACEI. In this setting, either an ARB or isosorbide dinitrate-hydralazine may be used as a substitute. If ACEIs are contraindicated due to renal failure, then isosorbide dinitrate-hydralazine is preferred.

Beta Blockers

Beta blockade is indicated in HF patients with LVSD except those who are dyspneic at rest with signs of congestion, hemodynamically unstable, or intolerant of beta blockers. Multiple trials including CIBIS-II, MERIT-HF, and COPERNICUS in symptomatic patients have demonstrated dramatic mortality benefits with bisoprolol, metoprolol succinate, and carvedilol.[39–41] Beta blockers have not been demonstrated to show benefit in patients with rest dyspnea and signs of congestion. Beta blockers should not be added as a rescue therapy for HF patients who are decompensating. The initial dosage level should be started and then doubled every 2 to 4 weeks until either the patient is unable to tolerate higher levels or the target dose is reached (see **Table 2**).

Beta blockers cannot be presumed to have a class effect on HF because at least 1 beta blocker has failed to reduce mortality in a randomized controlled trial.[42]

Table 2
Doses for major heart failure drugs

Drug Class and Generic Name	Brand Name	Starting Dose	Target Dose or Common Dose	Target/Common Dose 30 d Cost[a] Generic	Target/Common Dose 30 d Cost[a] Brand
ACEI[b]					
Drugs Demonstrated to Decrease Mortality and/or Improve Symptoms[b]					
Captopril	Capoten	6.25 mg tid (1/2 tab[c])	12.5–50 mg tid	$6–12	$81–300
Lisinopril	Zestril, Prinivil	5 mg daily	10–20 mg daily	$4–6	$41–46
Enalapril	Vasotec	2.5 mg bid	10 mg bid	$11–13	$147–188
Trandolapril	Mavik	1 mg daily	4 mg daily	$20	$47
Ramipril	Altace	1.25 mg bid	5 mg bid	n/a	$94
Fosinopril	Monopril	5–10 mg daily	40 mg daily	$8–15	n/a
Perindopril	Aceon	2 mg daily	8–16 mg daily	$40–60	$80–100
Quinapril	Accupril	5 mg bid	10–20 mg bid	$23	$67
Aldosterone Antagonist[b]					
Spironolactone	Aldactone	12.5 mg daily	25 mg daily	$4–7	$17–34
Eplerenone	Inspra	25 mg daily	50 mg daily	$98	$153
ARB[b]					
Candesartan	Atacand	4 mg daily	32 mg daily	n/a	$82–112
Valsartan	Diovan	40 mg bid	160 mg bid	n/a	$84–215

Beta Blocker[b]					
Bisoprolol	Zebeta	1.25 mg daily (1/4 tab[d])	10 mg daily	$25-29	$116
Metoprolol	Toprol XL	12.5 mg daily (1/2 tab)	200 mg daily	$15-68	$37-88
Carvedilol	Coreg	3.125 mg bid	25 mg bid	$17	$151
Vasodilator[b]					
Isosorbide dinitrate-hydralazine	BiDil (combination product)	20/37.5 mg tid	40/75 mg tid	n/a	$182-364
Isosorbide dinitrate	Isordil	20 mg tid	40 mg tid	$8-15	$31-63
Hydralazine	Hydralazine	37.5 mg tid	75 mg tid	$13-23	$21-42
Drugs for Symptomatic Therapy[c]					
Diuretics – Thiazide[e]					
Hydrochlorothiazide	HydroDiuril	25 mg daily	25-100 mg daily	$4-10	n/a
Metolazone	Zaroxolyn	2.5 mg daily	2.5-10 mg daily	$15-31	$82-326
Diuretics – Loop[e]					
Furosemide	Lasix	40 mg daily	40-400 mg daily-tid	$5-18	$25-128
Bumetanide	Bumex	1 mg daily	1-10 mg daily-tid	$10-38	n/a
Ethacrynic acid	Edecrin	25 mg daily	25-200 mg daily-bid	n/a	$112-222
Torsemide	Demadex	20 mg daily	20-100 mg daily-bid	$13-66	$60-216
Inotrope[b]					
Digoxin	Lanoxin	0.125 mg daily	0.125-0.375 mg daily	$8-14	$11-23

a Pricing information for brand drugs, Average Wholesale Price minus 10%. AWP from Amerisource Bergen Wholesale Catalog & Red Book Online 7/20/12. For generic drugs, Maximum Allowable Cost plus $3 from Michigan MAC List, 7/16/12.
b Although other drugs are available in these classes, they have not been demonstrated to decrease mortality or improve symptoms in patients with heart failure.
c Common doses.
d Tablet is scored for half tablet only.
e Diuretics have not been separately studied for target dose. Titrate as needed for symptom relief.

Although they differ pharmacologically, no evidence clearly demonstrates the overall superiority of any 1 of the 3 known efficacious beta blockers. One trial found carvedilol superior to metoprolol tartrate in prolonging survival in patients with symptomatic HF.[43] However, the dose and formulation of metoprolol in this comparison differed from the dose and formulation in the placebo-controlled trial in which metoprolol succinate was proved effective.

Aldosterone Antagonists

Landmark trials including RALES, EPHESUS, and EMPHASIS-HF demonstrated that aldosterone antagonism is indicated in all patients with LVSD and symptomatic HF and in patients following a recent myocardial infarction who develop LVSD with either manifest signs of HF or concomitant diabetes.[44–46] Aldosterone antagonists significantly reduced mortality and hospitalizations for HF. Aldosterone antagonists should be administered to patients with symptomatic HF and LVSD without renal dysfunction (serum creatinine level <2.5 mg/dL or a glomerular filtration rate >30 mL/min per 1.73 M2 of body surface area) and without baseline hyperkalemia (>5 mEq/L). After initiating an aldosterone antagonist, serum potassium levels should be closely monitored, especially in patients with mild symptoms.

The 2 available aldosterone antagonists, spironolactone and eplerenone, differ in potency and in other effects including their antiandrogenic effects. Spironolactone is twice as potent as eplerenone as an aldosterone antagonist, but spironolactone also produces gynecomastia in 7% of men when administered at a dose of 25 mg daily, a side effect not seen with eplerenone. The agents have been tested in different populations, spironolactone in patients with severe HF and eplerenone in patients with mild HF and in patients post-myocardial infarction.

Both spironolactone and eplerenone are potassium sparing diuretics and can cause hyperkalemia, especially when administered concomitantly with ACEIs or ARBs. In the trial of patients with severe HF, severe hyperkalemia was rare (2%). However, severe hyperkalemia was more common in the clinical trials of patients post-myocardial infarction (5.5%) and in patients with less severe HF (8%). In these clinical trial populations, selection criteria excluded patients with baseline renal dysfunction or baseline hyperkalemia. In presumably less selected populations, aldosterone antagonism has been associated with more frequent severe hyperkalemia and increased mortality.[47]

Angiotensin Receptor Blockers

ARBs have been tested as agents for use in place of or in addition to ACEI. Ample evidence supports the use and equivalence of ARB for patients who cannot tolerate ACEIs.[48,49] However, ACEIs have the advantage of lower cost and more patient experience and are still first line therapy.

The addition of ARBs to ACEIs is controversial. ARBs have been added safely and effectively to ACEIs to reduce persistent symptoms in a clinical trial of HF patients.[50] However, adverse events with this combination in another HF trial in patients receiving an ARB, ACEI, and beta blocker[51] and among non-HF patients have raised reservations about using these drugs in combination.[52] ACEIs, ARBs, and aldosterone antagonists may all increase potassium level and may represent a dangerous combination if used together.

Direct-acting Vasodilators

The combination of hydralazine and isosorbide dinitrate was an early intervention in the treatment of HF, and the combination represents the only direct-acting vasodilators to improve HF outcomes.[53] A subsequent trial demonstrated that ACEIs were superior to hydralazine and isosorbide.[54] In a post-hoc analysis of those trials, the combination of isosorbide dinitrate and hydralazine was particularly effective in African American patients.[55] A prospective trial demonstrated an improvement in mortality among African American patients when the combination was added to background therapy including ACEI or ARB, beta blocker, and aldosterone antagonist.[56] Patients in this trial self-identified as African American, but a substudy identified a genetic polymorphism more common among African Americans as the trait most likely to predict responsiveness to this drug combination.

Thus, the combination of isosorbide dinitrate and hydralazine may be used as tolerated by blood pressure in symptomatic HF patients who are African American and may be used as a substitute in any HF patient who is intolerant of ACEI and ARB. This combination may also be used in HF patients who are persistently symptomatic on ACEI, ARB, and/or beta blockade. Headache may develop and can become less problematic with continued use.

Diuretics

Diuretics are often required to manage volume overload acutely and chronically in patients with HF. The dose of loop diuretic will vary greatly between patients and will be determined by individual response.[57] Because diuretics may produce potassium and magnesium wasting, monitoring of these electrolytes is warranted.

Diuretic effect on mortality is not known. Although no large, controlled clinical studies of diuretics in the treatment of HF have been reported, most patients with HF received diuretics as part of baseline therapy in trials of ACEIs, ARBs, beta blockers, aldosterone antagonists, and digoxin.

All loop diuretics have similar efficacy when administered in appropriate doses. The most commonly used loop diuretic is furosemide. However, torsemide or bumetanide can be considered as alternatives, especially in patients who are frequently hospitalized for fluid accumulation. The biokinetics of the absorption of furosemide may decrease as patients begin to decompensate, resulting in decreased diuretic efficacy that may lead to increased fluid accumulation. Changes in drug absorption may be one of the factors that lead to frequent hospitalizations with individual patients. Torsemide's rate of absorption is not significantly altered when patients become decompensated.[58] Ethacrynic acid is an option for patients with allergies to furosemide, bumetanide, and torsemide.

Combination of a loop diuretic with a thiazide diuretic increases diuretic effect by minimizing distal tubular compensation.[59] Loop diuretics are most often used because of their diuretic potency, but are associated with acute and chronic distal tubular compensation (distal tubular hypertrophy), resulting in decreased urine output. Although adding a thiazide diuretic minimizes distal tubal compensation, the increase in diuretic response will likely result in an increase in the loss of potassium and magnesium.

The effect of a thiazide diuretic to increase diuretic responsiveness appears to be a class effect. Hydrochlorothiazide and metolazone are common thiazide diuretics used in combination with loop diuretics. Hydrochlorothiazide and metolazone differ in duration of action, and the long duration of action of metolazone may make it more effective than hydrochlorothiazide in some patients. No data support the sequential timing of loop and thiazide diuretics. Specifically, no data support the concept of administering the thiazide diuretic 30 minutes before a loop diuretic.

Digoxin

Digoxin should be considered in HF patients who remain symptomatic despite therapy with diuretics, ACEIs or ARBs, and beta blockers and in those who have atrial fibrillation. Digoxin may be used among patients on spironolactone with the caveat that spironolactone may increase digoxin levels by decreasing renal excretion. This effect has not been reported with eplerenone.

Digoxin improved symptoms and reduced hospitalization rates in symptomatic HF patients receiving diuretics and ACEIs in the DIG trial.[60] Digoxin had no effect on overall HF mortality. The usual dose range for digoxin is 0.125 to 0.25 mg/d adjusted for symptoms, other drugs, or renal impairment (see **Table 2**). Retrospective analysis of the DIG trial suggested that patients with serum levels less than 1 ng/mL when measured at least 6 to 8 hours after dosing had improved outcomes.[61] Digoxin may also be used to help control ventricular response rate in patients with HF and atrial fibrillation. Levels needed to control ventricular response rate may need to be greater than 1 ng/mL.

OTHER DRUGS
Calcium Channel Blockers

Currently, no evidence supports the use of calcium channel blockers (CCBs) for treatment of HF and LVSD. However, if CCBs are needed for management of hypertension, second generation agents appear to be safe. First generation agents (verapamil, diltiazem) were shown to have adverse outcomes in post-MI patients with LVSD.[62,63] Subsequent studies in ischemic and nonischemic HF NYHA III/IV with other CCBs (eg, amlodipine, felodipine) suggested their safety, but did not demonstrate their efficacy. A subgroup analysis of the first PRAISE trial found a 46% decrease in mortality in patients with nonischemic HF receiving amlodipine.[64] However, a second PRAISE trial demonstrated no mortality benefit from amlodipine in nonischemic cardiomyopathy.

Inotropes

Intravenous inotropic therapy with sympathomimetics (dobutamine or dopamine) or phosphodiesterase inhibitors (milrinone) may have a role in the treatment of patients hospitalized for acutely decompensated HF. Inotropic agents may increase cardiac output and decrease systemic and pulmonary vascular resistance.[65] Although these therapies may improve symptoms and decrease hospitalizations, they are associated with increased mortality.[66,67]

Intermittent bolus or continuous home infusion therapy for either dobutamine or milrinone is not recommended for the routine management of HF. Continuous intravenous inotropic therapy may have a role in palliation of patients with end-stage HF or as a bridge to transplantation.

Antiarrhythmic Drugs

Although arrhythmias such as atrial fibrillation and nonsustained ventricular tachycardia are common in HF patients, antiarrhythmic drugs do not improve survival. The use of device therapy (ICD) has supplanted the use of antiarrhythmic drugs for primary treatment of ventricular arrhythmias. However, antiarrhythmic therapy may be used in conjunction with device therapy in selected patients to suppress ventricular arrhythmias and minimize device firing.[26] Antiarrhythmic drugs that have potent negative inotropic effects (eg, flecainide) should be avoided in HF patients with or without device therapy.[68]

Lipid-Lowering Agents

The most common cause of LVSD is coronary artery disease. However, statins have not been beneficial in patients with HF and LVSD. Two large randomized trials of rosuvastatin in patients with symptomatic HF demonstrated no mortality benefit during

2.7 and 3.9 years of follow-up.[69,70] One trial enrolled only patients with ischemic HF, and the other trial enrolled patients with both ischemic and nonischemic HF. In these trials rosuvastatin lowered low-density lipoprotein levels by 45% and 27%, but ischemic events did not decrease, and there was no trend toward improved survival in any subgroup. Rosuvastatin did not cause safety problems.

Fish Oil

Supplementation with fish oils may be beneficial in patients with HF. Several cohort studies suggest that increased fish consumption is associated with a lower risk of developing HF. One large randomized study of n-3 polyunsaturated fatty acids supplementation in patients with symptomatic HF showed a small (8%) but significant reduction in mortality and cardiovascular hospitalizations.[71]

Antiplatelet Drugs

HF is not an indication for aspirin therapy. However, HF is also not a contraindication for aspirin in patients with coronary artery disease. Controversial data suggest that aspirin may interfere with ACEI effectiveness; however, the clinical relevance is not clear.[72,73] Aspirin therapy has also been associated with a controversial increase in hospitalization rates for HF.[74-76] With the limited data available, it is reasonable to administer aspirin to HF patients with coronary artery disease especially with a recent ischemic event history. In patients not able to tolerate aspirin therapy, clopidogrel therapy may be considered. Limited data suggest similar effects for aspirin and clopidogrel in HF patients regarding mortality, hospitalizations, and bleeding episodes.

Nonsteroidal Antiinflammatory Drugs/Cyclooxygenase 2 Inhibitors

Nonsteroidal antiinflammatory drugs (NSAIDs) and cyclooxygenase 2 (COX-2) inhibitors should be avoided in HF patients if possible. NSAIDs can interact with ACEIs and warfarin. NSAIDs may also have deleterious effects on renal function. Observational trials have demonstrated an increase in admissions for HF patients using NSAIDs or COX-2 inhibitors.[77,78]

VACCINATION
Influenza Vaccination

Influenza vaccination is recommended by the Centers for Disease Control for all individuals aged 6 months and older. In an observational study including more than 140,000 individuals aged 65 years or older, influenza vaccination was associated with 19% and 27% reductions in the risk of hospitalization for HF in consecutive years.[79]

Pneumococcal Vaccination

Pneumococcal vaccination is indicated for patients with HF. The incidence and mortality of pneumococcal disease are highest in older adults and in those with comorbidities.

COMPLEMENTARY AND ALTERNATIVE MEDICINE
Hawthorn (Crataegus)

In a randomized controlled trial of 2681 HF patients observed for 2 years, hawthorn was safe, but did not decrease mortality.[80] In one small study, hawthorn may have improved exercise capacity at high doses.[81] Overall, data do not support the routine use of hawthorn in treating HF.[82]

Mind-body Exercises (Tai Chi and Yoga)

Mind-body exercises represent an alternative exercise program that includes a meditative component. Small studies in stable HF patients have shown that Tai Chi may improve quality of life, mood, and sleep stability. Yoga may improve quality of life.

Chocolate

The benefit of chocolate for the treatment of HF is not known. In a prospective observational trial, intake of chocolate at a rate of 1 to 2 servings per week decreased the rate of incident HF or HF death among a group of 30,000 Swedish women without a history of coronary artery disease.[83] Intake at higher doses worsened outcomes.

Coenzyme Q10

Small trials of coenzyme Q10 in HF have shown variable results, and a meta-analysis of its effect on LVEF showed no benefit in the presence of ACEIs.[84,85] Adverse effects and drug interactions are not well defined but have included gastrointestinal complaints, elevated liver enzymes, and a possible interaction with warfarin.

Vitamin D

Several association studies link low vitamin D levels to increased total mortality, cardiovascular mortality, myocardial infarction, and HF.[86–88] In addition, low levels of vitamin D in patients with HF appear to independently predict poor outcomes.[89] However, the role of vitamin D supplementation to treat or prevent HF has not been established.

Alcohol

Given the potential risk of chronic alcohol consumption (including addiction, inappropriate risk taking, and disease progression), routine consumption of alcohol in patients with HF cannot be recommended. However, epidemiologic studies have suggested a protective effect of light to moderate alcohol intake against cardiovascular disease.[90] Among patients with HF and LVEF less than 35%, light to moderate alcohol consumption (1–14 drinks/wk) was associated with a 25% decrease in mortality, primarily among those with ischemic cardiomyopathy.[91,92]

SYSTEMS AIDING TREATMENT
Disease-based Management/Telemanagement

Hospitalization for HF is a powerful marker for subsequent rehospitalization and mortality. Patients with severe HF, repeated hospitalizations for HF, and possibly upon first hospitalization for HF, should be enrolled in an HF disease management program.

HF Disease Management Program

HF disease management programs substantially reduce mortality and HF hospitalizations. A 2004 meta-analysis of 29 trials including 5039 patients estimated that HF disease management reduced mortality and hospitalizations by 25% and 26%, respectively.[93] HF disease management programs should be multidisciplinary and should at least include intense patient support by HF-trained nurses, HF patient education, and facilitated access to physicians trained in HF.[94]

Telemanagement

In addition to HF disease management programs or as alternatives for patients who cannot gain access to an HF disease management program, different kinds of telemanagement have been tested including structured telephone support and semiautomated telemonitoring. Multiple trials of telemanagement yielded variable outcomes across heterogeneous interventions and populations. A Cochrane meta-analysis of 5613 patients included in trials through 2008 found that telemonitoring reduced all-cause mortality by 34% and that both telemonitoring and structured telephone support reduced HF hospitalizations by 21% and 23%, respectively.[95] However, a 2010 telemonitoring trial of 1652 patients in which daily data were transmitted to physicians rather than nurses showed no benefit.[96] Thus, the role of telemanagement in HF is controversial.

COMORBIDITIES
Kidney Disease

Acute kidney injury and chronic kidney disease (CKD) are common in patients with HF, especially in patients with more severe symptoms. More than 75% of patients hospitalized for HF have stage III, IV, or V CKD defined by a glomerular filtration rate of less than 60 mL/min. CKD may be a consequence of renal hypoperfusion from either an inadequate or a maldistributed cardiac output.[97] CKD may also represent intrinsic kidney disease or pharmacologic or other extrinsic toxicity. Regardless of the cause, CKD is associated with an increased risk of mortality and morbidity in patients with HF, especially in the presence of hypotension. For patients hospitalized with HF, the combination of a serum urea nitrogen level higher than 43 mg/dL, a serum creatinine level higher than 2.75 mmg/dL, and hypotension (defined by a systolic blood pressure <115 mm Hg) has been associated with a 25% in-hospital mortality rate.[98]

CKD can complicate treatment for patients with HF. CKD alters the pharmacokinetics of aldosterone antagonists and digoxin and can increase the risk of toxicity from these agents. CKD can impair the response to ACEIs and diuretics. Furthermore, diuretics, which are frequently necessary to control congestive symptoms, can concomitantly decrease glomerular filtration rates and contribute to additional diuretic resistance. Low-volume ultrafiltration has been recommended as an outpatient office procedure, but no large clinical trials are available to guide the role of this intervention. In end-stage kidney disease, dialysis or kidney transplantation can sometimes improve LVEF.[99]

To avoid kidney insufficiency, all nonsteroidal antiinflammatory drugs should be avoided in patients with HF. Adosterone antagonists should either be avoided or very closely monitored in patients with glomerular filtration rates less than 30 mL/min. Digoxin doses should be lowered in patients with kidney insufficiency.

Anemia

Anemia is common in patients with LVSD, especially in patients with severe HF symptoms. The anemia of HF is independently associated with increased mortality.[100] This anemia is often associated with blunted erythropoietin production and defective iron supply, and a small trial has demonstrated that treatment with subcutaneous erythropoietin and intravenous iron appears to improve symptoms, LVEF, and renal function.[101] Randomized controlled trials of intravenous iron in patients with HF and iron deficiency improved quality of life and functional capacity, but showed no improvement in mortality.[102] Administration of darbepoetin in anemic patients with HF has shown nonsignificant reductions in mortality and morbidity.[103,104] No controlled clinical trials have studied transfusion in patients with HF, but transfusion adversely affects outcomes in other, critically ill, anemic patients.

Atrial Fibrillation

Atrial fibrillation is common among patients with LVSD and is associated with higher mortality and an increased risk of hospitalization for HF.[105] Rapid ventricular rate responses to atrial fibrillation may worsen LVSD and HF symptoms and, in some cases, constitute the primary cause of the LVSD. Atrial fibrillation also increases the risk of thromboembolic events, especially stroke.

Strategies to convert and maintain sinus rhythm in patients with atrial fibrillation and LVSD are frequently unsuccessful, whether using antiarrhythmic medications (eg, amiodarone, dofetilide, etc) or performing electrophysiologic interventions (including atrial fibrillation ablation). Thus, ventricular rate control and anticoagulation are critical. Although strict rate control (<80 bpm at rest and <110 bpm with exercise) yielded equivalent outcomes to rhythm control, recent data in patients with normal systolic function suggest that lenient resting rate control (<110 bpm at rest) may provide equivalent or even superior benefit.[106,107] It is not known if these observations about lenient rate control can be extended to patients with LVSD. Beta blockers are more effective than digoxin in blocking exercise-induced increases in ventricular rate, although the combination of these agents may be especially efficacious. CCBs should be avoided as ventricular rate–controlling agents in patients with LVSD.

The primary indication for antithrombotics in HF patients is to prevent thromboembolic events associated with atrial fibrillation. Warfarin anticoagulation (INR 2–3) decreases the thromboembolic risk in patients with atrial fibrillation and CHADS2 scores greater than or equal to 2. HF patients with nonvalvular atrial fibrillation may be considered for alternative therapies other than warfarin. Newer agents include dabigatran (a direct thrombin inhibitor) and rivaroxaban and apixaban (direct factor Xa inhibitors). Compared with warfarin, they appear to be more efficacious (preventing stroke and systemic embolism), safer (causing less major and intracerebral hemorrhage), and more convenient (obviating the need for monitoring anticoagulation).[108–110] These newer agents will likely replace warfarin in many patients in the future. However, regardless of the antithrombotic agent, the risk of bleeding appears to increase with age, renal dysfunction, and through a variety of drug interactions.

Depression

Depression may occur in more than 20% of patients with HF and has been independently associated with increased mortality and morbidity. The most effective treatment of depression in patients with HF is not known. A recent, small, short-term randomized placebo controlled trial demonstrated that selective serotonin reuptake inhibitor therapy (sertraline) was safe in HF patients, but no more effective than placebo.[111] Tricyclic antidepressants should be used with extreme caution in HF patients, in part because of their effect on QT interval prolongation and association with increased cardiovascular events.

Diabetes

Approximately one-third of patients with HF have concomitant diabetes. HF patients with diabetes have poorer outcomes than patients without diabetes. HF is associated with insulin resistance and may contribute to diabetes and relative hyperglycemia. In addition, beta blockade can independently increase insulin resistance. The nonselective beta blocker, carvedilol, may have less effect on insulin resistance than the cardioselective beta blockers, metoprolol and bisoprolol. Secondary analyses from large prospective trials have shown that beta blockers are beneficial in patients with HF and diabetes.[112]

The optimal strategy to treat diabetes in patients with HF is not known. Metformin has been shown to improve outcomes in patients with diabetes. However, metformin use in patients with poor renal function has been historically discouraged because of the perceived risk of developing lactic acidosis. Retrospective reviews and recent observational study have suggested that metformin is safe in HF patients and may be associated with lower mortality rates.[113]

Thiazolidinediones can complicate the treatment of HF. A recent trial demonstrated that pioglitazone can significantly reduce heart attacks, strokes, and death in diabetics.[114] However, thiazolidinediones are associated with fluid retention and edema, especially in patients also receiving insulin. In addition, rosiglitazone may increase cardiovascular risk and pioglitazone may increase the risk of bladder cancer. Therefore, thiazolidinediones should be administered with caution in patients with HF, especially in patients whose fluid balance is tenuous.

Erectile Dysfunction

More than 60% of HF patients are estimated to report some degree of erectile dysfunction (ED). Small studies suggest that the use of PDE-5 inhibitors are effective in treating ED in HF patients and appear to be safe.[115,116] The use of PDE-5 inhibitors is contraindicated in patients taking nitrates.

Sleep Apnea

Sleep-disoriented breathing reportedly occurs in more than half of patients with HF approximately equally divided between obstructive sleep apnea and central sleep apnea. Obstructive apnea occurs more commonly in patients with the metabolic syndrome and is associated with hypertension, progressive LVSD, and a higher risk of death.

One small study demonstrated that continuous positive airway pressure can reduce blood pressure and improve LVSD. However, in HF patients with central sleep apnea the effects of positive airway pressure are ambiguous. The largest reported study demonstrated that continuous positive airway pressure decreased the degree of disordered breathing and marginally improved exercise capacity, but did not alter mortality or the need for heart transplantation.[117]

OLDER ADULTS AND PALLIATIVE CARE
Older Adults

Most patients with HF are older than 65 years. Most randomized controlled trials have included older adults, but not those older than 80 years.

Palliative Care

Discussions regarding advance directives with patients and family should occur in the context of HF management. Additionally, consultation with a hospice and palliative medicine physician may enhance symptom assessment and control in some patients. No definitive, evidence-based criteria exist for when to add palliative care to the multidisciplinary team caring for the patient with HF.[118] The Memorial Symptom Assessment Scale is used to measure symptoms to identify distressful symptoms related to impairment in quality of life as measured by the Multidimensional Index of Life Quality.[119]

REFERENCES

1. Roger VL, Go AS, Lloyd-Jones DM, et al. Heart disease and stroke statistics–2011 update: a report from the American Heart Association. Circulation 2011; 123:e18–209.
2. Butler J, Shapiro MD, Jassal D, et al. Comparison of multidetector computed tomography and two-dimensional transthoracic echocardiography for left ventricular assessment in patients with heart failure. Am J Cardiol 2007;99:247–9.
3. Hovland A, Staub UH, Bjornstad H, et al. Gated SPECT offers improved interobserver agreement compared with echocardiography. Clin Nucl Med 2010;35: 927–30.
4. Gitt AK, Wasserman K, Kilkowski C, et al. Exercise anaerobic threshold and ventilatory efficiency identify heart failure patients for high risk of early death. Circulation 2002;106:3079–84.
5. Bard RL, Gillespie BW, Clarke NS, et al. Combining peak oxygen consumption and ventilatory efficiency in the prognostic assessment of patients with heart failure. Int J Cardiol 2008;123:199–200.
6. Maisel AS, Krishnaswamy P, Nowak RM, et al. Rapid measurement of B-type natriuretic peptide in the emergency diagnosis of heart failure. N Engl J Med 2002;347:161–7.
7. Pfisterer M, Buser P, Rickli H, et al. BNP-guided vs symptom-guided heart failure therapy: the trial of intensified vs standard medical therapy in elderly patients with congestive heart failure (TIME-CHF) randomized trial. JAMA 2009;301:383–92.
8. Bielecka-Dabrowa A, Mikhailidis DP, Jones L, et al. The meaning of hypokalemia in heart failure. Int J Cardiol 2012;158(1):12–7.
9. Nicklas JM, Bleske BE, Brown M, et al. Nocturnal hypokalemia in patients with congestive heart failure treated with diuretics. Circulation 1998;98:I-24.
10. Cohn JN, Kower PR, Whelton PK, et al. New guideline for potassium replacement in clinical practice: a contemporary review by the National Council on Potassium in Clinical Practice. Arch Intern Med 2000;160:2429–36.
11. Powell LH, Calvin JE, Richardson D, et al. Self-management counseling in patients with heart failure: the heart failure adherence and retention randomized behavioral trial. JAMA 2010;304:1331–8.
12. Koelling TM, Johnson ML, Cody RJ, et al. Discharge education improves clinical outcomes in patients with chronic heart failure. Circulation 2005;111:179–85.
13. Bocchi EA, Cruz F, Guimaraes G, et al. Long-term prospective, randomized, controlled study using repetitive education at six-month intervals and monitoring for adherence in heart failure outpatients: the REMADHE trial. Circ Heart Fail 2008;1:115–24.
14. Davies EJ, Moxham T, Rees K, et al. Exercise training for systolic heart failure: cochrane systematic review and meta-analysis. Eur J Heart Fail 2010;12: 706–15.
15. O'Connor CM, Whellan DJ, Lee KL, et al. Efficacy and safety of exercise training in patients with chronic heart failure: HF-ACTION randomized controlled trial. JAMA 2009;301:1439–50.
16. Paterna S, Parrinello G, Cannizzaro S, et al. Medium term effects of different dosage of diuretic, sodium, and fluid administration on neurohormonal and clinical outcome in patients with recently compensated heart failure. Am J Cardiol 2009;103:93–102.
17. Allman KC, Shaw LJ, Hachamovitch R, et al. Myocardial viability testing and impact of revasculaization on prognosis in patients with coronary artery disease

and left ventricular dysfunction: a meta-analysis. J Am Coll Cardiol 2002;39: 1151–8.

18. Velazquez EJ, Lee KL, Deja MA, et al. Coronary-artery bypass surgery in patients with left ventricular dysfunction. N Engl J Med 2011;364:1607–16.

19. Bonow RO, Maurer G, Lee KL, et al. Myocardial viability and survival in ischemic left ventricular dysfunction. N Engl J Med 2011;364:1617–25.

20. Jones RH, Velazquez EJ, Michler RE, et al. Coronary bypass surgery with or without surgical ventricular reconstruction. N Engl J Med 2009;360:1705–17.

21. Wu AH, Aaronson KD, Bolling SF, et al. Impact of mitral valve annuloplasty on mortality risk in patients with mitral regurgitation and left ventricular systolic dysfunction. J Am Coll Cardiol 2005;45:381–7.

22. Moss AJ, Hall WJ, Cannom DS, et al. Improved survival with an implanted defibrillator in patients with coronary disease at high risk for ventricular arrhythmia. N Engl J Med 1996;335:1933–40.

23. Buxton AE, Lee KL, Fisher JD, et al. A randomized study of the prevention of sudden death in patients with coronary artery disease. N Engl J Med 1999; 341:1882–90.

24. Moss AJ, Zareba W, Hall WJ, et al. Prophylactic implantation of a defibrillator in patients with myocardial infarction and reduced ejection fraction. N Engl J Med 2002;346:877–83.

25. Kadish A, Dyer A, Daubert JP, et al. Prophylactic defibrillator implantation in patients with nonischemic dilated cardiomyopathy. N Engl J Med 2004;350: 2151–8.

26. Bardy GH, Lee KL, Mark DB, et al. Amiodarone or an implantable cardioverter-defibrillator for congestive heart failure. N Engl J Med 2005;352:225–37.

27. Bigger JT. Prophylactic use of implanted cardiac defibrillators in patients at high risk for ventricular arrhythmias after coromary-artery bypass graft surgery. N Engl J Med 1997;337:1569–75.

28. Hohnloser SH, Kuck KH, Dorian P, et al. Prophylactic use of an implantable cardioverter-defibrillator after acute myocardial infarction. N Engl J Med 2004; 351:2481–8.

29. Russo AM, Day JD, Stolen K, et al. Implantable cardioverter defibrillators: do women fare worse than men? gender comparison in the INTRINSIC RV trial. J Cardiovasc Electrophysiol 2009;20:973–8.

30. Santangeli P, PeLargonio G, Russo AD, et al. Gender differences in clinical outcome and primary prevention defibrillator benefit in patients with severe left ventricular dysfunction: a systematic review and meta-analysis. Heart Rhythm 2010;7:876–82.

31. Ghanbari H, Dalloul G, Hasan R, et al. Effectiveness of implantable cardioverter-defibrillators for the primary prevention of sudden cardiac death in women with advanced heart failure. Arch Intern Med 2009;169:1500–6.

32. Bristow MR, Saxon LA, Boehmer J, et al. Cardiac-resynchronization therapy with or without an implantable defibrillator in advanced chronic heart failure. N Engl J Med 2004;350:2140–50.

33. Cleland JG, Daubert JC, Erdmann E, et al. The effect of cardiac resynchronization on morbidity and mortality in heart failure. N Engl J Med 2005;352:1539–49.

34. Daubert C, Gold MR, Abraham WT, et al. Prevention of disease progression by cardiac resynchronization therapy in patients with asymptomatic or mildly symptomatic left ventricular dysfunction. J Am Coll Cardiol 2009;54:1837–46.

35. Goldenberg I, Hall WJ, Beck CA, et al. Reduction of the risk of recurring heart failure events with cardiac resynchronization therapy MADIT-CRT (Multicenter

Automatic Defibrillator Implantation Trial with Cardiac Resynchronization Therapy). J Am Coll Cardiol 2011;58:729–37.

36. The CONSENSUS Trial Study Group. Effects of enalapril on mortality in severe congestive heart failure: results of the Cooperative North Scandinavian Enalapril Survival Study (CONSENSUS). N Engl J Med 1987;316:1429–35.

37. The SOLVD Investigators. Effect of enalapril on survival in patients with reduced left ventricular ejection fractions and congestive heart failure. N Engl J Med 1991;325:293–302.

38. The SOLVD Investigators. Effect of enalapril on mortality and the development of heart failure in asymptomatic patients with reduced left ventricular ejection fractions. N Engl J Med 1992;327:685–91.

39. CIBIS II Investigators and Committees. The cardiac insufficiency bisoprolol study (CIBIS II): a randomised trial. Lancet 1999;353:9–13.

40. MERIT HF Study Group. Effect of metoprolol CR/XL in chronic heart failure: Metoprolol CR/XL: randomised intervention trial in congestive heart failure (MERIT-HF). Lancet 1999;353:2001–7.

41. Packer M, Coats AJ, Fowler MB, et al. Effect of carvedilol on survival in severe chronic heart failure. N Engl J Med 2001;344:1651–8.

42. The Beta-Blocker Evaluation of Survival Trial Investigators. A trial of the beta-blocker bucindolol in patients with advanced chronic heart failure. N Engl J Med 2001;344:1659–67.

43. Poole-Wilson PA, Swedberg K, Cleland JF, et al. Comparison of carvedilol and metoprolol on clinical outcomes in patients with chronic heart failure in the Carvedilol Or Metoprolol European Trial (COMET): randomised controlled trial. Lancet 2003;362:7–13.

44. Pitt B, Zannad F, Remme WJ, et al. The effect of spironolactone on morbidity and mortality in patients with severe heart failure. N Engl J Med 1999;341:709–17.

45. Pitt B, Remme W, Zannad F, et al. Eplerenone, a selective aldosterone blocker, in patients with left ventricular dysfunction after myocardial infarction. N Engl J Med 2003;348:1309–21.

46. Zannad F, McMurray JJ, Krum H, et al. Eplerenone in patients with systolic heart failure and mild symptoms. N Engl J Med 2011;364:11–21.

47. Juurlink DN, Mamdani MM, Lee DS, et al. Rates of hyperkalemia after publication of the randomized aldactone evaluation study. N Engl J Med 2004;351:543–51.

48. Pitt B, Poole-Wilson PA, Segal R, et al. Effect of losartan compared with captopril on mortality in patients with symptomatic heart failure: randomised trial—the losartan heart failure survival study ELITE II. Lancet 2000;355:1582–7.

49. Granger CB, McMurray JJ, Yusuf S, et al. Effects of candesartan in patients with chronic heart failure and reduced left-ventricular systolic function intolerant to angiotensin-converting-enzyme inhibitors: the CHARM-Alternative trial. Lancet 2003;362:772–6.

50. McMurray JJ, Ostergren J, Swedberg K, et al. Effects of candesartan in patients with chronic heart failure and reduced left-ventricular systolic function taking angiotensin-converting-enzyme inhibitors: the CHARM-Added trial. Lancet 2003;362:767–71.

51. Cohn JN, Tognoni G, Valsartan Heart Failure Trial Investigators. A randomized trial of the angiotensin-receptor blocker valsartan in chronic heart failure. N Engl J Med 2001;345:1667–75.

52. The ONTARGET Investigators, Yusuf S, Teo KK, Pogue J, et al. Telmisartan, ramipril, or both in patients at high risk for vascular events. N Engl J Med 2008;358:1547–59.

53. Cohn JN, Archibald DG, Ziesche S, et al. Effect of vasodilator therapy on mortality in chronic congestive heart failure results of a Veterans Administration cooperative study. N Engl J Med 1986;314:547–52.
54. Cohn JN, Johnson G, Ziesche S, et al. A comparison of enalapril with hydralazine-isosorbide dinitrate in the treatment of chronic congestive heart failure. N Engl J Med 1991;325:303–10.
55. Carson P, Ziesche S, Johnson G, et al. Racial differences in response to therapy for heart failure: analysis of the vasodilator-heart failure trials. J Card Fail 1999;5: 178–87.
56. Taylor AL, Ziesche S, Yancy C, et al. Combination of isosorbide dinitrate and hydralazine in blacks with heart failure. N Engl J Med 2004;351: 2049–57.
57. Brater DC. Diuretic therapy. N Engl J Med 1998;339:387–95.
58. Bleske BE, Welage LS, Kramer, et al. Torsemide administration in patients with decompensated and compensated congestive heart failure. J Clin Pharmacol 1998;38:708–14.
59. Jentzer JC, DeWald TA, Hernandez AF. Combination of loop diuretics with thiazide-type diuretics in heart failure. J Am Coll Cardiol 2010;56:1527–34.
60. The Digitalis Investigation Group. The effect of digoxin on mortality and morbidity in patients with heart failure. N Engl J Med 1997;336:525–33.
61. Rathore SS, Curtis JP, Wang Y, et al. Association of serum digoxin concentration and outcomes in patients with heart failure. JAMA 2003;289:871–8.
62. The Multicenter Diltiazem Postinfarction Trial Research Group. The effect of diltiazem on mortality and reinfarction after myocardial infarction. N Engl J Med 1988;319:385–92.
63. Goldstein RE, Boccuzzi SJ, Cruess D, et al. Diltiazem increases late-onset congestive heart failure in postinfarction patients with early reduction in ejection fraction. Circulation 1991;83:52–60.
64. Packer M, O'Connor CM, Ghali JK, et al. Effect of amlodipine on morbidity and mortality in severe chronic heart failure. N Engl J Med 1996;335:1107–14.
65. Amsallem E, Kasparian C, Haddour G, et al. Phosphodiesterase III inhibitors for heart failure. Cochrane Database Syst Rev 2005;(1):CD002230.
66. Tacon CL, McCaffrey J, Delaney A. Dobutamine for patients with severe heart failure: a systematic review and meta-analysis of randomised controlled trials. Intensive Care Med 2012;38:359–67.
67. Abraham WT, Adams KF, Fornarow GC, et al. In-hospital mortality in patients with acute decompensated heart failure requiring intravenous vasoactive medications: an anlysis from the Acute Decompensated Heart Failure Registry (ADHERE). J Am Coll Cardiol 2005;46:57–64.
68. Echt DS, Liebson PR, Mitchell B, et al. Mortality and morbidity in patients receiving encainide, flecainide, or placebo. The Cardiac Arrhythmia Suppression Trial. N Engl J Med 1991;324:781–8.
69. Kjekshus J, Apetrei E, Barrios V, et al. Rosuvastatin in older patients with systolic heart failure. N Engl J Med 2007;357:2248–61.
70. GISSI-HF Investigators, Tavazzi L, Maggioni AP, Marchioli R, et al. Effect of rosuvastatin in patients with chronic heart failure (the GISSI-HF trial): a randomized, double-blind, placebo-controlled trial. Lancet 2008;372:1231–9.
71. GISSI-HF Investigators, Tavazzi L, Maggioni AP, Marchioli R, et al. Effect of n-3 polyunsaturated fatty acids in patients with chronic heart failure(the GISSI-HF trial): a randomized, double-blind, placebo-controlled trial. Lancet 2008;372: 1223–30.

72. McAlister FA, Ghali WA, Gong Y, et al. Aspirin use and outcomes in a community-based cohort of 7352 patients discharged after first hospitalization for heart failure. Circulation 2006;113:2572–8.

73. Levy PD, Nandyal D, Welch RD, et al. Does aspirin use adversely influence intermediate-term postdischarge outcomes for hospitalized patients who are treated with angiotensin-converting enzyme inhibitors or angiotensin receptor blockers? Findings from Organized Program to Facilitate Life-Saving Treatment in Hospitalized Patients with Heart Failure (OPTIMIZE-HF). Am Heart J 2010; 159:222–30.

74. Cleland JG, Findlay I, Jafri S, et al. The warfarin/aspirin study in heart failure (WASH): a randomized trial comparing antithrombotic strategies for patients with heart failure. Am Heart J 2004;148:157–64.

75. Massie BM, Collins JF, Ammon SE, et al. Randomized trial of warfarin, aspirin, and clopidogrel in patients with chronic heart failure: the warfarin and antiplatelet therapy in chronic heart failure (WATCH) trial. Circulation 2009;119:1616–24.

76. Homma S, Thompson JL, Pullicino PM, et al. Warfarin and aspirin in patients with heart failure and sinus rhythm. N Engl J Med 2012;366:1859–69.

77. Gislason GH, Rasmussen JN, Abildstrom SZ, et al. Increased mortality and cardiovascular morbidity associated with use of nonsteroidal anti-inflammatory drugs in chronic heart failure. Arch Intern Med 2009;169:141–9.

78. Hudson M, Hugues R, Pilote L. Differences in outcomes of patients with congestive heart failure prescribed celecoxib, rofecoxib, or non-steroidal anti-inflammatory drugs: population based study. BMJ 2005;330:1370–5.

79. Nichol KL, Nordin J, Mullooly J, et al. Influenza vaccination and reduction in hospitalizations for cardiac disease and stroke among the elderly. N Engl J Med 2003;348:1322–32.

80. Holubarsch CJ, Colucci WS, Meinertz T, et al. The efficacy and safety of Crataegus extract WS 1442 in patients with heart failure: the SPICE trial. Eur J Heart Fail 2008;10:1255–63.

81. Tauchert M. Efficacy and safety of crataegus extract WS 1442 in comparison with placebo in patients with chronic stable New York Heart Association class-III heart failure. Am Heart J 2002;143:910–5.

82. Pittler MH, Guo R, Ernst E. Hawthorn extract for treating chronic heart failure. Cochrane Database Syst Rev 2008;(1):CD005312.

83. Mostofsky E, Levitan EB, Wolk A, et al. Chocolate intake and incidence of heart failure. A population-based prospective study of middle-aged and elderly women. Circ Heart Fail 2010;3:612–6.

84. Khatta M, Alexander BS, Krichten CM, et al. The effect of coenzyme Q10 in patients with congestive heart failure. Ann Intern Med 2000;132:636–40.

85. Sander S, Coleman CI, Patel AA, et al. The impact of coenzyme Q10 on systolic function in patients with chronic heart failure. J Card Fail 2006;12:464–72.

86. Giovannucci E, Liu Y, Hollis BW, et al. 25-Hydroxyvitamin D and risk of myocardial infarction in men: a prospective study. Arch Intern Med 2008; 168:1174–80.

87. Wang TJ, Pencina MJ, Booth SL, et al. Vitamin D deficiency and risk of cardiovascular disease. Circulation 2008;117:503–11.

88. Dobnig H, Pilz S, Scharnagl H, et al. Independent association of low serum 25-hydroxyvitamin D and 1,25-dihydroxyvitamin D levels with all-cause and cardiovascular mortality. Arch Intern Med 2008;168:1340–9.

89. Liu LC, Voors AA, van Veldhuisen DJ, et al. Vitamin D status and outcomes in heart failure patients. Eur J Heart Fail 2011;13:619–25.

90. Gaziano JM, Gaziano TA, Glynn RJ, et al. Light-to-moderate alcohol consumption and mortality in the Physicians' Health Study enrollment cohort. J Am Coll Cardiol 2000;35:96–105.
91. Cooper HA, Exner DV, Domanski MJ. Light-to-moderate alcohol consumption and prognosis in patients with left ventricular systolic dysfunction. J Am Coll Cardiol 2000;35:1753–9.
92. Padilla H, Michael Gaziano J, Dioussse L. Alcohol consumption and risk of heart failure: a meta-analysis. Phys Sportsmed 2010;38:84–9.
93. McAlister FA, Stewart S, Ferrua S, et al. Multidisciplinary strategies for the management of heart failure patients at high risk for admission. A systematic review of randomized trials. J Am Coll Cardiol 2004;44:810–9.
94. McDonagh TA, Blue L, Clark AL, et al. European Society of Cardiology heart Failure Association standards for delivering heart failure care. Eur J Heart Fail 2011;13:235–41.
95. Inglis SC, Clark RA, McAlister FA, et al. Structured telephone support or telemonitoring programmes for patients with chronic heart failure. Cochrane Database Syst Rev 2010;(8):CD007228.
96. Chaudhry SI, Mattera JA, Curtis JP, et al. Telemonitoring in patients with heart failure. N Engl J Med 2010;363:2301–9.
97. Heywood JT. The cardiorenal syndrome: lessons from the ADHERE Database and treatment options. Heart Fail Rev 2004;9:195–201.
98. Fonarow GC, Adams KF, Abraham WT, et al. Risk stratification for in-hospital mortality in heart failure using classification and regression tree (CART) methodology: analysis of 33,046 patients in the ADHERE registry. J Card Fail 2003; 9:S79.
99. Wali RK, Wang GS, Gottlieb SS, et al. Effect of kidney transplantation on left ventricular systolic dysfunction and congestive heart failure in patient with end-stage renal disease. J Am Coll Cardiol 2005;45:1051–60.
100. Groenveld HF, Januzzi JL, Damman K, et al. Anemia and mortality in heart failure patients. A systematic review and meta-analysis. J Am Coll Cardiol 2008;52: 818–27.
101. Silverberg DS, Wexler D, Sheps D, et al. The effect of correction of mild anemia in severe, resistant congestive heart failure using subcutaneous erythropoietin and intravenous iron: a randomized controlled study. J Am Coll Cardiol 2001; 37:1775–80.
102. Anker SD, Colet JC, Filippatos G, et al. Ferric carboxymaltose in patients with heart failure and iron deficiency. N Engl J Med 2009;361:2436–48.
103. Ghali JK, Anand IS, Abraham WT, et al. Randomized double-blind trial of darbepoetin alfa in patients with symptomatic heart failure and anemia. Circulation 2008;117:526–35.
104. Kotecha D, Ngo K, Walters JA, et al. Erythropoietin as a treatment of anemia in heart failure: systematic review of randomized trials. Am Heart J 2011;161(5): 822–31.
105. Dries DL, Exner DV, Gersh BJ, et al. Atrial fibrillation is associated with an increased risk for mortality and heart failure progression in patients with asymptomatic and symptomatic left ventricular systolic dysfunction: a retrospective analysis of the SOLVD trials. J Am Coll Cardiol 1998;32:695–703.
106. Wyse DG, Waldo AL, DiMarco JP, et al, The Atrial Fibrillation Follow-Up Investigation of Rhythm Management (AFFIRM) Investigators. A comparison of rate control and rhythm control in patients with atrial fibrillation. N Engl J Med 2002;347:1825–33.

107. Van Gelder IC, Groenveld HF, Crijns HJ, et al. Lenient versus strict rate control in patients with atrial fibrillation. N Engl J Med 2010;362:1363–73.
108. Connolly SJ, Ezekowitz MD, Yusuf S, et al. Dabigatran versus warfarin in patients with atrial fibrillation. N Engl J Med 2009;361:1139–51.
109. Patel MR, Mahaffey KW, Garg J, et al. Rivaroxaban versus warfarin in nonvalvular atrial fibrillation. N Engl J Med 2011;365:883–91.
110. Granger CB, Alexander JH, McMurray JJ, et al. Apixaban versus warfarin in patients with atrial fibrillation. N Engl J Med 2011;365:981–92.
111. O'Connor CM, Jiang W, Kuchibhatla M, et al. Safety and efficacy of sertraline for depression in patients with heart failure. J Am Coll Cardiol 2010;56:692–9.
112. Haas SJ, Vos T, Gilbert RE, et al. Are beta-blockers as efficacious in patients with diabetes mellitus as in patients without diabetes mellitus who have chronic heart failure? A meta-analysis of large-scale clinical trials. Am Heart J 2003;146: 848–53.
113. Aguilar D, Chan W, Bozkurt B, et al. Metformin use and mortality in ambulatory patients with diabetes and heart failure. Circ Heart Fail 2011;4:53–8.
114. Wilcox R, Kupfer S, Erdmann E, et al. Effects of pioglitazone on major adverse cardiovascular events in high-risk patients with type 2 diabetes: results from PROspective pioglitAzone Clinical Trial In macro Vascular Events (PROactive 10). Am Heart J 2008;155:712–7.
115. Katz SD, Parker JD, Glasser DB, et al. Efficacy and safety of sildenafil citrate in men with erectile dysfunction and chronic heart failure. Am J Cardiol 2005;95: 36–42.
116. Al-Ameri H, Kloner RA. Erectile dysfunction and heart failure: the role of phophodiesterase type 5 inhibitors. Int J Impot Res 2009;21:149–57.
117. Bradley TD, Logan AG, Kimoff RJ, et al. Continuous positive airway pressure for central sleep apnea and heart failure. N Engl J Med 2005;353:2025–33.
118. Low J, Pattenden J, Candy B, et al. Palliative care in advanced heart failure: an international review of the perspectives of recipients and health professionals on care provision. J Card Fail 2011;17:231–52.
119. Blinderman CD, Homel P, Billings JA, et al. Symptom distress and quality of life in patients with advanced congestive heart failure. J Pain Symptom Manage 2008;35:594–603.

Supraventricular and Ventricular Arrhythmias

Ramil Goel, MD[a], Komandoor Srivathsan, MD[a],
Martina Mookadam, MD[b],*

KEYWORDS

- Supraventricular tachycardia • Atrial fibrillation • Atrial flutter
- Multifocal atrial tachycardia • Ventricular arrhythmia

KEY POINTS

- Atrial fibrillation is the commonest persistent cardiac arrhythmia, affecting up to 5 million individuals in the United States, with the incidence expected to increase as the population ages. Pathophysiology, therapeutic options, and prevention strategies are discussed.
- Supraventricular tachycardias occur in structurally normal hearts as opposed to atrial fibrillation, atrial flutter, and mutifocal atrial tachycardia. They can cause significant morbidity in young individuals. Pathophysiology, acute, and long-term management are described.
- Ventricular arrhythmias have a wide variation in prognosis, from benign to risk of sudden cardiac death. Diagnosis and investigation as well as prevention are reviewed in this article.

ATRIAL FIBRILLATION

Atrial fibrillation (AF) is the most common persistent cardiac arrhythmia affecting up to 5 million individuals in the United States.[1] The incidence is expected to increase as the population ages.[2] The presence of AF doubles the risk of death.[3] The most common source of morbidity is stroke, which increases 5-fold in the presence of AF. The diagnosis is made by an irregular and usually rapid pulse on examination. The electrocardiogram (EKG) is characterized by chaotic, disorganized atrial activity. The disease usually shows a progressive course, with intermittent paroxysms that culminate in the permanent intractable form, which may be difficult to reverse. Many drugs and techniques to deal with AF have been developed but how and when these should

The authors have nothing to disclose.
[a] Department of Cardiovascular Disease, Mayo Clinic, 13400 East Shea Boulevard, Scottsdale, AZ 85259, USA; [b] Department of Family Medicine, Mayo Clinic, 13737 North 92nd Street, Scottsdale, AZ 85260, USA
* Corresponding author.
E-mail address: mookadam.martina@mayo.edu

be applied are unclear and marked by a lack of consensus. Evidence-based guidance recommends the need for both aggressive risk factor modification to prevent AF (eg, treating hypertension, diabetes, sleep apnea, and obesity) as well as anticoagulation for the prevention of stroke.

Epidemiology

AF has a prevalence of 1% to 2% in the general population.[4] Because AF can be asymptomatic, the prevalence is believed to be closer to the upper limits of this range. The prevalence increases with age and individuals older than 80 years have a prevalence of up to 15%.[5] An average 40-year-old individual has a 25% lifetime risk of developing AF.[6]

Classification of AF

The American College of Cardiology and American Heart Association (ACC/AHA) has divided AF into 4 categories by the temporal distribution of the disease[7]:

1. First detected episode: defined as the first diagnosed episode of AF regardless of duration or presence or absence of symptoms
2. Paroxysmal AF: defined as 2 or more episodes of AF that spontaneously terminate within 7 days (usually within 24 hours)
3. Persistent AF: characterized by an episode lasting longer than paroxysmal AF but not more than 1 year
4. Permanent: defined by AF episode lasting beyond 1 year

The category of lone AF defines that group of individuals with AF without any structural heart disease but this group is not a part of the classification by ACC/AHA. This classification is important, because it has implications with regards to the pathophysiology of the AF as well as the subsequent treatment options.

The European Society of Cardiology recently introduced a category: long-standing persistent AF, defined as more than 1 year in duration but in which rhythm control strategy is believed to be feasible.[8]

Risk Factors

The Framingham Heart Study population developed a model incorporating variables including age, gender, hypertension, treatment of hypertension, PR interval, significant cardiac murmur, heart failure, and body mass index (BMI, calculated as weight in kilograms divided by the square of height in meters) for predicting the development of AF over a 10-year period.[9] During a 38-year follow-up period, men were 1.5 times more likely to develop AF.[10] With each passing decade, the odds ratio for developing AF was 2.1 for men and 2.2 for women compared with the previous decade.[10]

Hypertension is associated with a relative risk of 1.42 for developing AF.[11] Even although this effect is modest, the high prevalence of hypertension in the general population makes hypertension the most common disorder associated with AF.

Coronary artery disease (CAD) burden does not cause AF by itself; however, in the setting of acute myocardial infarction with left ventricular dysfunction or in the presence of congestive heart failure (CHF), AF supervenes because of atrial stretch. In the CASS (Coronary Artery Surgical Study) registry, only 0.6% of the patients had AF.[12] Furthermore, the number of diseased coronary arteries was not associated with higher AF rates. A diagnosis of CAD was associated with a relative risk of 1.98 for developing AF over a period of 7 years,[12] mainly as a result of common risk factors of both CAD and AF.

Valvular heart disease is associated with increased risk for developing AF. In patients of rheumatic heart disease, those with combined valvular disease (mitral stenosis, mitral regurgitation [MR], and tricuspid regurgitation) had the highest prevalence of AF.[13]

Among patients with isolated valvular abnormalities, mitral stenosis (29%) had the highest prevalence of AF followed by MR (16%) and aortic valvular disease (1%).[13] Nonrheumatic valvular heart disease also confers a high risk of AF. In a study of Olmsted county patients retrospectively identified for their severe degenerative MR caused by flail leaflet or mitral valve prolapse,[14] the subsequent incidence of AF was 41% and 44% over 9 years, respectively. Because the outcomes of MR surgery are worse in the presence of AF, this study made the case for early surgery before AF supervenes.[14]

In patients with hypertrophic cardiomyopathy, the incidence of AF is as high as 28%, which may also worsen the mortality outcome of these patients.[15] The presence of atrial septal defect is associated with about 20% incidence of AF.[16] Some other congenital heart diseases are also associated with increased risk of AF. CHF of any cause, diagnosed clinically, has been associated with an odds ratio of 4.5 for men and 5.9 for women for developing AF.[10]

Pulmonary embolism and chronic obstructive pulmonary disease (COPD) are also at higher risk for AF.[17,18] Obstructive sleep apnea is also more common in patients with AF than those without (49% vs 32%, $P = .0004$), even after adjusting for age, gender, BMI, diabetes mellitus (DM), hypertension, and CHF.[19]

Obesity has been established as an independent risk factor for AF with a BMI greater than 30 (vs a BMI of <25) associated with a hazard ratio of 1.52 for men and 1.46 for women, as noted in the Framingham Heart Study.[20] Metabolic syndrome is also associated with AF, with a hazard ratio of 1.61.[21] Pericardial fat, which is emerging as a marker of visceral obesity, is also associated with higher rates of AF.[22]

Chronic kidney disease also confers higher risk of AF, with risk increasing as renal function declines, as shown in the Japanese Niigata preventive study.[23] The hazard ratios for AF were 1.32 (1.08–1.62) and 1.57 (0.89–2.77) for glomerular filtration rate 30 to 59 and less than 30 mL/min per 1.73 m², respectively.[23] The presence of AF in patients with normal renal function at entry also predicted development of renal failure during follow-up.[23]

The presence of family history was associated with a hazard ratio of 1.4 after adjusting for other AF risk factors when patients were followed for a duration of almost 4 decades.[24] Even although few individual gene mutations showing a Mendelian pattern of inheritance have been identified, most patients are believed to have polygenic inheritance.

Mechanism and Pathophysiology

AF is characterized by irregular chaotic atrial activity with cycle lengths usually less than 200 milliseconds (corresponding to an atrial rate of >300/min). Distinct atrial activity is difficult to discern on the surface EKG and is the hallmark of the diagnosis. The ventricular response is also irregular but slower, with the atrioventricular (AV) node acting as a filter, allowing only a proportion of the impulses to conduct. Uncommonly, in the presence of an accessory pathway with shorter refractory periods and higher rates of conduction, the ventricular rates may be higher and can culminate in ventricular fibrillation.

The electrophysiologic genesis of the rhythm takes place by 3 mechanisms[25]:

1. An irregular atrial response to a regularly firing ectopic atrial pacemaker
2. An irregular atrial response to a regular local reentrant circuit in the atrium
3. Multiple reentrant circuits in the atrium separated by time and space

Most paroxysmal AF is initiated and maintained by a rapidly firing atrial focus or local reentry in the atrial tissue surrounding and invaginating around 1 or more of the pulmonary veins.[26] This process forms the basis of pulmonary vein isolation to prevent the spread of these impulses to the rest of the atrial tissue. With time, as a result of progression of underlying cardiac disease and after multiple episodes of paroxysmal AF, the atrial tissue undergoes remodeling, which sustains longer-lasting AF.[27] This remodeling usually involves altered expression and function of ionic channels that support the sustenance of functional reentry substrates.[28] Worsening AF with longer and more frequent episodes further facilitates this process into a positive feedback loop in which AF begets AF. Initially, this remodeling is reversible, but with time, it becomes an irreversible permanent process involving structural changes, including fibrosis, which can create areas of slow conduction and promote reentry.[28] As the substrate for the development of AF becomes more complex, ablation procedures to interrupt these circuits become more challenging and less successful.

Apart from functional and structural changes in the atrial substrate, autonomic influences (parasympathetic and sympathetic tone) on the atrium also facilitate the initiation and sustenance of AF. Increases in both parasympathetic and sympathetic tone can facilitate AF.[29,30]

Once established, AF has 2 major clinical effects: decrease in the cardiac output and increased thromboembolic risk from left atrial thrombi. The cardiac output is decreased because of various mechanisms, including loss of atrial systolic function (which can contribute up to 20% of the normal stroke volume), irregular cardiac cycle length, rapid heart rates, and decreased coronary blood flow.[31]

Prolonged periods of increased ventricular rates (usually >120–130 beats/min) can lead to rate-related dilated cardiomyopathy. This phenomenon occurs more commonly in asymptomatic patients who do not seek medical attention despite being in AF for extended periods of time. The condition can develop as soon as 24 hours and peaks at about 5 weeks of being in AF.[32] Within 24 hours of rate control, the cardiomyopathy starts reversing itself and can resolve completely by 1 to 2 weeks after adequate ventricular rate control is achieved.[32]

The increased risk of left atrial thrombus formation is primarily related to the low flow state in the left atrium. The clots formed are rich in red blood cells and fibrin, which further attests to this proposition. Endothelial damage and hypercoagulability from the local inflammatory state are also contributors, making up the 2 remaining components of the Virchow triad.[33] The left atrial appendage is the site of thrombus in 90% of cases,[34,35] and thus exclusion of this structure is a potential target for mechanical approaches to prevent the thromboembolic complications of AF.

Clinical Features

The clinical presentation of AF is variable. Common symptoms include palpitations, dizziness, syncope, fatigue, dyspnea, and angina. There could be symptoms related to a thromboembolic event presenting as stroke, acute limb, and bowel ischemia. Often, AF manifests itself by decompensating the underlying cardiac disease, with subsequent symptoms of dyspnea, chest pain, and occasionally, cardiogenic shock. Many patients are diagnosed incidentally while being evaluated for associated conditions. Alcohol, caffeine, exercise, dehydration, anxiety, thyrotoxicosis, infection, and lung disease can precipitate AF in some patients.

The physical examination reveals an irregularly irregular cardiac rhythm, which may or may not be fast. Hypotension or hypoxia may be noted in sick patients with comorbidities. Increased irregular jugular venous pulsations can be noted. Cardiac auscultation may reveal a variable intensity of S1 and a loud P2, suggestive of high pulmonary pressures. Murmurs from associated valvular heart disease can frequently be auscultated. Lung auscultation may reveal related pulmonary processes, such as bronchospasm and congestion. The presence of lower extremity edema, hepato-megaly, and anasarca suggest underlying CHF.

Diagnosis and Investigations

Most patients are diagnosed with a 12-lead EKG or a rhythm strip (lasting at least 30 seconds) performed during the episode of the AF.[36] Occasionally, other arrhythmias such as frequent irregular premature atrial beats and atrial tachycardia (AT)/flutter with variable ventricular response can falsely give the impression of AF. A more careful exam-ination of the EKG, focusing on atrial activity, can be helpful in such cases. The use of vagal maneuvers or intravenous (IV) adenosine (in a monitored setting) can slow down the ventricular response rate and make the atrial activity seem more prominent.

Paroxysmal atrial fibrillation (PAF) may not be detected during the clinical visit. If PAF is suspected without an EKG to confirm the diagnosis, long-term and ambulatory moni-toring may be needed to establish the diagnosis. A 7-day Holter monitor or daily symptom-activated transtelephonic event monitoring can detect up to 70% of patients with recurrent AF.[36] However, even with these measures, the negative predictive value is about 25% to 40%.[36] When the index of suspicion for AF is high, an implantable loop recorder can extend the monitoring period for as long as 3 years, with higher sensitivity and negative predictive value, albeit at the cost of decreased specificity.[37]

Most patients require risk factor management and adjunctive diagnostic testing when diagnosed with AF. A transthoracic echocardiogram is essential for assessing cardiac structure and function. If cardioversion is being considered, a transesophageal echocardiogram to thoroughly scan the left atrial appendage for clots is considered an acceptable alternative to therapeutic anticoagulation of more than 3 weeks.[38] Blood tests to assess for DM, renal function, thyroid disorders, and lipid profile are reason-able in most patients. Many of these tests also help predict the risk of thromboembolic stroke in a patient with AF.

Testing for CAD may be reasonable when the clinical features (angina, left ventric-ular dysfunction, multiple cardiovascular risk factors) are present.

Polysomnography to evaluate for obstructive sleep apnea in the appropriate patient should be considered. Obstructive sleep apnea does not increase risk for AF but may predict the effectiveness of future treatment strategies.[39]

Management

The major goals of treatment in AF are symptom control, prevention of thromboem-bolic events, and tachycardia-induced cardiomyopathy. The 2 major strategies of management are rate control or rhythm control. The former entails ignoring the patient's atrial rhythm but slowing down the ventricular response rate by means of drugs or AV node ablation via catheter ablation. The rhythm control strategy, on the other hand, attempts to regulate the atrial rhythm by the use of antiarrhythmic agents or catheter ablation of atrial tissue to eliminate or isolate the arrhythmogenic foci. The rhythm control approach has a theoretic benefit in patients with symptoms related to irregular heart rate and impaired hemodynamics caused by irregular cardiac cycle length. However, in large randomized clinical trials (RACE [Rate Control Efficacy in Permanent Atrial Fibrillation] and AFFIRM [Atrial Fibrillation Follow-up Investigation of Rhythm Management]) neither strategy was found to be superior in terms of patient symptoms or clinical outcomes, including stroke risk, mortality, and echocardio-graphic parameters such as ejection fraction (EF).[40,41]

Regardless of the approach chosen for a particular individual, the need for adequate anticoagulation to prevent thromboembolic complications remains imperative.

Antithrombotic management

The most common and important thromboembolic complication of AF is cerebrovascular accident (CVA) or stroke. The guidelines for adequate anticoagulation in AF are based on individualized stroke risk. Best evidence has established that the major clinical factors associated with the risk of stroke are previous thromboembolic episode, poor left ventricular systolic function (EF <40%), hypertension (blood pressure >160/95 or use of antihypertensive agent), age older than 75 years, and DM.[42] The risk continues to increase with increasing number of risk factors present and is usually quantified in a user-friendly scoring system: the $CHADS_2$ (cardiac failure, hypertension, age, diabetes, stroke [doubled]) score. This scoring system evolved from the Stroke Prevention in Atrial Fibrillation (SPAF) investigators criteria.[43] The predicted risk of stroke in this model increases incrementally with increasing number of risk factors.

A score of more than 2 predicts a high risk of stroke at a level at which the risk for stroke is higher than the risk of major bleeding with the use of warfarin. Patients with a $CHADS_2$ score greater than 2 are candidates for anticoagulation with warfarin with a goal international normalized ratio (INR) of 2 to 3. Patients with a score of 0 are deemed to be at low risk and are prescribed aspirin based on physician discretion. A score equal to 1 to 2 is categorized as moderate risk and represents an area of uncertainty in terms of appropriate anticoagulation. Using the $CHADS_2$ score, almost 62% of the patients fall in this group. Aspirin use, at the least, is recommended for this group, even although this seems to be a heterogeneous group and there is a subset of patients who may derive benefit from warfarin therapy.[44] Additional risk factors such as vascular disease, age between 65 and 75 years, female gender, chronic kidney disease, proteinuria, and thyrotoxicosis have been identified that may influence stroke risk. A new scoring system incorporating some of these elements has been proposed to further stratify the moderate-risk group into a subset who may benefit from warfarin therapy.[44] The CHA_2DS_2-VASc score ascribes 2 points to age older than 75 years, and 1 point to age between 65 and 75 years. It also acknowledges the increased risk from vascular disease and female sex by ascribing 1 point each for the presence of these 2 factors.

Using warfarin can reduce the risk of stroke on an average by 68% compared with placebo.[45] Use of aspirin leads to an average reduction of 22% in the risk of thromboembolic stroke over placebo.[46] The use of warfarin is associated with higher risk of bleeding and requires close INR monitoring. Despite its limitations, warfarin was the only effective oral agent available for thromboprophylaxis in AF for more than 60 years.

In 2010, novel oral anticoagulant agents, approved for use, overcame some of the limitations posed by warfarin and were set to change the paradigm of anticoagulation in nonvalvular AF. Dabigatran, an oral direct thrombin inhibitor, and rivaroxaban, a direct factor X inhibitor, have been shown to be noninferior to warfarin in stroke thromboprophylaxis in nonvalvular AF.[47,48] The RE-LY (Randomized Evaluation of Long-Term Anticoagulation Therapy) trial compared dabigatran at a dose of 110 to 150 mg twice daily with dose-adjusted warfarin in 18,113 patients with nonvalvular AF (average $CHADS_2$ score = 2.1).[48] At the lower dose of dabigatran, there was no difference in event rate of CVAs compared with warfarin; however, the dabigatran group had fewer cases of major bleeding and intracranial hemorrhage. At the higher dose, dabigatran prevented more CVAs and intracranial hemorrhages but not other major bleeding events.

The ROCKET-AF (Rivaroxaban Once Daily Oral Direct Factor Xa Inhibition Compared with Vitamin K Antagonism for Prevention of Stroke and Embolism Trial in Atrial Fibrillation) was a double-blind randomized controlled trial to assess the efficacy of rivaroxaban 20 mg daily compared with dose-adjusted warfarin in patients with nonvalvular AF.[48] The mean $CHADS_2$ score was 3.5. Rivaroxaban was noninferior to dose-adjusted warfarin in achieving the primary end point. Bleeding complications were similar in both groups, but fatal and intracranial bleeding was reduced in the rivaroxaban group.

Another agent apixaban, also a direct factor X inhibitor, has been shown to be superior to warfarin both in terms of stroke prevention and bleeding risk. The ARISTOTLE (Apixaban for Reduction of Stroke and Other Thromboembolic Events in Atrial Fibrillation) trial compared apixaban 5 mg twice daily with dose-adjusted warfarin in 18,210 patients with AF or flutter for an average follow-up of 1.8 years.[49] Apixaban was superior to warfarin in terms of reaching the primary end point of ischemic or hemorrhagic stroke or systemic embolism (1.27% per year vs 1.6% per year, $P<.001$ for noninferiority and $P<.01$ for superiority). Risk of bleeding and hemorrhagic stroke was higher in the warfarin group ($P<.01$), although no significant difference was seen in all-cause mortality ($P = .047$). It was under consideration by the US Food and Drug Administration (FDA) for approval at the time of writing this article.[49]

Another nonpharmacologic approach that may become a viable option in future is the use of left atrial appendage occluders such as the WATCHMAN (Atritech, Plymouth, MN) device, which can be percutaneously implanted and positioned to block the entrance to the left atrial appendage. This procedure exploits the fact that the left atrial appendage is the source of most emboli in AF and isolating the appendage from the circulation may prevent formation of most emboli. This device was shown to be noninferior to vitamin K antagonists (warfarin and analogues) in the PROTECT AF (WATCHMAN Left Atrial Appendage System for Embolic protection in Patients with Atrial Fibrillation) trial.[50]

Rate control strategy
Available randomized trial data suggest no difference in clinical outcomes between the rate control and rhythm control strategies.[40,41] The intensity of rate control also does not seem to make a difference in terms of clinical parameters, including symptoms, quality of life, stroke, hospitalization, and death.[51,52] The strict rate control in this trial was defined as resting heart rate less than 80 beats per minute and heart rate during moderate exercise less than 110 beats per minute.[51,52] The lenient rate control criterion was a resting heart rate of less than 100 beats per minute.

Nonetheless, some patients have resting heart rates faster than the lenient heart rates as defined in the trial setting. These patients do qualify for pharmaceutical approaches for rate control. The mechanism of action of these agents relies on slowing down conduction through the AV node. The classes of agents used are β-blockers, nondihydropyridine calcium channel blockers, and digitalis. Digitalis has limited usefulness in patients with high adrenergic tone but may be of benefit in older or sedentary patients. Amiodarone can also occasionally serve as a rate control agent because of its β-blockade–type effect, in addition to being an antiarrhythmic. All of these agents can be used IV to achieve rapid rate control in an emergency setting, which can then be transferred to oral doses of the same or another agent (**Table 1**).

AV node ablation may be used as a last resort for rate control in patients in whom pharmacologic approaches fail. It is an invasive procedure and requires subsequent pacemaker implantation. Regardless of the approach used, considerations for stroke prophylaxis remain the same and form the most important component of therapy in patients for whom the rate control strategy has been chosen.

Rhythm control strategy
The main indication for opting for a rhythm control approach in AF is symptom control. Retrospective studies suggest beneficial effects for the maintenance of sinus rhythm

Table 1
Pharmaceutical agents used for rate control in AF

Drug	IV Dose	Oral Dose
Metoprolol	2.5–5 mg up to every 6 h	100–200 mg/d
Propranolol	0.5–1 mg over 1 min; may repeat, if necessary, up to a total maximum dose of 0.1 mg/kg	10–40 mg thrice daily
Atenolol	Not applicable	25–100 mg/d
Verapamil	2.5–5 mg initially followed by 5–10 mg every 30 min to a total maximum of 30 mg	240–480 mg/d in 3–4 divided doses
Diltiazem	5 mg bolus followed by 5–15 mg/h infusion	180–360 mg/d
Digoxin	0.25 mg every 2 h, up to 1.5 mg	0.125–0.375 mg/d
Amiodarone	5–7 mg/kg over 30–60 min, then 1.2–1.8 g/d continuous infusion or in divided oral doses until 10 g total	1.2–1.8 g/d in divided doses until 10 g total, then 200–400 mg/d

on quality of life and mortality when the adverse effects of antiarrhythmic agents are eliminated from the equation. However, randomized controlled studies on this issue are needed.

Cardioversion

Cardioversion allows the immediate termination of AF. It is indicated in patients with poor hemodynamic tolerance of an irregular rhythm or for whom a long-term rhythm control strategy has been chosen. The former can present as hypotension, angina, heart failure, and altered mental status from cerebral hypoperfusion. There are 2 important means of achieving this goal: electrical cardioversion and pharmacologic cardioversion.

Electrical cardioversion Direct current electrical cardioversion is effective at converting AF to sinus rhythm, with a success rate greater than 90%.[53] Administering 200 J of biphasic current applied in the anteroposterior orientation gives the highest success. Using 120 J may be appropriate in leaner patients and those with recent-onset AF. Complications associated with cardioversion includes a 1% to 2% risk of pericardioversion thromboembolic risk, which can be reduced by half with anticoagulation for 3 weeks before the procedure and 4 weeks after the procedure (as a result of atrial stunning). Transesophageal echocardiogram precardioversion to exclude left atrial thrombus obviates preprocedural anticoagulation but still requires postcardioversion anticoagulation.[38] Postcardioversion sinus arrest may occur in elderly patients with sinus node dysfunction but is usually transient, and allowing time for a suppressed sinus node to recover is all that is required in most instances. Skin burns and sedation complications are other known complications. Electrical cardioversion in patients who have been in AF for more than 3 months works better when premedicated with an antiarrhythmic agent.

Pharmacologic cardioversion In a stable patient, the inconvenience of an electric shock may be avoided by using a pharmacologic approach for the entire cardioversion. The success rate is lower than electrical cardioversion, but this approach obviates sedation and may also help in choosing an agent for long-term rhythm control in these patients.

Flecainide is an excellent agent to use in patients without CAD or structural heart disease. The rate of successful cardioversion with this agent is up to 90% in AF of less than 24 hours' duration. Propafenone has similar efficacy and is indicated for use in similar settings. Both drugs are class Ic agents and can effect cardioversion in a few hours. Flecainide has also been found to be effective when used as an as-needed self-directed treatment in a group of symptomatic patients with PAF (the so called pill-in-the-pocket approach).

Ibutilide, a class III agent, has about a 30% to 50% success rate of cardioversion but has a significant proarrhythmic effect and requires careful monitoring of the QT interval to prevent torsades de pointes.

Another class III agent, amiodarone, has an excellent safety profile and tolerability. However, it is of modest efficacy in converting AF to sinus rhythm.

Maintenance of sinus rhythm

Many patients with paroxysmal AF may spontaneously convert and stay in sinus rhythm for prolonged periods. Some patients with paroxysmal AF and most patients with persistent AF require cardioversion followed by an antiarrhythmic drug to maintain sinus rhythm.

Using long-term antiarrhythmic agents The use of antiarrhythmic agents can be helpful in certain patients, but in general, their use is marked by modest efficacy and poor side effect profile. Patients who are highly symptomatic from the arrhythmia rather than their heart rate or those in whom heart rate is difficult to control with AV node blocking agents are best suited to these agents. Antiarrhythmic agents can double the probability of being in sinus rhythm.[54] In a meta-analysis,[55,56] the number needed to treat AF with antiarrhythmic drugs was 2 to 9 for a year and the corresponding number needed to harm was 17 to 119. These agents may be proarrhythmic and should be used within strict clinical guidelines.

Flecainide is useful for maintaining sinus rhythm in patients without CAD or structural heart disease. Even in patients with grossly normal hearts, there is a defined risk of proarrhythmia. Periodic monitoring of the EKG for QRS duration when the drug is initiated or the dose increased is recommended. Drug cessation is advised when the QRS duration increases by 25% higher than baseline.

Propafenone is governed by similar considerations to flecainide but is less efficacious than flecainide.

Amiodarone is more effective at maintaining sinus rhythm when compared with flecainide, propafenone, and sotalol.[54] Amiodarone achieved freedom from AF in 65% versus 37% when compared with sotalol and propafenone by the end of 16 months. It may be used in the presence of CAD and structural heart disease; however, the QT interval should be monitored closely. Amiodarone is associated with important long-term extracardiac side effects, including hyperthyroidism and hypothyroidism, pulmonary fibrosis, hepatotoxicity, and optic neuritis/neuropathy.

Sotalol is another class III agent that has efficacy similar to amiodarone in maintaining sinus rhythm. It has a significant β-blocking action and should be used with caution in patients with bradycardia. Its proarrhythmic effect is more prominent in women, elderly individuals, and patients with heart failure, electrolyte abnormalities, and renal failure. A QT interval beyond 500 milliseconds warrants reduction or discontinuation of medication.

Dronedarone is an agent chemically and structurally similar to amiodarone but without the iodine moiety. The extracardiac side effects of amiodarone have been ascribed to the iodine atom. Although dronedarone has been found to be safer than amiodarone, it also has lower efficacy.[57] Patients with left ventricular dysfunction and advanced heart failure also suffer from higher mortality with dronedarone and it is contraindicated in such patients. The ATHENA (A Placebo-controlled, Double-blind, Parallel Arm Trial to Assess the Efficacy of Dronedarone 400 mg Twice a Day for the Prevention of Cardiovascular Hospitalization or Death From Any Cause in Patients with Atrial Fibrillation/Atrial Flutter) trial used dronedarone in patients with paroxysmal or persistent AF and atrial flutter at risk for thromboembolic complications and showed lower hospitalization rates in patients on dronedarone.[58] Improvement in a clinical parameter was unprecedented for any antiarrhythmic agent in the setting of AF. However, in the more recent PALLAS (Permanent Atrial Fibrillation Outcome Study Using Dronedarone on Top of Standard Therapy) trial, dronedarone was associated with increased rates of heart failure, stroke, and cardiovascular death.[59] The study population comprised high-risk patients in permanent AF who were at risk for major vascular events.

Catheter ablation The primary approach for rhythm control in qualifying patients has been the use of antiarrhythmic drugs. The efficacy of these agents in maintaining sinus rhythm is approximately 50% to 60% at the end of 1 year.[40] The drug-related side effects include death (0.5%), torsades de pointes (0.7%), neuropathy (5.0%), and thyroid dysfunction in 3.3%.[60] Catheter ablation of AF attempts to isolate or eliminate the foci of AF in the left atrium by the application of radiofrequency energy (radiofrequency ablation) or freezing (cryoablation) to destroy the atrial tissue. The most successful outcomes in terms of restoration of sinus rhythm are when the AF is paroxysmal and associated with distinct triggers of arrhythmia, around which ablation can be performed and propagation of electrical impulses to the rest of the atrium can be blocked. In more long-standing AF, when the entire atrial myocardium gets remodeled and the foci for AF are more widespread in the atrial tissue, isolation may not be possible. In some such cases, targeting the individual areas of arrhythmia origin may improve the chances of success.

Several trials have shown the superiority of ablation over antiarrhythmic drug therapy in terms of maintenance of sinus rhythm. In a trial of 146 patients who had chronic AF (defined as 6 months of continuous AF), 77 were assigned to the ablation arm and 69 to the drug therapy arm; 74% of patients in the ablation group and 58% of those in the control group were free of recurrent AF or flutter without antiarrhythmic drug therapy at 1 year ($P = .05$). Because this was an intention-to-treat trial, 32% of patients in the ablation arm underwent repeat ablation and 77% of patients in the drug arm crossed over to undergo ablation because of recurrent AF.[61] Recent meta-analysis has shown a success rate of 77% with multiple ablation treatments with or without drugs compared with 52% with drugs only.[60] In drug-resistant AF, the relative efficacy of the ablative procedure is even more impressive.

Catheter ablation (radiofrequency and cryoablation) for paroxysmal AF is approved by the FDA. The use of ablation in persistent AF is off-label. The ACC/AHA/Heart Rhythm Society guidelines suggest the use of ablation in paroxysmal drug-resistant AF (failing 1 antiarrhythmic drug) as a class 1 indication (upgraded from class IIa). Meanwhile, the use of ablation in symptomatic persistent AF is now a new recommendation at class IIa level.[3]

Summary

AF is a highly prevalent arrhythmia associated with significant morbidity and mortality. The therapeutic options for this condition are not perfect and are controversial. AF is a heterogeneous condition, with variable effects on different patients; hence an individualized approach as to the goals of treatment should be tailored accordingly.

Prevention of this arrhythmia is better than an attempt at cure. Because at least half of all patients with AF having underlying cardiovascular risk factors,[62] this situation represents an important opportunity for aggressive modification of the risk factors as a viable preventive strategy.

ATRIAL FLUTTER

Atrial flutter is characterized by regular but rapid and organized atrial activity formed by a macroreentrant circuit, usually in the right atrium. It is the most common arrhythmia after AF. The epidemiology of atrial flutter is poorly characterized because it has been studied in combination with AF. Its prevalence is difficult to estimate because it is unusual for patients to sustain atrial flutter for long periods, because most patients either convert to sinus rhythm or may degenerate into AF as a result of shared risk factors between the 2 arrhythmias.[63]

Epidemiology

The incidence of atrial flutter as assessed from data from a single-center study, derived from the Marshfield Epidemiologic Study Area (MESA) cohort, over a 4-year period was 88/100,000 person-years.[63] The risk of developing atrial flutter is higher in men by a factor of 2.5. The risk in patients with heart failure and COPD is higher by a factor of 3.5 and 1.9 times, respectively.[63] The risk factors for development of atrial flutter are identical to those for AF, and this arrhythmia affects a similar population of patients. In the analysis of the MESA subset, 58% of the patients with atrial flutter had at least 1 episode of AF.[63] One population group who have a unique predilection for atrial flutter is the subset of patients with previous history of endocardial scarring either from previous ablation procedures or cardiac surgery causing block in a critical location, which serves as a substrate for development of reentry. Mortality risk in patients affected with atrial flutter is 1.7 times that of the control group.[64]

Pathophysiology

Atrial flutter develops as a macroreentrant rhythm around a site of anatomic or functional block. The typical atrial flutter (also called type 1 flutter) develops in the right atrium around the tricuspid annulus, with the crista terminalis and the opening of the inferior cava forming an anatomic-functional block. The narrow band of atrial tissue bound by the inferior vena cava posteriorly and the tricuspid annulus anteriorly, called the cavotricuspid isthmus, often forms the critical path of slow conduction,[65] which is a suitable target for ablation. Usually, the direction of impulse propagation is counterclockwise around the tricuspid annulus, with impulses traveling up in the interatrial septum. Ninety percent of typical atrial flutters are counterclockwise, reflected as negative flutter waves in the inferior leads and positive atrial deflections in the anterior precordial leads.[66] The clockwise circuit propagates in the opposite direction, with opposite flutter wave direction on the EKG. The cycle length of a typical atrial flutter rhythm is characteristically at 200 to 240 milliseconds (corresponding to rates of 250–300 beats/min). The ventricular rate is usually slower, with the atrial activity being variably blocked at the level of the AV node at a ratio of 2:1 to 4:1. The ventricular rates are usually a whole number factor of 300 beats/min, often providing a clue to the presence of underlying atrial flutter when the flutter waves may not be clearly evident or are fused with the ventricular complexes. A conduction ratio of less than 4:1 is usually a sign of AV nodal disease.

Atypical atrial flutter, on the other hand, does not use these circuits, traveling through the cavotricuspid isthmus. The atypical atrial flutters are often scar-related from previous surgical incisions, such as right atriotomy scar formed after postcardio-pulmonary bypass or from other cardiac surgeries involving atrial tissue, including congenital heart surgery. A narrow area of tissue between the scar and an anatomic barrier like tricuspid annulus or inferior vena cava then forms a critical slow zone in the atypical flutter circuit. Previous endocardial ablation procedures leaving behind areas of conduction block can also form substrates for atypical atrial flutter formation and propagation. With AF ablation procedures becoming more common, the development of left atrial flutter as a result of incomplete scar lines around the pulmonary veins is also emerging as an important cause of atypical atrial flutter.

The clinical effects of atrial flutter are similar to AF. Long-term presence of atrial flutter can lead to tachycardia-induced cardiomyopathy. Long-term atrial flutter also comes with thromboembolic risks, but the risk attributable to atrial flutter alone is difficult to quantify because most patients have coexisting AF.[63] The ACC/AHA recommend that chronic or recurrent atrial flutter be treated identical to AF with regards to stroke prophylaxis.[67] The CHADS$_2$ and CHADS$_2$-VASc scores can be applied to patients with atrial flutter when determining stroke risk.[68]

Clinical Features

The symptoms related to atrial flutter include palpitations, shortness of breath, angina, and dizziness (occasionally, syncope). Hemodynamic effects of flutter can also lead to exercise intolerance and worsening of CHF.

On examination, no specific feature points to a diagnosis of atrial flutter. Tachycardia may be evident from rapid ventricular response rates. Features of underlying cardiac and noncardiac comorbidities may be noted. Cannon waves suggestive of atrial contraction during tricuspid valve closure may be present.

Diagnosis and Investigations

The diagnosis of atrial flutter is confirmed on EKG by the presence of repetitive fast atrial activity faster than 240 beats/min (cycle length <250 milliseconds) and no isoelectric line (some isoelectric line between discernible p waves may be seen in atypical flutters and under the influence of antiarrhythmic medication if the slow zone occupies nearly 70% of the circuit and surface EKG does not record any activity when conduction occurs through this area) between the atrial complexes, because some part of the atrium is always being activated. The EKG shows atrial activity commonly as flutter waves (sawtooth pattern).

Investigations such as echocardiogram to diagnose associated cardiac conditions and other blood tests are similar to those for AF.

Management

The management issues with atrial flutter are similar to AF and involve addressing the rate, rhythm, and anticoagulation both acutely and over the long-term. The important differences are mentioned in the following sections.

Rate control agents slow down conduction at the AV node to decrease ventricular rate response to atrial flutter. AV node ablation for pure atrial flutter is rarely recommended for patients refractory to or intolerant of such agents. In elderly patients with multiple comorbidities and concurrent AF, AV node ablation may be the best clinical option.

Electrical cardioversion, indicated for unstable patients, is successful in almost 100% of patients and usually requires less energy than is required for AF (50–100 J vs 120–200 J).

Atrial flutter in the short-term is a stable rhythm and difficult to convert pharmacologically. IV-administered class III agents such as ibutilide and dofetilide prolong the action potential and increase the refractory period of the tissue in the slow zone, which can interrupt the reentrant circuit.

Pharmacologic control of atrial flutter over the long-term involves administration of antiarrhythmic agents to prevent atrial flutter. The success rates for various agents are in the range of 50% and are affected by issues of drug-related toxicity.

Rhythm control and conversion to sinus rhythm are different by virtue of the relative ease and efficacy of catheter ablation for atrial flutter. Catheter ablation of typical flutter has a success rate of more than 90%, with a major complication rate of less than 0.5%. The latter includes inadvertent heart block, tamponade, and phrenic nerve paralysis. Catheter ablation in typical atrial flutter involves ensuring a bidirectional block across the cavotricuspid isthmus, which, as mentioned earlier, forms the narrowest area of the circuit for arrhythmia sustenance. Catheter ablation when feasible is the definitive treatment choice for typical atrial flutter.

Summary

Atrial flutter is a common arrhythmia, which shares many clinical and therapeutic features with AF and coexists with AF in many patients. However, it has a distinct pathophysiology in that it occurs as a result of a macroreentrant circuit, which provides an opportunity to interrupt the circuit using currently available catheter ablation techniques.

MULTIFOCAL AT

Multifocal AT (MAT) is characterized by a rapid irregular atrial rhythm. It differs from AF in that the atrial rate is slower (but >100 beats/min by definition) and the organized atrial activation is seen on the EKG in the form of discernible P waves. MAT is characterized by the presence of more than 3 distinct P waves on a 12-lead EKG.

It is mostly seen as a secondary condition complicating underlying pulmonary disease or metabolic/electrolyte derangements. In addition, CHF and right atrial enlargement also predispose to MAT. Some agents used in the treatment of pulmonary diseases, such as aminophylline and albuterol, also contribute to MAT.

Epidemiology

This arrhythmia is most commonly seen in hospitalized patients, with an incidence of 0.05% to 0.32%.[69] MAT may occur in almost 20% of patients with acute respiratory failure[70] and is associated with a mortality of up to 45%.[69] However, the high mortality represents the underlying severe comorbidities of these patients rather than a consequence of the arrhythmia itself.

Mechanism and Pathophysiology

MAT develops as a result of increased irritability of the atrial tissue, giving rise to multiple ectopic foci of automaticity in the atrial tissue. The most likely mechanism seems to be delayed after depolarizations, which are caused by a calcium overload in the myocytes. The excess calcium in the cells is a consequence of catecholamine excess, acidosis, and hypoxemia.[71]

Most cases of MAT are transient, with most patients converting to a sinus rhythm or degenerating into AF or flutter.[72]

Clinical Features

The clinical features in affected patients are dominated by the underlying disease condition, usually decompensated pulmonary disease with severe respiratory distress and hypoxia. MAT does not seem to cause any clinical consequences of its own. Even at rapid rates, unlike AF, there is no evidence that MAT leads to hypotension or CHF exacerbation.

Management

The definitive management is treatment of the underlying condition, elimination of stimuli such as hypoxia, acidemia, electrolyte disturbances, and hyperadrenergic state. However, this goal may not be easy to achieve under the clinical circumstances in which this arrhythmia occurs.

Directed treatment to convert the rhythm to sinus is rarely warranted and only when there is risk of myocardial ischemia from rapid ventricular response rate.[69] However, rhythm conversion to sinus is almost never effective without treating the underlying disease state, and antiarrhythmic agents are notoriously ineffective in MAT.[73] Guidelines emphasize treatment of the underlying pulmonary and electrolyte abnormalities.[74]

Slowing down the rate using AV node blocking agents may be more successful. β-Blockers are often contraindicated, because of the usual presence of bronchospasm. Digoxin has occasionally been implicated in the formation of MAT and is not a good choice. Nondihydropyridine calcium channel blockers are usually recommended as the drug of first choice for rate control in MAT.

Administration of high-dose magnesium may be helpful, even with normal magnesium levels, but outside its use in patients with hypomagnesemia, its usefulness is debatable.[75]

SUPRAVENTRICULAR TACHYCARDIA

Supraventricular tachycardia (SVT) is defined as any arrhythmia originating above the bundle of His and associated with atrial rates higher than 100 beats/min. This broad definition therefore encompasses AF, atrial flutter, and MAT. However, from the clinical perspective, these conditions are addressed separately because of their distinct presentation and mechanisms of formation.

The SVTs described later are characterized by their ability to occur in structurally normal hearts and in the absence of cardiopulmonary disease, as opposed to AF, atrial flutter, and MAT, which usually present in patients with underlying cardiopulmonary disease states.

Because of their similar clinical presentations and consequences, the SVTs are divided by mechanism of formation as AV nodal reentrant tachycardia (AVNRT), AV reentrant tachycardia (AVRT), and AT.

Epidemiology

The prevalence of SVT is approximately 2.3/1000 in the general population,[76] with AVNRT accounting for 60% of all cases,[77] whereas AVRT constitutes 30% and AT accounts for 10%.[77]

Mechanisms and Pathophysiology

The most common mechanism of SVT is reentry, which is seen in both AVNRT and AVRT. The basic requirements of a reentrant circuit are the presence of an anatomic or functional area of no conduction or of poor conduction, around which a propagating impulse has to travel in 2 distinct paths. A reentrant circuit develops when the 2 pathways have different refractory periods and different velocities of propagation. An oncoming impulse, when timed correctly, may propagate via only 1 path and return via the second pathway in a circuitous fashion. By the time it returns, the original path is ready to be activated and can therefore transmit the impulse repeatedly, thereby setting up a continuous self-propagating circuit.

In AVNRT, the 2 limbs of circuit are the fast and slow pathways of bringing impulses to the AV node from the rest of the atrium. The impulse usually travels down the slow pathway and returns via the fast pathway (slow-fast or typical AVNRT). Occasionally the impulse goes in the opposite direction, giving rise to fast-slow or atypical AVNRT (**Figs. 1** and **2**).

In AVRT, an accessory AV conduction pathway and either the AV node or another accessory pathway form the 2 limbs of the circuit. The impulse traverses down the accessory pathway and returns via the AV node (antidromic conduction) or may travel in the opposite direction (orthodromic conduction). AVRT occasionally coexists with Wolff-Parkinson-White (WPW) syndrome, in which case the accessory pathway conducts antegradely faster than the AV node, shortening the PR interval.

As opposed to the reentrant mechanisms causing AVNRT and AVRT, AT is caused by increased automaticity of an ectopic atrial focus. Atrial tissue in the crista terminalis and pulmonary veins is particularly susceptible to the development of increased auto- maticity, causing AT.

The result of these aberrant conduction mechanisms is the development of episodic rapid narrow complex rhythm, with rates reaching up to 250 beats/min. Some patients are asymptomatic during these episodes but most experience palpitations, near syncope, and occasionally syncope. The syncope usually is a result of extremely fast ventricular rates, leading to incomplete ventricular filling and ejection. A sinus pause after the termination of an SVT episode can also cause syncope, as can the precipitation of a vasovagal event from tachycardia.[78,79] Because most episodes are paroxysmal or transient and terminate spontaneously, there are usually no long- term effects of this arrhythmia. One rule to this exception is a special form of AVRT, called permanent junctional reentrant tachycardia, which involves a slow retrogradely conducting accessory pathway, which may be sustained for long periods.[80] The

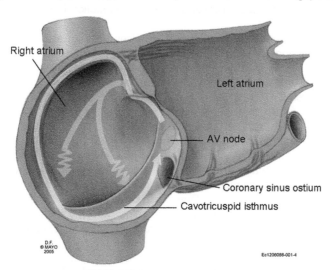

Fig. 1. Cross-section of the right atrium in the anterior projection. This is a schematic diagram of the typical atrial flutter going around the IVC and crista terminalis in an anti- clockwise direction. At times, the circuit involves the atrial tissue above the superior vena cava. Occasionally the circuit is inferior to the SVC and is termed lower loop atrial flutter (depicted in a *lighter shade*). Copyright © 2005 Mayo Clinic.

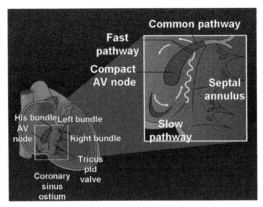

Fig. 2. Cross section of the heart in the right anterior oblique projection. This view shows the location of the AV node in the interatrial septum. The inset shows the fast pathway (*continuous curved arrow*) and slow pathway (*wavy line*) in relation to the AV node.

relative durability of this tachycardia increases the propensity for tachycardia-induced cardiomyopathy. However, the slow conduction through the pathway also limits the rate of the tachycardia.

A special scenario in patients prone to SVT is the presence of an accessory pathway causing a preexcitation syndrome or WPW syndrome. In these patients, the accessory pathway competes with the AV node for anterograde conduction of the atrial impulses from the atrium to the ventricle. These pathways often do not share the decremental conduction properties of the AV node and can conduct at very fast rates with short refractory periods. Hence, in the presence of an accessory pathway conduction, patients with AT or AF can conduct at excessively fast rates to the ventricle, potentially leading to ventricular fibrillation. Blocking AV node conduction in such situations may depress AV node conduction, further enhancing conduction through the accessory pathway.

AT results from increased discharge of impulses from an ectopic atrial location outside the sinus node. The mechanism is enhanced automaticity, triggered activity, or reentry. If it is reentry, all the components of the reentrant circuit are located entirely within the atrium, unlike AVNRT or AVRT, and do not involve the AV node or ventricular tissue, respectively.

Clinical Features

Symptoms are related to the episodic tachycardia and include palpitations, abnormal neck pulsations, anxiety, presyncope, and occasionally syncope. In many patients, a provoking factor such as caffeine or other stimulants, stress, and exercise can be identified. The physical examination reveals rapid heart rate during the episode but may be normal between episodes. During episodes of AVNRT caused by the atrial activation immediately after initiation of ventricular systole, the atrium may contract on a closed AV valve, giving rise to cannon waves in the jugular venous pulse.

Diagnosis and Investigations

The diagnosis of SVT rests on identifying a narrow complex tachycardia rhythm on EKG or telemetry. Occasionally, the QRS may be wide because of an underlying aberrant intraventricular conduction or preexcitation arrhythmia arising from an accessory pathway. Frequently, episodes of SVT may not be detected during routine EKG. In such cases, 24-hour to 48-hour Holter monitoring, or, if infrequent, an event monitor, may provide a longer window of opportunity to diagnose the SVT. Episodes that are even rarer may be diagnosed by using an implantable loop recorder.

Thyroid function tests may be helpful to diagnose an underlying thyrotoxic state contributing to increased atrial ectopy. Transthoracic echocardiogram is indicated to rule out any coexisting structural heart disease.

Management

Acute management

The management priority in a patient presenting with tachycardia acutely is rate control to prevent adverse symptoms of hypotension and cardiac ischemia. Rarely, patients may be unstable, and resuscitation in the form of ensuring airway patency and adequate ventilation and treating shock takes priority. In these patients, DC cardioversion to achieve a sinus rhythm is a reasonable option.[81] A synchronized shock of 50 to 100 J delivered in biphasic waveform is usually adequate to achieve conversion to sinus rhythm.

However, most patients remain hemodynamically stable, allowing for a detailed assessment with a brief history, physical examination, and 12-lead EKG. After an appropriate diagnosis is made and it is decided that blocking the AV node is safe, a variety of vagal maneuvers can be applied to try to slow the ventricular response rate and, in some cases of AV node-dependent tachycardias (AVRT and AVNRT), even break the arrhythmia. The most effective and widely recommended vagal maneuver is carotid massage, but others include the Valsalva maneuver, breath holding (Mueller maneuver), water immersion, and gagging. Carotid sinus massage (CSM) is contraindicated in patients with significant ipsilateral carotid stenosis and recent stroke (<3 months, except when stenosis has been ruled out).[82] CSM is safe and can be prescribed to patients for self-application, when the arrhythmia has been well characterized. It involves the application of deep pressure over the carotid bulb at the level of the thyroid cartilage for 5 to 10 seconds. If adequate pressure on 1 side does not cause a vagal response, pressure on the contralateral side maybe applied. No particular side is superior for effective vagal stimulation. When performed in a medical facility, the maneuver should be performed in a monitored setting with an eye on the rhythm and vital signs. The expected response is a transient sinus bradycardia or pause and slowed AV conduction. Uncommonly, complete AV nodal block, hypotension, and occasionally AF may occur.

The AV nodal block elicited by the vagal maneuvers can slow down conduction to the ventricle, allowing for better visualization of atrial activity on the EKG. In cases of AV node-dependent tachycardia (AVRT, AVNRT), it may also terminate the arrhythmia by interrupting the circuit. The same effect can be obtained by using IV adenosine, which blocks the AV node by acting on A_1 adenosine receptors. Although adenosine is vasodilatory and can cause hypotension, the half-life of this agent is less than 10 seconds, making any adverse effects transient. Acute bronchospasm can be precipitated by adenosine via stimulation of A_2 receptors on bronchi, and caution is advised in asthmatics. The standard dose is 6 mg, with 12 to 18 mg being the usual dose to attain the desired clinical result.

Nondihydropyridine calcium channel blockers such as verapamil and diltiazem can be used to achieve a longer-lasting AV nodal blockade in hemodynamically stable patients. Occasionally, β-blockers can be used in the same role.

Pharmacologic cardioversion is rarely indicated, but when it is considered, procainamide is the drug of choice.

Patients with preexcitation are usually treated in the same fashion, except when the accessory pathway is a bystander (ie, not integral to the arrhythmia circuit, like in AT, flutter, or fibrillation). In this situation, administering an AV nodal blocking agent paradoxically increases the rate of conduction through the accessory pathway and leads to excessively fast ventricular rates, precipitating ventricular fibrillation.

Long-term management

In patients with recurrent episodes of symptomatic SVT, prophylactic treatment to decrease or eliminate future events is indicated. Catheter-based invasive techniques have emerged as options for first-line therapy in pathway-mediated SVT. This recommendation is based on increasing safety and efficacy of catheter-based technologies. Both AVRT and AVNRT can be treated with ablation of accessory AV connections and the slow pathway, resulting in cure rates greater than 95%. The incidence of major complications, including AV node block requiring pacemaker or tamponade, is approximately 3%, and death is rare, at less than 0.2%.[83]

Catheter ablation for recurrent symptomatic AVRT or AVNRT is a class I indication by the ACC/AHA guidelines.[84]

Drug therapy is only modestly effective in preventing SVT but may be the only available option for AT. In patients with AVRT and AVNRT, procainamide, propafenone, and flecainide can be effective in those unwilling or unable to undergo catheter ablation.[84] Sotalol has also been used with some success. AV nodal blocking agents, although useful, should be used with caution and are relatively contraindicated in AVRT (especially in patients prone to AF or AT), because of the risk of accessory pathway conduction, which may result in rapid ventricular rates. Amiodarone is also an effective agent but is rarely used for this indication given its multiple extracardiac side effects with long-term use.

Summary

SVTs are a heterogeneous group of arrhythmias that occur above the Hisian conduction system and can cause significant morbidity in young and active individuals, even in the absence of structural heart disease. Although the underlying mechanisms of the various SVTs are markedly different, the clinical presentation may be similar. The acute management of most of these arrhythmias is similar as well. The primary focus is to ameliorate symptoms by focusing on rate control using AV nodal blocking agents. In less stable patients, after initial resuscitative efforts, pharmacotherapy can be attempted, and for unstable patients, synchronized cardioversion can be performed. One important caveat is that in the presence of an accessory pathway when there is a risk for AF or AT, AV node blocking agents can precipitate rapid accessory pathway conduction and ventricular fibrillation, cardiovascular collapse, or death. The long-term management of choice is catheter ablation in patients with recurrent symptoms. Antiarrhythmic drugs have a lower efficacy and have potentially toxic side effects.

VENTRICULAR ARRHYTHMIAS
Premature Ventricular Beats

Premature ventricular beats (PVBs) or complexes (PVCs) are common in the general population. A community-based study of 15,792 unselected subjects (45–65 years), using a 2-minute continuous EKG recording, showed a 6% prevalence.[85] In a 24-hour Holter study of 50 medical students, the incidence of PVCs was 50%.[86] The incidence of PVCs seems to increase proportionately with age, with a 34% increase for each 5-year age increment.[85] Male gender, African American ethnicity, structural heart disease, and recent myocardial infarction are also risk factors for developing PVCs.

In the absence of structural heart disease (hypertrophic, dilated, nonischemic or ischemic cardiomyopathy), the presence of PVCs does not portend a worse prognosis.[87] However, recent data suggest that apparently healthy individuals with PVCs have a 2-fold higher risk of dying from CAD even after adjustment for other cardiovascular risk factors,[88] but specific guidance on the management of these patients beyond cardiovascular risk is lacking. Exercise-induced PVCs or PVCs occurring during recovery phase after exertion are of uncertain significance and require no treatment. Highly trained athletes are also at a higher risk for development of PVCs, even at rest. In the absence of underlying structural heart disease, no specific treatment or restriction from exercise is recommended.[89]

A subset of patients with frequent (>16% burden), monomorphic PVCs on 24-hour Holter monitoring can develop a reversible nonischemic dilated cardiomyopathy.[90] Once the causative role of the PVCs in the development of cardiomyopathy is suspected, antiarrhythmic therapy or catheter-based ablation procedures to decrease PVC burden can improve myocardial function. The diagnosis is usually made in retrospect if a reduction in PVC burden results in an improvement EF.

In the setting of myocardial infarction, the incidence of PVCs may be as high as 93% and is associated with worse prognosis if: (1) the frequency of PVCs is greater than 10 beats/min, (2) they occur more than 48 hours after the acute event, and (3) they are associated with a large infarct or low EF.[91,92] Suppression of PVCs after acute myocardial infarction using antiarrhythmic agents has been associated with worse prognosis and is not recommended.[93] The reason is the proarrhythmic effect of these agents in the presence of structural heart disease or CAD. Instead, the focus should be on electrolyte correction and reduction in ischemia by drugs or revascularization.

All patients with PVCs need a transthoracic echocardiogram to evaluate left ventricular structure and function. Those with no evidence of underlying abnormalities usually do not need further workup or treatment.

If an underlying myocardial disease such as dilated cardiomyopathy, regional wall motion abnormalities with scar, arrhythmogenic right ventricular cardiomyopathy, or noncompaction syndrome is identified, then further investigation and treatment pertinent to the specific diagnosis are warranted.

Suppression of PVCs in asymptomatic patients has not been studied and is not recommended because of the high risk of antiarrhythmic agents, which may outweigh any potential benefits. Occasional patients with symptomatic PVCs (usually palpitations) are candidates for β-blocker therapy.

Nonsustained Ventricular Tachycardia

Nonsustained ventricular tachycardia (NSVT) is defined as a series of more than 3 consecutive PVCs occurring at a rate of more than 100/min but lasting less than 30 seconds. NSVT occurs with an incidence of up to 4% in the general population.[94] Similar to PVCs, the prognosis of NSVT depends on the presence of underlying structural heart disease. When structural heart disease has been diligently excluded, NSVT is not associated with an increase in mortality.[95] However, when only clinical criteria (by history) are used to exclude CAD, NSVT was associated with an up to 2-fold increase in all-cause mortality and myocardial infarction.[96] Exercise-induced NSVT also does not seem to portend a poor prognosis in the absence of structural heart disease.[97]

Because of its transient nature, NSVT is well tolerated and only rarely causes symptoms. β-Blockers are the first line of therapy for symptomatic patients. Antiarrhythmic agents are rarely indicated and their use is guided by considerations similar to those for ventricular tachycardia (VT), as discussed later.

NSVT in the presence of underlying structural heart disease or channelopathies is dealt with by managing the underlying cardiac disease. Some considerations are discussed later, but details are beyond the scope of this article.

VT

Sustained VT, defined by a ventricular rhythm at a rate greater than 100/min for more than 30 seconds, is usually poorly tolerated and can be fatal, especially because these arrhythmias mostly occur in the setting of underlying structural heart disease. The annual incidence of sudden cardiac death (VT and ventricular fibrillation) in the United States is 450,000.[98]

CAD is present in 70% of these patients. Other predisposing factors for malignant VT include dilated nonischemic cardiomyopathy, valvular heart disease, congenital heart disease, sarcoidosis, and other cardiomyopathies.

Idiopathic VT occurs in the absence of underlying structural heart disease, is usually monomorphic, and is associated with a benign prognosis. A thorough workup to exclude arrhythmogenic right ventricular dysplasia, subtle cardiomyopathy, or infiltration is necessary before invoking this diagnosis. Idiopathic VTs account for 10% of all patients seen for VT and are discussed later.[99]

Clinical features

The symptoms of VT depend on the rate of the tachycardia, presence of underlying myocardial dysfunction and valvular abnormalities, location and origin of the tachycardia (which may affect sequence of ventricular activation), and the degree of AV dissociation. Short episodes of slow VT can cause presyncope, syncope, angina, and cardiogenic shock. Sufficiently long and fast VTs, especially in the presence of underlying cardiac disease, can cause hemodynamic instability and poor myocardial perfusion, causing further ventricular arrhythmias, which may culminate in cardiac arrest.

The physical examination may reveal a marked tachycardia, weak pulse, and hypotension. Cannon waves may be present in the jugular veins because of AV dissociation. On auscultation, variable intensity of first heart sound, variable splitting of first or second heart sound, and the occasional presence of an S3 or an S4 heart sound may be noted.

Diagnosis and investigations

VT when presenting as a nonemergent condition is usually suspected on an EKG during the episode. VT is characterized by the presence of wide ventricular complexes greater than 120 milliseconds. Usually, the ventricular complexes are wider than 140 milliseconds, and in this situation, the diagnosis is almost always VT. However, when the width of the QRS complex is between 120 and 140 milliseconds, the differential diagnosis can include a supraventricular rhythm with aberrant ventricular conduction. Evidence of AV dissociation may also be present, but because of constant high-voltage activity from a fast ventricular rhythm, the p waves from the atrial activation may not be easily discernible. When in doubt, especially in a patient with underlying structural heart disease, it may be safer to treat a wide complex tachycardia as you would as VT.

After the diagnosis of VT is established or suspected, possible reversible causes and acute precipitating factors for VT, including electrolyte imbalance, sepsis, and drug effects, should be identified. After the acute management and stabilization, a thorough investigation for a predisposing cardiac condition should be undertaken.

An echocardiogram to diagnose structural myocardial and valvular heart disease is necessary. Cardiac computed tomography or cardiac magnetic resonance imaging are recommended when echo images are unrevealing or may be used as an adjunct to delineate myocardial scar or anatomic abnormalities. These imaging modalities are also helpful when a specific diagnosis of VT, like arrhythmogenic right ventricular dysplasia, is suspected and needs confirmation.

Exercise stress testing may help identify CAD when suspected; if the pretest probability for CAD is high, it may be reasonable to go directly to coronary angiography.

Electrophysiologic studies are not routinely recommended but may be useful when the diagnosis of VT is in doubt. They may also help elucidate the mechanism of VT when ablation is being considered for drug-resistant arrhythmias or for idiopathic VT. For patients with cardiomyopathy, EP studies are no longer used for risk stratification for primary prophylaxis purposes. The EP study in this setting has limited ability to predict future risk of ventricular arrhythmias, because the underlying substrate is prone to remodeling with time and thus the risk is subject to change.[100] They may have a role in identifying the need for an implantable cardioverter defibrillator (ICD) for primary prophylaxis in patients with cardiomyopathy and EF between 35% and 40% (a subgroup that has not been specifically studied in trials, as discussed later).

Management

Primary prevention Life-threatening VT usually affects a small group of patients with underlying myocardial dysfunction. This situation allows for primary prevention efforts to be focused on a select group of patients. Drug therapy with various antiarrhythmic agents is not effective for primary prevention of VT. The primary prevention of VT has been revolutionized by randomized controlled trials proving the efficacy of ICD devices for primary prevention in patients with decreased left ventricular systolic function.

The implantation of an ICD for primary prevention in patients with cardiomyopathy depends on several factors, including:

1. The extent of systolic dysfunction (as measured by the EF)
2. The cause of cardiomyopathy (ischemic vs nonischemic)
3. The functional status of the patient

The important trials with regards to primary prevention in cardiomyopathy are summarized in **Table 2**. These studies excluded New York Heart Association class IV patients. The bulk of the data show clear evidence of benefit of ICD implantation compared with medical therapy in the patient groups studied and have led to a paradigm shift in the management of these patients over the last decade.

Secondary prevention A meta-analysis of 3 major trials (AVID [Antiarrhythmics versus Implantable Defibrillator], CASH [Cardiac Arrest Study Hamburg], and CIDS [Canadian Implantable Defibrillator Study]) showed a hazard ratio of 0.72 ($P = .0006$) and 0.5 ($P<.0001$) for ICD over medical therapy with regards to overall mortality and arrhythmia-related mortality, respectively.[101]

Drug therapy is inferior to ICD implantation but may have a role in patients with high arrhythmias burden and suffering from excessive ICD discharges, in whom it is used as an adjunct to reduce the number of defibrillator shocks. Radiofrequency ablation may have a dramatic effect in scar-related arrhythmias but in nonischemic cardiomyopathy, in which the substrate is more diffuse, no advantage has been shown.

Idiopathic VT

A specific class of VT that occurs in younger patients without any structural cardiac defects and is associated with freedom from malignant ventricular arrhythmias and an excellent prognosis is termed idiopathic VT.

Table 2
Landmark trials showing the efficacy of ICDs in the primary prevention of sudden cardiac death

Trial	ICD Compared with	EF Requirement (%)	Cause of Cardiomyopathy/No. of Patients/Follow-up Period	Associated Feature Required	Relative Risk of Overall Mortality with ICD (CI)
Multicenter Automatic Defibrillator Implantation Trial (MADIT) (14)	Conventional medical therapy	<35	Ischemic/196 patients/average follow-up 27 mo	NSVT or positive electrophysiology study	0.46 (0.26–0.82)
Multicenter Unsustained Tachycardia Trial (MUSTT) (15)	Conventional medical therapy and no therapy	<40	Ischemic/707 patients/median follow-up 39 mo	NSVT or positive electrophysiology study	0.42 (0.29–0.6)
Multicenter Automatic Defibrillator Implantation Trial II (MADIT II) (16)	Conventional medical therapy	<30	Ischemic/1232 patients/average follow-up 20 mo	None	0.69 (0.51–0.93)
Sudden Cardiac Death in Heart Failure Trial (SCD-HeFT) (17)	Conventional medical therapy	<35	Ischemic (52%), rest nonischemic/2521 patients/median follow-up 45.5 mo	None	0.77 (0.62–0.96)

Abbreviation: CI, confidence interval.

VT in patients without any gross structural abnormalities but with underlying genetic channelopathies, such as long QT syndrome, Brugada syndrome, and catecholaminergic polymorphic VT, are associated with fatal ventricular arrhythmias and are not included in this classification.

The most common idiopathic VT is right ventricular outflow tract VT, which can manifest itself by showing salvos of PVCs and NSVT on the EKG or telemetry. The morphology of the ventricular complexes is marked by left bundle branch morphology and inferior axis. However, an increase in adrenergic discharge while exercising can provoke longer episodes of NSVT or even VT. The condition occurs because of a genetic defect leading up to a gain of function in the cyclic adenosine monophosphate activity, causing calcium overload and triggered arrhythmias. Symptomatic patients respond well to calcium channel blockers like verapamil and also to β-blockers. Intractable cases can be treated effectively with RF ablation.

Another common form of idiopathic VT is idiopathic fascicular left ventricular VT. This arrhythmia can be associated with palpitations and presyncope, but cardiac arrest is rare. The pathogenesis of this tachycardia comprises a reentrant circuit involving the fascicular fibers of the left bundle branch of His. The ventricular complexes thus typically have a right bundle branch morphology and are narrow because of their origin close to the His-Purkinje system. Calcium channel blockers (verapamil) are highly effective for the acute and long-term management of this condition. Radiofrequency ablation of the tachycardia circuit is another highly effective therapeutic option.

Summary

Ventricular arrhythmias are not infrequently encountered in the primary care setting. The prognosis of the arrhythmia can range from innocuous in patients with PVCs or NSVT or in idiopathic VT to significant morbidity and mortality in high-burden PVCs, in which cardiomyopathy, cardiovascular collapse, and sudden cardiac death may result when associated with underlying structural heart disease or channelopathy-related arrhythmias. In all cases, further evaluation is recommended to recognize the origin and mechanism of the arrhythmia and to better elucidate the underlying myocardial substrate. Depending on the outcome of investigations, management strategies vary from observation to β-blockers or calcium channel blockers for specific arrhythmias to ICDs. In a select group of patients, an ICD is warranted solely from risk alone for primary prevention. Recognizing this subset of patients and their timely referral are critical.

REFERENCES

1. Feinberg WM BJ, Laupacis A, Kronmal R, et al. Prevalence, age distribution, and gender of patients with atrial fibrillation: analysis and implications. Arch Intern Med 1995;155:469–73.
2. Miyasaka Y, Barnes ME, Gersh BJ, et al. Secular trends in incidence of atrial fibrillation in Olmsted County, Minnesota, 1980 to 2000, and implications on the projections for future prevalence [Erratum, Circulation 2006;114(11):e498.]. Circulation 2006;114:119–25.
3. Fuster V RL, Cannom DS, Crijins HJ, et al. 2011 ACCF/AHA/HRS focused updates incorporated into the ACC/AHA/ESC 2006 Guidelines for the management of patients with atrial fibrillation: a report of the American College of Cardiology Foundation/American Heart Association Task Force on Practice Guidelines developed in partnership with the European Society of Cardiology

and in collaboration with the European Heart Rhythm Association and the Heart Rhythm Society. J Am Coll Cardiol 2011;57:e101–98.

4. Stewart S, Hart CL, Hole DJ, et al. Population prevalence, incidence, and predictors of atrial fibrillation in the Renfrew/Paisley study. Heart 2001;86:516–21.

5. Naccarelli GV, Varker H, Lin J, et al. Increasing prevalence of atrial fibrillation and flutter in the United States. Am J Cardiol 2009;104:1534–9.

6. Lloyd-Jones DM, Wang T, Leip EP, et al. Lifetime risk for development of atrial fibrillation: the Framingham Heart Study. Circulation 2004;110:1042–6.

7. Wann LS, Curtis AB, January CT, et al. 2011 ACCF/AHA/HRS focused update on the management of patients with atrial fibrillation (Updating the 2006 Guideline): a report of the American College of Cardiology Foundation/American Heart Association Task Force on Practice Guidelines. J Am Coll Cardiol 2011;57(2): 223–42.

8. European Heart Rhythm Association, European Association for Cardio-Thoracic Surgery, Camm AJ, Kirchhof P, Lip GY, et al. Guidelines for the management of atrial fibrillation: the Task Force for the Management of Atrial Fibrillation of the European Society of Cardiology (ESC). Eur Heart J 2010;31(19):2369–429.

9. Schnabel RB, Sullivan LM, Levy D, et al. Development of a risk score for atrial fibrillation (Framingham Heart Study): a community-based cohort study. Lancet 2009;373(9665):739–45.

10. Benjamin EJ, Levy D, Vaziri SM, et al. Independent risk factors for atrial fibrillation in a population-based cohort: the Framingham Heart Study. JAMA 1994; 271:840–4.

11. Krahn AD, Manfreda J, Tate RB, et al. The natural history of atrial fibrillation: incidence, risk factors, and prognosis in the Manitoba Follow-Up Study. Am J Med 1995;98(5):476–84.

12. Cameron A, Schwartz M, Kronmal RA, et al. Prevalence and significance of atrial fibrillation in coronary artery disease (CASS Registry). Am J Cardiol 1988;61(10): 714–7.

13. Diker E, Aydogu S, Ozdemir M, et al. Prevalence and predictors of atrial fibrillation in rheumatic valvular heart disease. Am J Cardiol 1996;77(1):96–8.

14. Grigioni F, Avierinos JF, Ling LH, et al. Atrial fibrillation complicating the course of degenerative mitral regurgitation: determinants and long-term outcome. Am Coll Cardiol 2002;40(1):84–92.

15. Cecchi F, Olivotto I, Montereggi A, et al. Hypertrophic cardiomyopathy in Tuscany: clinical course and outcome in an unselected regional population. J Am Coll Cardiol 1995;26(6):1529–36.

16. Tikoff G, Schmidt AM, Hecht HH. Atrial fibrillation in atrial septal defect. Arch Intern Med 1968;121(5):402–5.

17. Weber DM, Phillip JH Jr. A re-evaluation of electrocardiographic changes accompanying acute pulmonary embolism. Am J Med Sci 1966;251(4):381–98.

18. Buch P, Friberg J, Scharling H, et al. Reduced lung function and risk of atrial fibrillation in the Copenhagen City Heart Study. Eur Respir J 2003;21(6):1012–6.

19. Gami AS, Pressman G, Caples SM, et al. Association of atrial fibrillation and obstructive sleep apnea. Circulation 2004;110(4):364–7.

20. Wang TJ PH, Levy D, D'Agostino RB Sr, et al. Obesity and the risk of new-onset atrial fibrillation. JAMA 2004;292(20):2471–7.

21. Grundy SM, Cleeman JI, Daniels SR, et al, American Heart Association, National Heart, Lung, and Blood Institute. Diagnosis and management of the metabolic syndrome: an American Heart Association/National Heart, Lung, and Blood Institute Scientific Statement. Circulation 2005;112(17):2735–52.

22. Chekakie MO, Welles CC, Metoyer R, et al. Pericardial fat is independently associated with human atrial fibrillation. J Am Coll Cardiol 2010;56(10):784–8.
23. Watanabe H, Watanabe T, Sasaki S, et al. Close bidirectional relationship between chronic kidney disease and atrial fibrillation: the Niigata preventive medicine study. Am Heart J 2009;158(4):629–36.
24. Lubitz SA, Yin X, Fontes JD, et al. Association between familial atrial fibrillation and risk of new-onset atrial fibrillation. JAMA 2010;304(20):2263–9.
25. Nattel S. New ideas about atrial fibrillation 50 years on. Nature 2002;415(6868): 219–26.
26. Haissaguerre M, Jais P, Shah DC, et al. Spontaneous initiation of atrial fibrillation by ectopic beats originating in the pulmonary veins. N Engl J Med 1998;339: 659–66.
27. de Vos CB, Pisters R, Nieuwlaat R, et al. Progression from paroxysmal to persistent atrial fibrillation clinical correlates and prognosis. J Am Coll Cardiol 2010; 55:725–31.
28. Nattel S, Burnstein B, Dobrev D. Atrial remodeling and atrial fibrillation: mechanisms and implications. Circ Arrhythm Electrophysiol 2008;1:62–73.
29. Kneller J, Zou R, Vigmond EJ, et al. Cholinergic atrial fibrillation in a computer model of a two-dimensional sheet of canine atrial cells with realistic ionic properties. Circ Res 2002;90:E73–87.
30. Gould PA, Yii M, McLean C, et al. Evidence for increased atrial sympathetic innervation in persistent human atrial fibrillation. Pacing Clin Electrophysiol 2006;29:821–9.
31. Naito M, David D, Michelson EL, et al. The hemodynamic consequences of cardiac arrhythmias: evaluation of the relative roles of abnormal atrioventricular sequencing, irregularity of ventricular rhythm and atrial fibrillation in a canine model. Am Heart J 1983;106:284–91.
32. Shinbane JS, Wood MA, Jensen DN, et al. Tachycardia-induced cardiomyopathy: a review of animal models and clinical studies. J Am Coll Cardiol 1997;29:709–15.
33. Watson T, Shantsila E, Lip GY. Mechanisms of thrombogenesis in atrial fibrillation: Virchow's triad revisited. Lancet 2009;373:155–66.
34. Alberg H. Atrial fibrillation: a study of atrial thrombus and systemic embolism in a necropsy material. Acta Med Scand 1969;185:373–9.
35. Stoddard MF, Dawkins PR, Price CR, et al. Left atrial appendage thrombus is not uncommon in patients with acute atrial fibrillation and a recent embolic event: a transesophageal echocardiographic study. J Am Coll Cardiol 1995;25:452–9.
36. Kirchhof P, Auricchio A, Bax J, et al. Outcome parameters for trials in atrial fibrillation: executive summary. Eur Heart J 2007;28:2803–17.
37. Hindricks G, Pokushalov E, Urban L, et al. Performance of a new leadless implantable cardiac monitor in detecting and quantifying atrial fibrillation–results of the XPECT trial. Circ Arrhythm Electrophysiol 2010;3:141–7.
38. Klein AL, Grimm RA, Murray RD, et al. Assessment of cardioversion using transesophageal echocardiography investigators: use of transesophageal echocardiography to guide cardioversion in patients with atrial fibrillation. N Engl J Med 2001;344:1411–20.
39. Matiello M, Nadal M, Tamborero D, et al. Low efficacy of atrial fibrillation ablation in severe obstructive sleep apnoea patients. Europace 2010;12(8):1084–9.
40. Wyse DG, Waldo AL, DiMarco JP, et al, Atrial Fibrillation Follow-up Investigation of Rhythm Management (AFFIRM) Investigators. A comparison of rate control and rhythm control in patients with atrial fibrillation. N Engl J Med 2002;347: 1825–33.

41. Van Gelder IC, Hagens VE, Bosker HA, et al. A comparison of rate control and rhythm control in patients with recurrent persistent atrial fibrillation. N Engl J Med 2002;347:1834–40.
42. Stroke Risk in Atrial Fibrillation Working Group. Independent predictors of stroke in patients with atrial fibrillation: a systematic review. Neurology 2007;69(6):546–54.
43. Gage BF, Waterman AD, Shannon W, et al. Validation of clinical classification schemes for predicting stroke: results from the National Registry of Atrial Fibrillation. JAMA 2001;285:2864–70.
44. Lip GY, Nieuwlaat R, Pisters R, et al. Refining clinical risk stratification for predicting stroke and thromboembolism in atrial fibrillation using a novel risk factor-based approach: the Euro Heart Survey on atrial fibrillation. Chest 2010;137:263–72.
45. Risk factors for stroke and efficacy of antithrombotic therapy in atrial fibrillation. Analysis of pooled data from five randomized controlled trials. Arch Intern Med 1994;154(13):1449–57.
46. Hart RG, Benavente O, McBride R, et al. Antithrombotic therapy to prevent stroke inpatients with atrial fibrillation: a meta-analysis. Ann Intern Med 1999;131:492–501.
47. Connolly SJ, Ezekowitz MD, Yusuf S, et al. Dabigatran versus warfarin in patients with atrial fibrillation. N Engl J Med 2009;361(12):1139–51.
48. Patel MR, Mahaffey KW, Garg J, et al. Rivaroxaban versus warfarin in nonvalvular atrial fibrillation. N Engl J Med 2011;365(10):883–91.
49. Granger CB, Alexander JH, McMurray JJ, et al. Apixaban versus warfarin in patients with atrial fibrillation. N Engl J Med 2011;365(11):981–92.
50. Holmes DR, Reddy VY, Turi ZG, et al. Percutaneous closure of the left atrial appendage versus warfarin therapy for prevention of stroke in patients with atrial fibrillation: a randomised noninferiority trial. Lancet 2009;374:534–42.
51. Groenveld HF, Crijns HJ, Rienstra M, et al, RACE investigators. Does intensity of rate control influence outcome in persistent atrial fibrillation? Data of the RACE study. Am Heart J 2009;158(5):785–91.
52. Van Gelder IC, Groenveld HF, Crijns HJ, et al. Lenient versus strict rate control in patients with atrial fibrillation. N Engl J Med 2010;362:1363–73.
53. Alegret JM, Vinolas X, Sagristá J, et al, REVERSE Study Investigators. Predictors of success and effect of biphasic energy on electrical cardioversion in patients with persistent atrial fibrillation. Europace 2007;9(10):942–6.
54. McNamara RL, Bass EB, Miller MR, et al. Management of new onset atrial fibrillation (evidence report/Technology assessment). In: Agency for Healthcare Research and Quality 2001: Publication No. AHRQ 01–E026.
55. Lafuente-Lafuente C, Mouly S, Longas-Tejero MA, et al. Antiarrhythmics for maintaining sinus rhythm after cardioversion of atrial fibrillation. Cochrane Database Syst Rev 2007;(4):CD005049.
56. Roy D, TM, Dorian P, et al. Amiodarone to prevent recurrence of atrial fibrillation. Canadian Trial of Atrial Fibrillation Investigators. N Engl J Med 2000;342(13):913–20.
57. Piccini JP, Hasselblad V, Peterson ED, et al. Comparative efficacy of dronedarone and amiodarone for the maintenance of sinus rhythm in patients with atrial fibrillation. J Am Coll Cardiol 2009;54:1089–95.
58. Hohnloser SH, Crijns HJ, van Eickels M, ATHENA Investigators. Effect of dronedarone on cardiovascular events in atrial fibrillation. N Engl J Med 2009;360:668–78.

59. Connolly SJ, Camm AJ, Halperin JL, et al. Dronedarone in high-risk permanent atrial fibrillation. N Engl J Med 2011;365(24):2268–76.
60. Calkins H, Reynolds MR, Spector P, et al. Treatment of atrial fibrillation with anti-arrhythmic drugs or radiofrequency ablation: two systematic literature reviews and meta-analyses. Circ Arrhythm Electrophysiol 2009;2:349–61.
61. Oral H, Pappone C, Chugh A, et al. Circumferential pulmonary-vein ablation for chronic atrial fibrillation. N Engl J Med 2006;354:934–41.
62. Huxley RR, Lopez FL, Folsom AR, et al. Absolute and attributable risks of atrial fibrillation in relation to optimal and borderline risk factors: the Atherosclerosis Risk in Communities (ARIC) Study. Circulation 2011;123:1501–8.
63. Granada J, Uribe W, Chyou PH, et al. Incidence and predictors of atrial flutter in the general population. J Am Coll Cardiol 2000;36(7):2242–6.
64. Vidaillet H, Granada JF, Chyou PH, et al. A population-based study of mortality among patients with atrial fibrillation or flutter. Am J Med 2002;113(5): 365–70.
65. Tai CT, Chen SA, Chiang CE. Characterization of low right atrial isthmus as the slow conduction zone and pharmacological target in typical atrial flutter. Circulation 1997;96:2601–11.
66. Cosio FG, Arribas F, López-Gil M, et al. Atrial flutter mapping and ablation. I. Studying atrial flutter mechanisms by mapping and entrainment. Pacing Clin Electrophysiol 1996;19:841–53.
67. Fuster V, Ryden LE, Cannom DS, et al. ACC/AHA/ESC 2006 guidelines for the management of patients with atrial fibrillation a report of the American College of Cardiology/American Heart Association Task Force on Practice Guidelines and the European Society of Cardiology Committee for Practice Guidelines (Writing Committee to Revise the 2001 Guidelines for the Management of Patients with Atrial Fibrillation). J Am Coll Cardiol 2006;48(4):e149–246.
68. Parikh MG, Aziz Z, Krishnan K, et al. Usefulness of transesophageal echocardiography to confirm clinical utility of CHA2DS2-VASc and CHADS2 scores in atrial flutter. Am J Cardiol 2012;109(4):550–5.
69. McCord J, Borzak S. Multifocal atrial tachycardia. Chest 1998;113(1):203–9.
70. Hudson LDKT, Petty TL, Genton E. Arrhythmias associated with acute respiratory failure in patients with chronic airway obstruction. Chest 1973;63(5):661–5.
71. Adamantidis MM, Caron JF, Dupuis BA. Triggered activity induced by combined mild hypoxia and acidosis in guinea pig Purkinje fibers. J Mol Cell Cardiol 1986; 18:1287–99.
72. Wang K, Goldfarb B, Gobel FL, et al. Multifocal atrial tachycardia: a clinical analysis in 41 cases. Arch Intern Med 1977;137:161–4.
73. Kastor J. Multifocal atrial tachycardia. N Engl J Med 1990;322(24):1713–7.
74. Blomström-Lundqvist C, Scheinman MM, Aliot EM, et al. ACC/AHA/ESC guidelines for the management of patients with supraventricular arrhythmias–executive summary. A report of the American College of Cardiology/American Heart Association Task Force on Practice Guidelines and the European Society of Cardiology Committee for Practice Guidelines (Writing Committee to Develop Guidelines for the Management of Patients with Supraventricular Arrhythmias) developed in collaboration with NASPE-Heart Rhythm Society. J Am Coll Cardiol 2003;42(8):1493–531.
75. Iseri LT, Fairshter R, Hardeman JL, et al. Magnesium and potassium therapy in multifocal atrial tachycardia. Am Heart J 1985;110:789–94.
76. Orejarena LA, Vidaillet H Jr, DeStefano F, et al. Paroxysmal supraventricular tachycardia in the general population. J Am Coll Cardiol 1998;31(1):150–7.

77. Ko JK, Deal BJ, Strasburger JF, et al. Supraventricular tachycardia mechanisms and their age distribution in pediatric patients. Am J Cardiol 1992;69(12): 1028–32.

78. Brembilla-Perrot B, Marcon F, Bosser G, et al. Paroxysmal tachycardia in children and teenagers with normal sinus rhythm and without heart disease. Pacing Clin Electrophysiol 2001;24(1):41–5.

79. Leitch J, Klein G, Tee R, et al. Neurally mediated syncope and atrial fibrillation [letter]. N Engl J Med 1991;324(7):495–6.

80. Meiltz A, Weber R, Halimi F, et al, Réseau Européen pour le Traitement des Arythmies Cardiaques. Permanent form of junctional reciprocating tachycardia in adults: peculiar features and results of radiofrequency catheter ablation. Europace 2006;8(1):21–8.

81. Zimetbaum P, Josephson M. Evaluation of patients with palpitations. N Engl J Med 1998;338(19):1369–73.

82. Moya A, Sutton R, Ammirati F, et al, Task Force for the Diagnosis and Management of Syncope, European Society of Cardiology (ESC), European Heart Rhythm Association (EHRA), Heart Failure Association (HFA), Heart Rhythm Society (HRS). Guidelines for the diagnosis and management of syncope (version 2009). Eur Heart J 2009;30(21):2631–71.

83. Calkins H, Yong P, Miller JM, et al. Catheter ablation of accessory pathways, atrioventricular nodal reentrant tachycardia, and the atrioventricular junction: final results of a prospective, multicenter clinical trial. The Atakr Multicenter Investigators Group. Circulation 1999;99:262–70.

84. Blomström-Lundqvist C, Scheinman MM, Aliot EM, et al. ACC/AHA/ESC guidelines for the management of patients with supraventricular arrhythmias–executive summary: a report of the American College of Cardiology/American Heart Association Task Force on Practice Guidelines and the European Society of Cardiology Committee for Practice Guidelines (Writing Committee to Develop Guidelines for the Management of Patients with Supraventricular Arrhythmias). Circulation 2003;108(15):1871–909.

85. Simpson RJ Jr, Cascio WE, Schreiner PJ, et al. Prevalence of premature ventricular contractions in a population of African American and white men and women: the Atherosclerosis Risk in Communities (ARIC) study. Am Heart J 2002;143(3):535–40.

86. Brodsky M, Wu D, Denes P, et al. Arrhythmias documented by 24 hour continuous electrocardiographic monitoring in 50 male medical students without apparent heart disease. Am J Cardiol 1977;39(3):390–5.

87. Kennedy HL, Whitlock J, Sprague MK, et al. Long-term follow-up of asymptomatic healthy subjects with frequent and complex ventricular ectopy. N Engl J Med 1985;312:193–7.

88. Massing MW, Simpson RJ, Rautaharju PM, et al. Usefulness of ventricular premature complexes to predict coronary heart disease events and mortality (from the Atherosclerosis Risk In Communities cohort). Am J Cardiol 2006; 98(12):1609–12.

89. Zipes DP, Garson A. 26th Bethesda conference: recommendations for determining eligibility for competition in athletes with cardiovascular abnormalities. Task Force 6: arrhythmias. J Am Coll Cardiol 1994;24:892–9.

90. Hasdemir C, Ulucan C, Yavuzgil O, et al. Tachycardia-induced cardiomyopathy in patients with idiopathic ventricular arrhythmias: the incidence, clinical and electrophysiologic characteristics, and the predictors. J Cardiovasc Electrophysiol 2011;22:663–8.

91. Bigger JT Jr, Dresdale FJ, Heissenbuttel RH, et al. Ventricular arrhythmias in ischemic heart disease: mechanism, prevalence, significance, and management. Prog Cardiovasc Dis 1977;19(4):255–300.
92. Mukharji J, Rude RE, Poole WK, et al. Risk factors for sudden death after acute myocardial infarction: two-year follow-up. Am J Cardiol 1984;54(1):31–6.
93. Echt DS, Liebson P, Mitchell LB, et al. Mortality and morbidity in patients receiving encainide, flecainide, or placebo. The Cardiac Arrhythmia Suppression Trial. N Engl J Med 1991;324:781–8.
94. Kinder C, Tamburro P, Kopp D, et al. The clinical significance of nonsustained ventricular tachycardia: current perspectives. Pacing Clin Electrophysiol 1994; 17(4 Pt 1):637–64.
95. Fleg JL, Lakatta EG. Long-term prognostic significance of ambulatory electrocardiographic findings in apparently healthy subjects greater than or equal to 60 years of age. Am J Cardiol 1992;70(7):748–51.
96. Bikkina M, Larson MG, Levy D. Prognostic implications of asymptomatic ventricular arrhythmias: the Framingham Heart Study. Ann Intern Med 1992;117(12): 990–6.
97. Fleg JL, Lakatta EG. Prevalence and prognosis of exercise-induced nonsustained ventricular tachycardia in apparently healthy volunteers. Am J Cardiol 1984;54(7):762–4.
98. Centers for Disease Control and Prevention (CDC). State-specific mortality from sudden cardiac death–United States, 1999. MMWR Morb Mortal Wkly Rep 2002;51(6):123.
99. Brooks R, Burgess J. Idiopathic ventricular tachycardia. A review. Medicine (Baltimore) 1988;67(5):271.
100. Buxton AE, Lee K, Fisher JD, et al. A randomized study of the prevention of sudden death in patients with coronary artery disease. Multicenter Unsustained Tachycardia Trial Investigators. N Engl J Med 1999;341(25):1882–90.
101. Connolly SJ, Hallstrom AP, Cappato R, et al. Meta-analysis of the implantable cardioverter defibrillator secondary prevention trials. AVID, CASH and CIDS studies. Antiarrhythmics vs Implantable Defibrillator study. Cardiac Arrest Study Hamburg. Canadian Implantable Defibrillator Study. Eur Heart J 2000;21(24): 2071–8.

Management of Venous Thromboembolism

Bruce Burnett, MD

KEYWORDS

- Venous thromboembolism • Pulmonary embolism • Deep vein thrombosis
- Anticoagulation therapy

KEY POINTS

- Risk factors for venous thromboembolism (VTE) are important to understand for both the work-up and management of patients. A clinician should consider the effect of combined environmental and inherent factors in determining the risk of disease.
- Incorrectly diagnosing or missing the diagnosis of VTE can pose serious risk to patients. Tools that can help validate clinician evaluation include pretest probability, D-dimer, venous ultrasound, and computed tomography pulmonary angiography. These tools are particularly useful for diagnostic work-up of lower-extremity deep venous thrombosis and pulmonary embolism.
- Length of initial anticoagulation treatment of an acute VTE is usually 3 to 6 months. Treatment beyond this point is for secondary prevention of VTE.

INTRODUCTION

Venous thromboembolism (VTE) has an annual incidence of 1 to 3 in 1000 patients.[1,2] Its most significant complication, pulmonary embolism (PE), is responsible for most of the 1% to 2% of acute deaths associated with this disease.[1]

The most effective way of reducing VTE-associated mortality is prevention.[3] However, early, accurate diagnosis and appropriate treatment significantly reduces both the morbidity and mortality.[4] This article reviews the diagnostic and therapeutic tools available to achieve this goal.

RISK FACTORS FOR VTE

Understanding the risk factors that can be related to VTE is important both for the initial evaluation of patients with suspected VTE and for decision making regarding the long-term use of antithrombotic agents to prevent recurrent episodes.

The author has nothing to disclose.
Park Nicollet Health Services, Thrombosis Clinic, 6600 Excelsior Boulevard, Suite 131, St Louis Park, MN 55426, USA
E-mail address: burneb@parknicollet.com

Prim Care Clin Office Pract 40 (2013) 73–90
http://dx.doi.org/10.1016/j.pop.2012.11.004   **primarycare.theclinics.com**

A thrombus materializes primarily through 3 stimulating factors first described by Virchow[5] in 1856: blood flow change (stasis), vessel wall injury, and changes in blood composition (hypercoagulability). Venous thrombus formation depends more on stasis and hypercoagulability, whereas arterial thrombosis develops more via changes in the vessel wall. Given these differing pathophysiologic mechanisms, risk factors for venous thrombosis are distinct from those seen in arterial disease.

Risk factors for VTE can be categorized as acquired or inherent. Risks are further defined as those that are transient versus persistent. Up to 25% of patients can present with idiopathic VTE.[6] These unprovoked patients presumably have a persistent, inherent tendency toward future episodes of VTE.

Acquired risks include environmental factors such as immobilization, surgery, trauma, and female hormonal therapies. Other patient states associated with VTE include age, pregnancy, puerperium, malignancy, myeloproliferative disorders, antiphospholipid syndrome, and inflammatory bowel disease.[7]

Inherent factors associated with VTE include several genetic disorders with varying degrees of prevalence in the population and varying levels of thrombogenicity. Protein C deficiency, protein S deficiency, antithrombin deficiency, and dysfibrinogenemia are rare disorders with a significant risk for VTE. Heterozygous factor V Leiden and prothrombin 20210A mutations are identified more commonly but carry an overall lower risk of VTE. Combined heterozygous genetic disorders or homozygous states are occasionally seen and are associated with stronger VTE risk. Some other factors that are associated with VTE but less well defined include increases of clotting factors VIII, IX, XI, and hyperhomocysteinemia. **Table 1** lists some of the recognized risk factors.

Rather than looking at any single causative factor for VTE, a clinician should consider the effect of combined environmental and inherent factors in determining the risk of disease. For instance, a woman taking oral contraceptives or who is heterozygous for factor V Leiden might have a 3-fold to 5-fold relative risk for VTE. The combined risk of heterozygous factor V Leiden and oral contraceptive use translates to a 15-fold risk.[8,9]

DIAGNOSIS OF VTE

Using clinical acumen alone to make the diagnosis of VTE is considered inadequate.[10] Only 1 in 5 patients with a suspected VTE are eventually confirmed positive for this disease. In addition, diagnostic radiologic tools such as venous ultrasound or computed tomography (CT) pulmonary angiogram can lack both sensitivity and specificity in certain circumstances, leading to false-negative and false-positive results if radiologic evaluation is the only method of investigating a patient's symptoms.

The consequences of inaccurate evaluations are significant. Missing the diagnosis of VTE can lead to short-term morbidity and mortality as well as long-term risks of recurrent disease.

However, incorrectly diagnosing a patient with significant venous thrombosis exposes them to the short-term risk of antithrombotic therapy and the longer-term risk of mislabeling a patient with a diagnosis that carries both financial and psychological consequences.

Over the past 2 decades, much work has been done to develop tools and processes that significantly increase a clinician's confidence of either confirming or excluding the diagnosis of VTE. These tools have been validated by well-designed studies and are now a part of the standard approach to evaluate many patients with suspected VTE.

This article describes the 4 tools most commonly used to evaluate patients with suspected VTE. It then outlines a diagnostic approach to patients who present with

Table 1
Risk factors for venous thromboembolism

	Relative Risk[a]
Genetic	
Antithrombin deficiency	15–20
Protein C deficiency	15–20
Protein S type I deficiency	15–20
F5 R506Q	5–7
F2 G20210A	2–3
Non-O blood group	1.5–1.8
Factor XIII val34leu	1.2–1.5
Recently discovered SNPs	1.1–1.4
Acquired	
Increasing age	1–∞
Malignancy	7–20
Lupus anticoagulant	3–10
Systemic lupus erythematosus	3–8
Inflammatory bowel disease	3–4
Hyperthyroid disease	1.5–3
HIV	3–10
Nephrotic syndrome	3–10
Renal transplant recipients	3–8
Chronic kidney disease	1.3–1.7
Microalbuminuria	1.5–2.5
Overweight and obesity	2–3
Environmental	
Surgery, trauma, immobilization	5–50
Pregnancy and puerperium	3–5
Oral contraceptives	4–7
Hormone replacement therapy	2–5
Air travel	1.5–3
Transient infectious disease	1.0–3.0
Mixed	
Low free protein S levels	5–10
High factor VIII	3–5
APC resistance	3–5
High factor IX	2–3
High factor XI	1.5–2.5
High TAFI	1.5–2.5
Hyperhomocysteinemia	1.5–2.5
Hypofibrinolysis	1.5–2.5
Enhanced thrombin generation	1.5–2.5
Not well established	
Air pollution	1.1–2.0
High CRP	1.2–1.8
Abnormal interleukin levels	1.0–2.5

(continued on next page)

Table 1 (continued)	
	Relative Risk[a]
High factor VII	1.0–2.5
Hypertension	0.7–2.0
Diabetes mellitus	0.7–2.0
Male sex	0.8–1.5
Smoking	0.8–1.5
Dyslipidemia	0.8–1.5

Abbreviations: APC, activated protein C; CRP, C-reactive protein; HIV, human immunodeficiency virus; SNPs, single nucleotide polymorphisms; TAFI, thrombin activatable fibrinolysis inhibitor.
[a] Risk for first venous thrombosis compared with the general population.
Data from Lijfering WM, Rosendaal FR, Cannegieter SC. Risk factors for venous thrombosis–current understanding from an epidemiologic point of view. Br J Haematol 2010;149:825.

symptoms that suggest the 2 most common forms of VTE: lower-extremity deep venous thrombosis (DVT) and PE.

Clinical Evaluation and Pretest Probability

Although clinical assessment alone can be inadequate in its ability to make the diagnosis of venous thrombosis, a clinician must never bypass the clinical history and physical. This initial evaluation can quickly eliminate the need for further testing when an assessment reveals no significant likelihood of VTE and/or an obvious alternative diagnosis. An over-the-phone evaluation of a patient with no assessment of clinical findings can result in misinterpretation of symptoms. Testing based on these data can lead to undesired consequences for patients.

When a clinician determines a suspicion for VTE, the clinical assessment is key to developing a pretest probability (PTP) of disease that can be used to stratify the patient's risk into lower or higher probability of disease. Along with other testing, this risk stratification improves the clinician's confidence of either a negative or positive diagnostic work-up.

PTP uses a combination of history and objective examination findings to determine the patient's likelihood of having VTE. Patients are scored according to number of risk factors and findings as well as the presence of alternative diagnoses. Criteria developed by Wells and colleagues[11,12] are added to a total score that aligns with a certain level of disease likelihood.

With these initial clinical assessments, clinicians can effectively use objective tests to more accurately diagnose or exclude the diagnosis of VTE in a patient. More detailed information on PTP scoring systems for DVT and PE are presented later in this article.[13]

D-Dimer

Another useful tool in the initial evaluation of patients with suspected VTE is the D-dimer assay. This blood test is a measure of the cross-linked fibrin degradation products and thus reflects a level of clotting activity in the blood.

D-dimer has a sensitive association with acute thromboembolism and thus has a high negative predictive value. However, this test is not specific and can be increased in multiple other circumstances, including surgery, acute injury, hemorrhage, illness, pregnancy, and prolonged hospitalization.[14] An increased D-dimer cannot be used as the sole indicator of VTE, making the D-dimer a helpful rule-out test but a poor rule-in test.

D-dimer assays can be divided into moderate sensitivity and high sensitivity. Moderate-sensitivity qualitative tests can have faster turnaround times and are less expensive but often require visual inspection and reader interpretation. High-sensitivity quantitative tests can further enhance a D-dimer's ability to rule out active VTE at the expense of more false-positives.

Venous Ultrasound

Venous Doppler ultrasound has essentially replaced venography in the evaluation of most patients with suspected DVT. This technique identifies venous vessels using real-time imaging often aided by Doppler color flow visualization. As opposed to arteries, veins are usually compressible under pressure when not filled with solid thrombus. The diagnostic criterion for a venous thrombosis is the inability to compress an identified vein.[15,16] Other factors such as a lack of color flow or visualization of echogenicity may be helpful but cannot be used as identification of thrombus without associated lack of compressibility at that site.

Lower-extremity DVT is the most common presenting finding in patients with VTE. Lower-extremity veins can be categorized as deep or superficial as well as proximal or distal. Deep veins are defined as those lying beneath the muscularis fascia closer to the skeletal system. Superficial veins lie above this demarcation in the subdermal layers. Proximal veins are located in the pelvic and thigh regions caudad to the popliteal trifurcation behind the knee. Distal (calf) veins are below this level. These definitions are important because they are often used to determine the necessity for aggressive treatment versus clinical follow-up. **Fig. 1** shows the venous distribution of the lower extremity.

Venous ultrasound is most sensitive and specific when evaluating the femoral and popliteal regions; more proximal iliac and distal calf veins are less easily identified by ultrasound, which lowers both the sensitivity and specificity of findings in these regions.[17] Another limitation of ultrasound is the inability to accurately distinguish acute from chronic findings. Although recannulization and calcifications might indicate older disease, these findings cannot be relied on in patients with acute symptoms. Comparison with older studies can sometimes help with interpretation. These shortfalls of venous ultrasound make it essential that a clinician interpret ultrasound findings in context with the patient's clinical evaluation.

Ultrasound can be performed on the proximal and distal portions of the lower extremity or only in the proximal region of the leg from the popliteal trifurcation caudad. The advantages of whole-leg ultrasound include the ability to evaluate for positive calf findings; the caveat is less sensitivity and specificity.[18] The controversy of treatment of distal calf-vein thrombosis is discussed later in this article.

In addition to its use in evaluating patients with suspected lower-extremity DVT, venous ultrasound is used in the evaluation of patients with upper-extremity and abdominal symptoms when DVT is suspected in these areas. Ultrasound has also been used as an adjuvant test in the evaluation of patients with suspected PE.

CT Pulmonary Angiography

CT pulmonary angiogram has replaced ventilation perfusion scanning in most institutions as the standard radiologic evaluation for PE. Intravenous (IV) contrast is given by bolus with a rapidly performed computerized scan of the thorax. Pulmonary arteries are identified and evaluated for any filling defects that suggest intraluminal thrombus. The CT pulmonary angiogram has high sensitivity and specificity for thrombi identified

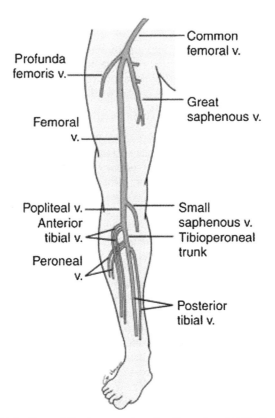

Fig. 1. Venous distribution of the lower extremity. (*From* Scoutt LM, Cruz J, Hamper UM. Ultrasound diagnosis of lower extremity venous thrombosis. In: Pellerito JS, Polak JF, editors. Introduction to Vascular Ultrasonography. 6th edition. Philadelphia: Elsevier Saunders; 2012. p.379; with permission.)

in the proximal pulmonary arteries. However, in the peripheral (segmental and subsegmental) vessels, sensitivity and specificity of CT pulmonary angiogram declines.[19,20]

CT pulmonary angiogram carries the advantage of identifying other intrathoracic diseases that might be a cause for the patient's symptoms. Disadvantages include exposure to radiation as well as the possibility of dye reactions and renal injury. Because of its heightened sensitivity, nonspecific findings can be generated. It is common to find pulmonary nodules unrelated to the patient's symptoms. Such findings require further follow-up, with unclear benefit to patients. These caveats show the need to be certain of a reasonable suspicion of PE before exposing a patient to testing.

This article discusses the use of these tools in an approach to evaluate the 2 most common presentations of VTE: DVT and PE. Although looking at these variables in different circumstances can seem complex, the underlying concept is intuitive:

- The less suggestive a patient's initial findings, the more a clinician can trust negative testing but should question positive results.
- The more suggestive a patient's initial findings, the more a clinician can trust positive testing but should question negative results.

Diagnostic Work-up of Suspected Lower-extremity DVT

Lower-extremity DVT is the most common presenting finding in patients with VTE. Presenting symptoms for lower-extremity DVT include calf pain (often described by patients as a charley horse that does not get better), heaviness, warmth, and swelling. Symptoms are often dependent even when venous obstruction occurs higher up in the thigh or groin. Clinical findings include edema, pain along the distribution of the deep venous systems, and occasionally with calf dorsiflexion (Homans sign), erythema, and engorged superficial veins.

When a clinician is suspicious of a patient having lower-extremity DVT, a PTP score (DVT-PTP) can be generated to help direct further work-up (**Table 2**). To help facilitate this, the author's affiliated institution has incorporated the Wells PTP score into the standard orders form for venous ultrasound.

Table 3 outlines the approach to patients with suspected lower-extremity DVT.

In patients with an unlikely PTP score, D-dimer evaluations can be performed before any further radiologic evaluation. If D-dimer testing is negative, the likelihood of an active thrombosis is small. In this circumstance, it is acceptable to stop further evaluation for a venous thrombosis unless a clinician's gestalt prompts them to pursue the diagnosis. It is also important to evaluate for alternative diagnoses and follow the patient clinically at this stage.

In patients with an unlikely PTP and positive D-dimer, ultrasound evaluation is recommended. However, if ultrasound is negative in these patients, the likelihood of disease is low enough to stop work-up at this point and follow the patient clinically.

If PTP is high, further objective testing is recommended. D-dimer and ultrasound can be performed at the same time. In those patients with high PTP but negative D-dimer and ultrasound, overall likelihood of active disease is low, and further testing is not required. However, in patients with both high PTP and positive D-dimer, a clinician should be suspicious of a possible false-negative ultrasound result. Suspicion of distal calf deep vein thrombosis warrants follow-up ultrasound in 1 to 2 weeks. When

---

Table 2
Simplified clinical model for assessment of DVT[a]

Clinical Variable	Score
Active cancer (treatment ongoing, within previous 6 mo, or palliative)	1
Paralysis, paresis, or recent plaster immobilization of the lower extremities	1
Recently bedridden for 3 d or more, or major surgery within the previous 12 wk requiring general or regional anesthesia	1
Localized tenderness along the distribution of the deep venous system	1
Entire leg swelling	1
Calf swelling at least 3 cm larger than that on the asymptomatic leg (measured 10 cm below the tibial tuberosity)	1
Pitting edema confined to the symptomatic leg	1
Collateral superficial veins (nonvaricose)	1
Previously documented DVT	1
Alternative diagnosis at least as likely as DVT	−2

[a] ≥ 2, probability of DVT is likely; ≤ 1, probability for DVT is unlikely. Alternatively, <1 is low probability, moderate is 1 or 2, and high is >2.

Reprinted from Wells PS. Integrated strategies for the diagnosis of venous thromboembolism. J Thromb Haemost 2007;5(Suppl 1):42; with permission.

Table 3
Diagnostic algorithm for patients with suspected lower-extremity DVT

DVT-PTP	D-Dimer	Ultrasound	DVT?
Unlikely (score ≤ 1)	–	N/A	No
	+	–	No
	+	+	Yes
Likely (score ≥ 2)	–	–	No
	–	+	Yes
	+	+	Yes
	+	–	? DVT[a]

Abbreviation: N/A, not applicable.

[a] Patients with a likely DVT-PTP and positive D-dimer should have follow-up testing if initial ultrasound is negative. Consider repeat ultrasound in 1 week if distal DVT is suspected or CT venogram if proximal (iliac vein) DVT is suspected.

Adapted from Wells PS. Integrated strategies for the diagnosis of venous thromboembolism. J Thromb Haemost 2007;5(Suppl 1):43; with permission.

more proximal obstruction in the iliac vein is suspected (as is seen in May Thurner syndrome),[21] CT venography can be performed.

Diagnostic Work-up of PE

About 30% of patients with VTE present initially with signs and symptoms of PE.[22] Although most of these emboli are thought to have originated in the lower extremities, patients may have few or no leg symptoms at the time of presentation. Symptoms suggesting PE may include dyspnea, chest pain (which is usually pleuritic but can be generalized in nature), and tachycardia. Other symptoms include fatigue, fever, anxiety, cough, and hemoptysis. Patients with more dramatic presentation might present with syncope, seizure, or hypotension.

Depending on a patient's initial findings, a clinician may decide on a carefully planned evaluation in stable lower-risk patients or emergent evaluation with early treatment in unstable patients with a strong likelihood of PE. In stable patients in whom the likelihood of PE is lower, an approach similar to that for DVT has been effective.[11] When patients present in extreme duress and unstable clinical condition, clinicians need to act quickly to both identify and treat a patient with suspected pulmonary emboli. These emergent cases are beyond the scope of this article.

Stable patients are first evaluated clinically. Patients who have little or no likelihood of having pulmonary emboli should not be included in a diagnostic work-up. Sensitive tests such as D-dimer can be falsely positive in this group and promote further clinical evaluation in patients who do not require it.[23]

Table 4 shows a strategy for the evaluation of PE. In stable patients with suspected PE, initial clinical evaluation can be used to generate a PTP score for PE (PE-PTP) (**Table 5**). D-dimer testing is done for patients with less likely PTP score.

A combination of PTP showing a less likely score and a negative D-dimer can be used to exclude patients from further radiologic evaluation.

In patients with more likely PTP, CT pulmonary angiogram is recommended irrespective of D-dimer results. Even if CT pulmonary angiogram is negative in these patients, the clinician should consider follow-up testing such as lower-extremity ultrasound to avoid missing a patient with active VTE.

Additional Insights on the Diagnostic Process

It is important to keep patients informed when going through this sometimes prolonged diagnostic work-up. Make patients aware that you are evaluating them for

Table 4
A strategy for the evaluation of stable patients with suspected PE

PE-PTP	D-Dimer	CTPA	US	PE?
Unlikely (score ≤1)	−	N/A[a]	N//A	No
	+	−	N/A	No
	+	+	+	Yes
	+	+	−	? PE[b]
LIKELY (score ≥2)	N/A[c]	+	N/A	Yes
	N/A	−	+	Yes
	N/A	−	−	No

Abbreviations: CTPA, CT pulmonary angiogram; US, ultrasound.
   [a] Unlikely PE-PTP and negative D-dimer do not require further testing.
   [b] Unlikely PE-PTP and positive D-dimer should have clinical correlation, scan review, and further testing if false-positive scan suspected.
   [c] For likely PE-PTP, CTPA and, if negative, ultrasound should be performed irrespective of D-dimer.
   Adapted from Wells PS. Integrated strategies for the diagnosis of venous thromboembolism. J Thromb Haemost 2007;5(Suppl 1):46; with permission.

a significant problem but also reassure them that this approach has been shown to give reliable answers for most patients with their symptoms. You should clarify with the patient when and how you will be communicating with them for test results. This approach goes a long way to compelling your patient to follow up with testing and subsequent examinations that are required to adequately confirm or eliminate the diagnosis of venous thrombosis. The American College of Chest Physicians (ACCP) consensus recommends that patients with a high likelihood of DVT or PE be covered with parenteral anticoagulation if further diagnostic evaluation is delayed.[4]

VTE OCCURRING IN OTHER SITES

VTE can present less commonly in sites other than the lower extremity and lung. These areas of thrombosis may need different approaches to evaluation and also may have different treatment regimens. The most significant 3 other sites are discussed later.

Table 5
Variables used to determine patient PE-PTP[a]

Clinical Variable	Score
Clinical signs and symptoms of DVT (minimum of leg swelling and pain with palpation of the deep veins)	3
PE as likely or more likely than an alternative diagnosis	3
Heart rate greater than 100 bpm	1.5
Immobilization or surgery in the previous 4 wk	1.5
Previous DVT/PE	1.5
Hemoptysis	1
Malignancy (on treatment, treated in the last 6 mo, or palliative)	1

Abbreviation: bpm, beats per minute.
   [a] >4, probability of PE is likely; ≤4, probability for PE is unlikely. Alternatively, <2 is low probability, moderate is 2 to 6, and high is >6.
   Reprinted from Wells PS. Integrated strategies for the diagnosis of venous thromboembolism. J Thromb Haemost 2007;5(Suppl 1):44; with permission.

Upper-Extremity DVT

DVT can occur in the upper extremity from the proximal jugular, subclavian, and axillary areas to the more distal brachial, basilic, and cephalic veins. Symptoms are usually related to vascular congestion and include pain and swelling of the arm with the associated appearance of prominent superficial vein collaterals.

An increasing number of patients have upper-extremity thrombosis related to more frequent use of IV catheters and central lines. Other associated causes for upper-extremity deep vein thrombosis include trauma and thoracic outlet obstruction with impingement of the proximal subclavian vein as it passes over the first rib at the neck. Patients with chronic overuse and thoracic outlet often have positional symptoms with pain and numbness of the arm when raised above 90° and findings that included a diminished arterial pulse when the arm is elevated.[24]

Upper-extremity thrombosis is usually evaluated and diagnosed through ultrasonography.[25] Again, a combination of poor flow, intraluminal thrombus, and, most importantly, poor compressibility of accessible veins is used to make the diagnosis. In general, patients with more proximal disease involving jugular, subclavian, and axillary regions are candidates for antithrombotic therapy. More distal disease involving the brachial, basilic, and cephalic veins often can be monitored and managed without anticoagulation. If persistent obstruction occurs because of thoracic outlet syndrome, angioplasty or first-rib resection have been used.

Cerebral Vein Thrombosis

Thrombosis can occur in the major cerebral veins and sinuses of the cranium.[26] Most frequently, it involves the transverse sinuses and/or as the superior sagittal sinuses. Most patients' symptoms are related to central venous obstruction with associated cerebral edema as well as venous infarction. Associated symptoms include persistent severe headache, obtundation, and, less frequently, focal neurologic symptoms or seizure. Spontaneous cerebral vein thrombosis occurs with patients who have risk factors for VTE in general. Other associated provoking causes include mastoid and ethmoid sinusitis as well as central nervous system surgery, trauma, jugular vein catheterization, and lumbar puncture. Diagnosis is usually made by contrast CT or magnetic resonance imaging (MRI). Treatment is similar to that given for DVT and PE. Patients with cerebral vein thrombosis can have associated cerebral hemorrhage, which most likely is related to vascular congestion. Often, the cerebral hemorrhage does not negate the need for anticoagulation therapy.

Abdominal Vein Thrombosis

Venous vessels in the abdomen can thrombose, causing nonspecific symptoms. Veins involved can include the mesenteric, renal, and portal veins. Diagnosis is suggested from a contrast CT, ultrasound, and sometimes MRI evaluations.

Renal vein thrombosis can occur in individuals with trauma, tumor invasion, or nephrotic syndrome. Most patients present with chronic findings often found incidentally.[27] Acute presenting symptoms include flank pain, hematuria, and renal failure. MRI and ultrasound can be diagnostic. Patients with acute renal vein thrombosis respond well to thrombolytic therapy. Anticoagulation is associated with improved outcomes in these patients.

Mesenteric vein thrombosis presents as severe abdominal pain, vomiting, and diarrhea, and often shows peritoneal signs on an abdominal examination. Thrombosis results in hemorrhagic infarction of bowel that sometimes leads to the need for bowel resection. Anticoagulation therapy can prevent extension and recurrence.

Portal vein thrombosis presents as portal hypertension with associated ascites and variceal bleeding, and bowel ischemia. It is often associated with underlying cirrhosis or pancreatitis. Hepatic vein thrombosis (Budd-Chiari syndrome) presents in a similar fashion to portal vein thrombosis with hepatomegaly. It is strongly associated with myeloproliferative disorder, tumors, and other hypercoagulable states. Thrombolytic therapy for acute disease or various shunts for chronic obstruction relief have been used. Long-term anticoagulation is of questionable benefit in these patients, given increased bleeding risk from esophageal varices.

VTE TREATMENT IN THE INITIAL 3 TO 6 MONTHS

Acute proximal DVT and PE require treatment, usually with anticoagulation therapy. Upper-extremity DVT, abdominal vein thrombosis, and cerebral vein thrombosis often require anticoagulation therapy.[4] However, distal (beyond the axillary vein) upper-extremity venous thrombosis or incidentally found abdominal vein thrombosis do not require anticoagulation in most circumstances.[4]

Patients with isolated symptomatic distal (calf) DVT are at low risk for PE but have a 20% to 30% risk for propagation of thrombus to the proximal system. The ACCP consensus recommends that clinicians consider anticoagulation treatment, similarly to other patients with VTE, in patients with calf-vein thrombosis that is acutely symptomatic, and especially that carries risks for propagation.[4] These risks include length greater than 5 cm, proximity to the popliteal trifurcation, a positive D-dimer, and persistent risk such as immobilization or cancer.[4] In patients who are poor candidates for anticoagulation therapy or if findings are not associated with symptoms that suggest acute DVT, it is considered appropriate to follow patients with serial ultrasound over a 2-week period to look for signs of propagation.[4]

Anticoagulation

Anticoagulation therapy is described in detail by Ansell elsewhere in this issue and is only briefly discussed here. Anticoagulation therapy significantly reduces the risk of propagation and thromboembolism in VTE. Anticoagulants are effective in arresting the formation of new thrombus while allowing the patient's own thrombolytic system to resorb the existing clot.

Traditional treatment of acute venous thrombus with anticoagulants usually requires initial parenteral anticoagulation therapy followed by chronic oral anticoagulation with vitamin K antagonists.[4,28] This is because, after oral vitamin K antagonists are started, it takes 4 to 5 days for circulating clotting factors to fully diminish in the bloodstream. Parenteral anticoagulants inhibit prothrombotic clotting factors immediately and negate this lag effective of oral vitamin K antagonists.

Since the 1990s, low-molecular-weight heparins (LMWHs), a purified form of unfractionated heparin, have been used with success in treating patients with both DVT and PE.[29] These drugs offer the advantage of reliable anticoagulant response without the need for monitoring. More recently, fondaparinux (a synthesized pentasaccharide analogue) has been shown to have even fewer side effects and equal efficacy to treatment of patients with VTE.[30,31] These agents have also allowed earlier discharge from the hospital or even de novo outpatient treatment of patients with uncomplicated VTE.

IV unfractionated heparin is still used in certain circumstances in which more immediate interruption of therapy may be anticipated. In unstable patients who may require interventions such as thrombolytic therapy, inferior vena cava filter placement, or surgical procedures, IV unfractionated heparin allows transient interruption in therapy to minimize bleed risk. Moreover, patients who have a significant bleeding risk related to anticoagulation therapy may be started on unfractionated heparin until it is documented that they can safely tolerate this therapy.

Several large studies have shown that patients who have cancer benefit from therapy with LMWH or fondaparinux as their sole therapy rather than the use of vitamin K antagonists.[4,32]

Superficial thrombophlebitis is often treated with local measures and antiinflammatory medications. However, extensive disease, especially in the greater saphenous vein and close to the deep system at the saphenofemoral junction, often prompts treatment. Recent trials have shown that a 6-week course of prophylactic fondaparinux and LMWH can be effective in treating patients with superficial vein thrombosis.[33,34]

Outpatient Treatment of VTE

Patients who are clinically stable and meet other criteria can be treated in the outpatient arena for both DVT and PE.[35–37] **Box 1** presents patient criteria and provider needs to accomplish this treatment safely. It is important that patients are willing participants in initial therapy because it can be laborious for them to complete laboratory testing and make dose adjustments. Patients who do not fully meet these safety criteria are often initially treated in the hospital and discharged when it is thought to be safe for them to continue anticoagulation therapy as an outpatient. Family and home health services are often recruited to help patients who are challenged with this difficult task. Anticoagulation dosing services and thrombosis clinics have greatly improved the ability to safely monitor and manage patients on anticoagulation, especially in this initiation phase of warfarin therapy.

Length of Initial Anticoagulation Therapy

It is now generally accepted that most patients with an acute venous thromboembolic event require only 3 months of anticoagulation therapy for that event. Therapy for 6 months is given to patients who have persistent transient risk factors or significant

---

Box 1
Criteria for outpatient treatment of DVT and PE

Patient criteria

- Medically stable
- Good cardiorespiratory reserve
- No recent history of bleeding peptic ulcer disease or major surgery
- Compliant/accepting
- Support at home
- Access to emergent evaluation

Outpatient DVT treatment needs

- Careful screening for eligibility
- Dedicated expert team for outpatient management
- High-quality patient education
- Daily patient contact and international normalized ratio (INR) for first 5 days
- On-call provider (24 hours)
- Detailed tracking system

residual thrombus after initial DVT treatment.[38] Beyond this initial phase of 3 to 6 months of anticoagulation, any further therapy is given to prevent a recurrent (new second) episode in patients at high risk.

The most effective approach is to focus attention on a patient's acute recovery and treatments in the first 3 to 6 months of therapy. Further discussion and evaluation for risk of recurrence should take place after this initial treatment period.

MANAGEMENT OF OTHER PATIENT ISSUES

In addition to anticoagulation therapy, clinicians should also focus on helping the patient recover from tissue injury related to their acute thrombus.

Postthrombotic Syndrome

In lower-extremity deep vein thrombosis, more than 30% of patients develop some form of postthrombotic syndrome. Patients can develop long-term venous stasis with associated leg swelling, pain, rash, and eventually skin breakdown. This injury is related to both passive congestion from residual thrombus and venous valve destruction.[39] Several studies have shown that early use of compression stockings can help alleviate acute symptoms and diminish long-term risk for postthrombotic syndrome. Stockings are fitted to achieve a compression of 30 to 40 mm Hg.[40] Usually knee-high stockings are acceptable unless the patient has extensive upper leg swelling that requires thigh-high compression.[41] Stockings are put on in the morning and worn while the patient is ambulatory through the day, then taken off at night. We also promote early reinstitution of physical activity because this has been associated with better outcomes.[42]

At the end of a patient's initial course of therapy, clinicians should always perform a follow-up ultrasound as a posttreatment baseline reference to document whether there are residual thrombotic changes.

Pulmonary Complications

Patients who have significant sequelae from PE also require close clinical follow-up. Ongoing management of pulmonary infarction and effusions are part of this requisite monitoring. Chronic pulmonary hypertension can be a devastating sequel of PE. For good operative candidates with residual central disease, pulmonary thromboendarterectomy can be performed at an experienced center.

Many patients are seen in the emergency room shortly after discharge from either DVT or PE. This visit relates to ongoing symptoms in the leg or thorax from the original injury. In stable patients, analgesic therapies, use of compression stocking, education, and careful follow-up help alleviate many of these patients' concerns and decrease the number of emergency room visits that can occur in the first several weeks after diagnosis.

SECONDARY PREVENTION OF VTE

After 3 to 6 months of treatment, a patient has successfully completed a course of therapy for that VTE event. Any continuation of anticoagulation from this point is designed to prevent a new recurrent episode of VTE. A clinician's determination of a patient's risk for recurrence takes into account many factors. One of the major predictors of a patient's risk for recurrence involves whether the initial VTE event was related to a transient risk factor.

Patients who develop VTE in relation to a transient provocation generally have a low likelihood of recurrent VTE. Provocations can be defined as strong (eg, major surgery, prolonged hospitalization and illness) versus weak (eg, oral contraception, postmenopausal estrogen, or prolonged immobilization [>6 hours] from travel). In general, unless a patient and clinician think there is a significant ongoing risk factor associated with the patient's VTE, anticoagulation therapy is usually stopped after the initial 3 to 6 months in this patient population.[4] Other circumstances associated with a low risk of recurrent VTE include distal (calf) lower-extremity DVT, superficial thrombophlebitis, and upper-extremity DVT related to catheters.

Although the baseline risk for recurrent VTE after an initial transient provoked episode is small, patients are still at higher risk of future VTE than the age-adjusted population risk. With this in mind, these patients should be counseled on modifying risks by weight loss, increased exercise and activity levels, and avoidance of estrogen therapy. Patients should be advised on prophylactic measures that can be used if they have future hospitalizations or surgeries that might put them at risk.

A markedly higher risk of recurrent disease occurs among patients whose first proximal DVT, PE, or other more significant VTE was (1) idiopathic (unprovoked) or (2) related to ongoing risk factors such as cancer or inflammatory bowel disease. In multiple studies performed in the last 2 decades, patients with unprovoked episodes had risks of recurrence ranging from 20% to 30% over a 5-year period.[43]

The ACCP consensus recommends these patients be considered for ongoing anticoagulation therapy beyond the initial 3 to 6 months to prevent recurrent disease. However, a final decision needs to take into account an individual patient's safety while on chronic anticoagulation therapy and their own preferences as to risks associated with recurrent VTE versus risks and inconveniences associated with ongoing anticoagulation.

Several factors can influence a patient's overall risk of recurrence and strengthen a clinician's recommendation for a patient to remain on anticoagulation therapy. A known strong thrombophilia, persistently increased D-dimer on treatment, male gender, postthrombotic syndrome, and obesity are all associated with a higher risk of recurrence. Residual pulmonary hypertension, heart failure, and severe postthrombotic syndrome influence the patient's risk for worsened morbidly or mortality if a recurrence does occur. A patient whose first unprovoked episode of VTE is a PE is more likely (60%) to present with a PE on the second episode.[6] Patients with recurrent VTE can have an even higher risk of recurrence and should be strongly advised to remain on anticoagulation.

A logical approach to patients with an unprovoked event is to allow them the initial 3 to 6 months anticoagulation to recover and determine how well they tolerate oral anticoagulation therapy. If patients are regarded as good candidates for oral vitamin K therapy, the clinician can then discuss the estimated risk of recurrence and ask the patient whether they are in agreement with staying on anticoagulation therapy. However, some patients choose to discontinue anticoagulation and/or look further into a more individualized risk of recurrence before making their final decision. The author always warns patients that, even in the best of circumstances, with posttreatment D-dimer and thrombophilia testing negative, they will still carry a minimal of 5% to 10% risk of recurrent disease when they are no longer taking anticoagulation therapy.

Posttreatment D-Dimer Testing

Patients who choose to discontinue warfarin therapy can be further evaluated by performing a posttreatment D-dimer assay, usually conducted 1 month after discontinuing warfarin therapy. In multiple studies, posttreatment D-dimer and thrombin testing have been helpful in differentiating very high from moderate risk of recurrence.

Patients who have a normal D-dimer level after discontinuation of warfarin usually have one-third the risk of recurrent VTE compared with those who have an increased D-dimer level.[44]

Thrombophilia Testing

Clinicians and patients may elect to undergo thrombophilia testing if they suspect the presence of an inherited or acquired defect. Indicators for suspicion of thrombophilia include spontaneous VTE in younger individuals, strong family history of VTE, recurrent VTE, or VTE in unusual sites.

We promote a light-of-day approach to this testing, addressing this issue with patients after their initial course of therapy ends. Early testing does not change the patient's initial therapy, and several tests (eg, protein S, protein C, antithrombin, lupus anticoagulant) can have erratic results because of the acute VTE event or anticoagulant therapy. Clinicians should inform patients about the pros and cons of this testing, including genetic counseling, before they are performed.

Strong thrombophilic factors such as deficiencies in protein C, protein S, and antithrombin, as well as antiphospholipid antibody syndrome and combine or homozygous states, are associated with increased risk for recurrent disease. Identifying less thrombogenic states, such as heterozygous factor V Leiden and prothrombin mutation, has not been as helpful in predicting recurrence risks.[45]

Recurrent VTE Prediction Rules

Several risk-stratification tools are currently being developed to help identify patients with unprovoked VTE who might be at a low enough risk of recurrent disease (usually considered less than 5%) to be excluded from warfarin therapy. Further study is required, however. Validation studies may show that these tools could be of some help in identifying patients with a low enough recurrence risk not to require ongoing anticoagulation.

Aspirin for Secondary Prevention of VTE

A recently published report showed that 100 mg of aspirin, when given to unprovoked patients with VTE after an initial 6 months of anticoagulation therapy, was associated with a 40% risk reduction of recurrent VTE compared with placebo.[46] The absolute risk of VTE was ~11% in the placebo and ~6% in the aspirin group at 2 years from warfarin cessation. Although this risk level does not come close to the 80% to 90% risk reduction associated with warfarin therapy, patients who choose to discontinue warfarin therapy for their first unprovoked event are candidates to start on low-dose aspirin for secondary prevention. Although it has not been studied, patients who discontinue warfarin because of a low risk for recurrent disease could sensibly initiate aspirin therapy for further reduction in their risk of recurrence. However, aspirin is still not considered an adequate treatment of patients with acute VTE. In addition, adding aspirin in combination with chronic oral anticoagulation therapy can produce a significant (2-fold to 3-fold) increase in a patient's risk for bleeding, with little added benefit.

NEW ANTITHROMBOTICS

New direct thrombin inhibitors and direct factor Xa inhibitors are described in Ansell's article on anticoagulation therapy. Both rivaroxaban and dabigatran were found to be as effective as traditional anticoagulation in the initial treatment of an acute DVT or PE, as well as for secondary prevention of VTE.[47–49] Just recently, rivaroxaban has been approved in Europe and the United States for treatment and secondary prevention of VTE. Rivaroxaban is given twice daily for 3 weeks then once daily. No bridging with parenteral anticoagulants or INR monitoring is required.

These new medications will greatly change how many patients are managed in the future. Although innovative, these agents, like parenteral anticoagulants and warfarin, carry a similar bleeding risk. Patients with prohibitive bleed risks or renal insufficiency may not be ideal candidates because these new agents are irreversible and sensitive to renal clearance.

The same thoughtful approach to diagnosing and treating patients for VTE needs to be considered for patients when using these new agents. Patients will continue to have concerns about the underlying cause for their VTE, treatment of acute injury related to their event, and long-term risks and benefits of antithrombotic therapies for secondary prevention. Much of the knowledge that has been developed in making decisions with patients will still apply with the advent of these new antithrombotic therapies.

ACKNOWLEDGMENTS

The author wishes to acknowledge Jeanne Mettner for her technical assistance in preparing this article. This article is dedicated to John R. Burnett MD Cpt. Ret. USN, 1943–2012: a brother, mentor, and my inspiration to become a physician.

REFERENCES

1. Anderson FA, Wheeler HB, Golberg RJ, et al. A population based perspective of the hospital incidence and case fatality rates of deep vein thrombosis and pulmonary embolism; the Worcester DVT Study. Arch Intern Med 1991;151:933–8.
2. Nordström M, Lindblad B, Bergqvist D, et al. A prospective study of the incidence of deep vein thrombosis within a defined urban population. J Intern Med 1992;232:155–60.
3. Guyatt GH, Eikelboom JW, Gould MK, et al. Approach to outcome measurement in the prevention of thrombosis in surgical and medical patients: antithrombotic therapy and prevention of thrombosis, 9th edition: American College of Chest Physicians Evidence-Based Clinical Practice Guidelines. Chest 2012;141(Suppl 2):e185S–94S.
4. Kearon C, Akl EA, Comerota AJ, et al. Antithrombotic therapy for VTE disease. Chest 2012;141(Suppl 2):e419S–94S.
5. Virchow R. Gesammalte Abhandlungen zur wissenschaftlichen Medtzin. Frankfurt (Germany): Medinger Sohn; 1856. p. 219–732.
6. Heit JA, O'Fallon WM, Petterson TM, et al. Relative impact of risk factors for deep vein thrombosis and pulmonary embolism: a population-based study. Arch Intern Med 2002;162(11):1245–8.
7. Rosendaal FR. Risk factors for venous thrombosis: prevalence, risk and interaction. Semin Hematol 1997;34:171–87.
8. Rosendaal FR, Vessey M, Rumley A, et al. Hormonal replacement therapy, prothrombotic mutations and the risk of venous thrombosis. Br J Haematol 2002;116:851–4. http://dx.doi.org/10.1046/j.0007-1048.2002.03356.
9. Vandenbroucke JP, Koster T, Briët E, et al. Increased risk of venous thrombosis in oral-contraceptive users who are carriers of factor V Leiden mutation. Lancet 1994;344:1453–7.
10. Hirsh J, Hull RD, Rashkob GE. Clinical features and diagnosis of venous thrombosis. J Am Coll Cardiol 1986;8:114B–27B.
11. Wells PS, Anderson DR, Rodger M, et al. Evaluation of D-dimer in the diagnosis of suspected deep-vein thrombosis. N Engl J Med 2003;349:1227–35.

12. Wells PS, Anderson DR, Rodger MA, et al. Excluding pulmonary embolism at the bedside without diagnostic imaging: management of patients with suspected pulmonary embolism presenting to the emergency department by using a simple clinical model and D-dimer. Ann Intern Med 2001;135(2):98–107.
13. Wells PS. Integrated strategies for the diagnosis of venous thomboembolism. J Thromb Haemost 2007;5(Suppl 1):41–50.
14. Stein PD, Hull RD, Patel KC, et al. D dimer for the exclusion of acute venous thromboembolism: a systemic review. Ann Intern Med 2004;140:589–602.
15. Polak JF, Culter SS, O'Leary DH. Deep veins of the calf: assessment with color Doppler flow imagery. Radiology 1989;171:481–5.
16. Lensing AN, Prandoni P, Brandjes D, et al. Detection of deep vein thrombosis by real-time B-mode ultrasonography. N Engl J Med 1989;320:342–5.
17. Cogo A, Lensing AW, Koopman MM, et al. Compression ultrasonography for diagnostic management of patients with clinically suspected deep vein thrombosis: prospective cohort study. Br Med J 1998;320:324–5.
18. Simons GR, Skibo LK, Polak JF, et al. Utility of leg ultrasound in suspected symptomatic isolated calf thrombosis. Am J Med 1995;99:43–7.
19. Hayashino YE. Ventilation perfusion scan and helical CT in suspected pulmonary embolism: meta-analysis of diagnostic performance. Radiology 2005;234:740–8.
20. Perrier A. Multidetector-row computed tomography in suspected pulmonary embolism. N Engl J Med 2005;352:1760–8.
21. Fazel R, Froehlich JB, Williams DM, et al. Clinical problem-solving. A sinister development–a 35-year-old woman presented to the emergency department with a 2-day history of progressive swelling and pain in her left leg, without antecedent trauma. N Engl J Med 2007;357(1):53.
22. White RH. The epidemiology of venous thromboembolism. Circulation 2003;107: I4–8.
23. Chopra N, Doddamreddy P, Grewal H, et al. An elevated D-dimer value: a burden on our patients and hospitals. Int J Gen Med 2012;5:87–92.
24. Machleder H. Neurovascular compression syndromes of the thoracic outlet. In: Lascalzo J, Creager M, Dzau V, editors. Vascular medicine. Boston: Little, Brown; 1996. p. 1187–208.
25. Prandoni P, Poliisterna P, Bernardi E, et al. Upper-extremity deep vein thrombosis. Risk factors, diagnosis and complications. Arch Intern Med 1997;157:57–62.
26. Stam J. Thrombosis of the cerebral veins and sinuses. N Engl J Med 2005;352: 1791–8.
27. Llach F, Papper S, Massery SC. The clinical spectrum of renal vein thrombosis, acute and chronic. Am J Med 1980;69:819–27.
28. Barritt DW, Jordan SC. Anticoagulant drugs in the treatment of pulmonary embolism: a controlled trial. Lancet 1960;1(7138):1309–12.
29. Gould MK, Dembitzer AD, Doyle RL, et al. Low-molecular-weight heparins compared with unfractionated heparin for treatment of acute deep venous thrombosis. A meta-analysis of randomized, controlled trials. Ann Intern Med 1999;130(10):800.
30. Büller HR, Davidson BL, Decousus H, et al. Fondaparinux or enoxaparin for the initial treatment of symptomatic deep venous thrombosis: a randomized trial. Ann Intern Med 2004;140(11):867–73.
31. Büller HR, Davidson BL, Decousus H, et al. Subcutaneous fondaparinux versus intravenous unfractionated heparin in the initial treatment of pulmonary embolism. N Engl J Med 2003;349(18):1695–702.
32. Lee AY. The effects of low molecular weight heparins on venous thromboembolism and survival in patients with cancer. Thromb Res 2007;120(Suppl 2):S121–7.

33. Decousus H, Prandoni P, Misimetti P, et al, Calisto Study Group. Fondaparinux for the treatment of superficial vein thrombosis in the legs. N Engl J Med 2010; 363(13):1222–32.
34. Lozanno FS, Almazan A. Low-molecular-weight heparin versus saphenofemoral disconnection for the treatment of above-knee greater saphenous thrombophlebitis: a prospective study. Vasc Endovascular Surg 2003;37(6):415–20.
35. Boccalon H, Elias A, Chailé JJ, et al. Clinical outcome and cost of hospital vs home treatment of proximal deep vein thrombosis with low-molecular weight heparin. The Vascular Midi-Pyrenees Study. Arch Intern Med 2000;16012: 1769–73.
36. Aujesky D, Roy PM, Verschuren F, et al. Outpatient versus inpatient treatment for patients with acute pulmonary embolism: an international, open label, randomized, noninferiority trial. Lancet 2011;378:41–8.
37. Koopman MM, Prandoni P, Plovella F, et al. The Tasman Study Group treatment of deep vein thrombosis with intravenous unfractionated heparin in the hospital as compared with low molecular weight heparin administered at home. N Engl J Med 1996;334(11):682–7.
38. Carrier M, Rodger MA, Wells PS, et al. Residual vein obstruction to predict the risk of recurrent venous thromboembolism in patients with deep vein thrombosis: a systemic review and meta-analysis. J Thromb Haemost 2011;9:119–25.
39. Stain M, Schonauer V, Minar E, et al. The post thrombotic syndrome: risk factors and impact on the course of thrombotic disease. J Thromb Haemost 2005;3(12): 2671–6.
40. Brandjes DP, Buller HR, Heijboer H, et al. Randomised trial of effect of compression stockings in patients with symptomatic proximal-vein thrombosis. Lancet 1997;349(9054):759–62.
41. Prandoni P, Lensing AW, Prims MH, et al. Below the knee elastic compression stockings to prevent the post thrombotic syndrome; a randomized, controlled trial. Ann Intern Med 2004;141(4):249–56.
42. Kahn SR, Shrier I, Kearon C. Physical activity in patients with deep vein thrombosis: a systemic review. Thromb Res 2008;122(6):763–73.
43. Prandoni P, Lensing AW, Cogo A, et al. The long-term clinical course of acute deep venous thrombosis. Ann Intern Med 1996;125(1):1–7.
44. Palareti G, Cosmi B, Legnani C, et al. D-dimer testing to determine the duration of anticoagulation therapy. N Engl J Med 2006;355(17):1780–9.
45. Crowther MA, Kelton JG. Congenital thrombophilic states associated with venous thrombosis: a qualitative overview and proposed classification system. Ann Intern Med 2003;138(2):128–34.
46. Becattini C, Agnelli G, Schenone A, et al. Aspirin for preventing the recurrence of venous thromboembolism. N Engl J Med 2012;366:1959–67.
47. The EINSTEIN–PE Investigators. Oral rivaroxaban for the treatment of symptomatic pulmonary embolism. N Engl J Med 2012;366:1287–97.
48. The EINSTEIN Investigators. Oral rivaroxaban for symptomatic venous thromboembolism. N Engl J Med 2010;363:2499–510.
49. Schulman S, Kearon C, Kakkar AK, et al. Dabigatran versus warfarin in the treatment of acute venous thromboembolism. N Engl J Med 2009;361:2342–52.

Heart Valve Disease

Adam S. Helms, MD[a],*, David S. Bach, MD[b]

KEYWORDS

- Aortic stenosis • Mitral regurgitation • Heart valve disease • Valve lesion

KEY POINTS

- Soft (1–2/6) midsystolic murmurs at the upper sternal border that do not increase with Valsalva maneuver and are not associated with cardiac symptoms do not require further testing; all other murmurs warrant echocardiography for further evaluation.
- The presence of symptoms (usually dyspnea) caused by a severe valve lesion is almost always an indication for valve intervention.
- Patients with valve disease should be educated about symptoms that may be attributable to their valve lesion and that the development of symptoms is a reason for immediate clinical evaluation.
- Asymptomatic patients with severe valve disease may warrant surgical intervention if lesion-specific guideline criteria of ventricular remodeling are met, determined primarily from echocardiography.
- Echocardiography provides invaluable information in nearly all cases of valve disease, but inherent limitations in determining the precise severity of valve disease mandate careful clinical correlation.

INTRODUCTION

Heart valve disease is most often characterized by a prolonged asymptomatic period that lasts for years and presents primary care physicians with an opportunity to detect disease before irreversible heart failure or other cardiac complications develop. Alternatively, acute valvular disease can masquerade as a respiratory illness or present with nonspecific systemic symptoms, and an astute physical examination by a primary care physician can quickly direct appropriate urgent care. Therefore, an understanding of the common pathologies and presentations of valvular heart disease is critical. This review focuses on the 2 most common valve lesions, aortic stenosis and mitral regurgitation, in addition to providing an overview of other valve disease topics.

---

[a] Department of Internal medicine, University of Michigan Health System, Medical Science Research Building III, 1150 West Medical Center Drive, Room 7301, Ann Arbor, MI 48109-5644, USA; [b] Department of Internal medicine, University of Michigan, 1500 East Medical Center Drive, CVC Room 2147, SPC 5853, Ann Arbor, MI 48109-5853, USA
* Corresponding author.
E-mail address: adamhelm@med.umich.edu

Prim Care Clin Office Pract 40 (2013) 91–108
http://dx.doi.org/10.1016/j.pop.2012.11.005
0095-4543/13/$ – see front matter © 2013 Elsevier Inc. All rights reserved.
primarycare.theclinics.com

PHYSICAL EXAMINATION

Cardiac auscultation can reveal a multitude of insights regarding the nature and severity of heart valve disease. In the modern era, however, the most important point is to identify which auscultatory signs are indicative of pathology and warrant more definitive investigation with echocardiography versus those that require no further testing. During auscultation, special care should be given to discriminating systolic murmurs, which may or may not need further evaluation, from diastolic murmurs, which always warrant echocardiographic imaging. The carotid pulse should be palpated to confirm the diastolic versus systolic timing of the murmur. In general, a soft (1–2/6) midsystolic murmur at the upper sternal border that does not increase with Valsalva maneuver does not require further testing in the absence of cardiac symptoms.[1]

Common characteristic murmurs are reviewed in **Table 1**. Other key findings on physical examination that should usually lead to echocardiographic imaging include elevation of the jugular venous pressure, rales, peripheral edema, hepatomegaly, abdominal distension, peripheral edema, and widened pulse pressure.

AORTIC STENOSIS
Causes

Aortic stenosis is the most commonly encountered valve lesion. The primary cause is either bicuspid aortic valve or calcific degeneration in the elderly, with only a small

Table 1
Common murmurs and auscultatory characteristics

Cardiac Pathology	Murmur Characteristics
Physiologic flow murmur	1–2/6 Early- to mid-peaking systolic murmur at the upper sternal border that does not change with Valsalva maneuver
Aortic stenosis	≥3/6 Mid- to late-peaking murmur at the right upper sternal border with diminished second heart sound and decreased carotid upstroke
Aortic insufficiency	Early, soft decrescendo diastolic murmur at the right upper sternal border best heard leaning forward with end-expiratory breath hold
Mitral stenosis	Low-pitched, soft, rumbling mid–late diastolic murmur at the apex, sometimes with associated early diastolic opening snap
Mitral regurgitation	Variable intensity blowing systolic murmur at the apex that may be holodiastolic and can radiate to the sternal border, axilla, or back. If due to mitral valve prolapse, may increase with Valsalva and squat-to-stand maneuvers and may be late systolic (after a click).
Hypertrophic obstructive cardiomyopathy	Mid- to late-peaking systolic murmur at the right sternal border that increases with Valsalva or squat-to-stand maneuvers.

Data from American College of Cardiology/American Heart Association Task Force on Practice Guidelines, Society of Cardiovascular Anesthesiologists, Society for Cardiovascular Angiography and Interventions, Society of Thoracic Surgeons, Bonow RO, Carabello BA, Kanu C, et al. ACC/AHA 2006 guidelines for the management of patients with valvular heart disease: a report of the American College of Cardiology/American Heart Association Task Force on Practice Guidelines (writing committee to revise the 1998 Guidelines for the Management of Patients With Valvular Heart Disease): developed in collaboration with the Society of Cardiovascular Anesthesiologists: endorsed by the Society for Cardiovascular Angiography and Interventions and the Society of Thoracic Surgeons. Circulation 2006;114(5):e84–231.

minority of cases due to rheumatic heart disease or congenital (nonbicuspid) aortic stenosis.

Bicuspid Aortic Valve

Patients with a bicuspid aortic valve typically present in middle age but can present at any time from infancy to advanced age. The bicuspid valve can be due to either the formation of only 2 sinuses of Valsalva at the root of the aorta or a lack of separation of 2 of the 3 leaflets during cardiac development (**Fig. 1**). Clinically, however, these entities carry the same risk of complications and are managed the same way. Although the genetic underpinnings of the bicuspid aortic valve are not yet fully elucidated, direct evidence of heritability has been demonstrated, warranting clinical screening of first-degree relatives.[2]

The primary complications and associated conditions related to bicuspid aortic valve are

- Aortic stenosis (most common)
- Aortic insufficiency
- Aortic valve endocarditis
- Aortic aneurysm and dissection
- Concurrent aortic coarctation (upper extremity hypertension in a young person with a bicuspid valve is strongly suggestive)

The presenting symptoms of a bicuspid aortic valve are dependent on the specific complication affecting the valve. In addition to follow-up of the valve disease, screening for an ascending aortic aneurysm is critical (annual echocardiography generally is adequate if the ascending aorta is well visualized) as is as screening for aortic coarctation (thoracic CT or MRI) if hypertension or diminished lower extremity pulses are present.[1] Aortic aneurysm is now understood to be due to a concomitant connective tissue pathology and not poststenotic dilation. Therefore, this screening should take place regardless of the presence of aortic stenosis.

Calcific Aortic Valve

Calcific aortic stenosis typically presents in older individuals (ages 70–90 years) and affects 2.6% of the population over age 75.[3] The course of aortic stenosis is inevitably

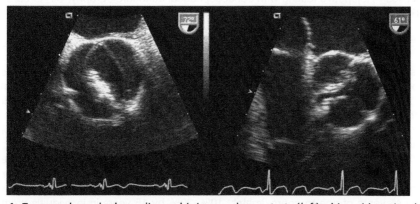

Fig. 1. Transesophageal echocardiographic images demonstrate (*left*) a bicuspid aortic valve with 2 equal aortic valve cusps and a central, ellipsoid-shaped opening, with moderate aortic stenosis and (*right*) a tricuspid aortic valve with heavy calcification and restricted opening consistent with severe aortic stenosis.

progressive, with an average narrowing of the valve area by 0.1 cm^2 per year; progression may be more rapid, particularly in the presence of heavy aortic valve calcification or aortic regurgitation (see **Fig. 1**).[4–7]

Presentation and Natural History

Aortic stenosis may present with either an isolated murmur on routine cardiac examination (see **Table 1**) or 1 or more of the following symptoms:

- Angina (due to subendocardial demand ischemia)
- Syncope (typically exertional, due to inability to augment cardiac output)
- Heart failure

These symptoms do not occur until aortic stenosis is severe. An absence of symptoms typically is associated with a low risk of cardiac complications. The development of symptoms in the presence of severe aortic stenosis, however, heralds a dramatic increase in mortality, with an average survival of only 2 to 3 years and a substantial mortality rate from sudden death.[8–10]

Grading Aortic Stenosis Severity

Accurate grading of aortic stenosis is both highly important and often difficult. The physical examination remains of great value, because clinical evidence of severe aortic stenosis (late-peaking murmur, diminished carotid pulse, and diminished second heart sound) should always prompt clinicians to be skeptical of diagnostic testing that may underestimate the true severity. Nonetheless, echocardiography has proved an extremely useful tool for grading the severity of aortic stenosis. The ability to visualize the stenotic valve as well as measure blood flow velocity (used to calculate both pressure gradients and valve area) allows stratification of stenosis severity in most cases. Common pitfalls of echocardiography include underestimation of the gradients and overestimation of the valve area if the ultrasound beam is not aligned parallel to the stenotic jet and underestimation or overestimation of the valve area if the left ventricular (LV) outflow tract is not accurately measured.[11] In the occasional case when the clinical presentation and echocardiography results are discrepant, cardiac catheterization can be performed for direct pressure measurements. Routine cardiac catheterization is no longer needed, however, in the majority of cases.[1] Adjunctive testing with transesophageal echocardiography, CT, or cardiac MRI may be useful in select cases for clearer visualization of the valve orifice.

Management of Aortic Stenosis

No medication has proved to have an impact on the progression of or adverse prognosis associated with aortic stenosis. Initial enthusiasm for statin therapy to slow progression of calcific aortic stenosis was tempered by the negative simvastatin and ezetimibe in aortic stenosis (SEAS) trial, which showed no benefit of lipid lowering with simvastatin and ezitimibe in patients with mild or moderate aortic stenosis.[12] Although some speculation remains that earlier up-front statin therapy in aortic sclerosis might be of benefit, no prospective evidence supports this practice.

The most important aspect of management is the timing of valve replacement surgery. Because bioprosthetic tissue valves uniformly undergo structural degeneration (ranging from approximately 50% degeneration rate by 10 years in individuals less than 45 years of age to approximately 10%–20% by 15 years in individuals greater than 65 years of age) and mechanical valves require lifelong anticoagulation with warfarin, a valve replacement is not really a cure, but an exchange of one disease for another chronic medical condition.[1] Although surgery should not be performed too early, waiting too long places patients at excessive risk for sudden death or irreversible cardiomyopathy. The timing of intervention can require significant clinical judgment, and consultation with a specialist in heart valve disease is reasonable for any patient with significant aortic stenosis.

Although cardiology referral is appropriate for moderate or severe aortic stenosis, primary care physicians, who often have a closer relationship with patients than the subspecialist, continue to have a critical role in the surveillance for symptomatic progression. Patients must be reminded of these symptoms at each visit. Echocardiography plays a pivotal role in follow-up to verify that LV size and function remain normal. **Table 2** summarizes recommendations for routine follow-up.

The American College of Cardiology (ACC)/American Heart Association (AHA) class I and class IIA indications for surgery for aortic stenosis include the following[1]:

- Severe aortic stenosis with symptoms of angina, syncope, or dyspnea (class I recommendation)
- Severe aortic stenosis and LV systolic dysfunction (ejection fraction $\leq$50%)
- Severe (class I) or moderate (class IIA recommendation) aortic stenosis and cardiac surgery for another reason (bypass surgery, aorta surgery, or other valve surgery)

Additional class IIB (lower level of evidence) recommendations include asymptomatic aortic stenosis that is very severe (eg, aortic valve area $\leq$0.6 cm^2), is rapidly progressing ($\geq$0.3 cm^2 decrease in valve area over 12 months), or is associated with symptoms on exercise stress testing. Among 116 patients in a prospective trial, 5% of patients with asymptomatic but very severe aortic stenosis died suddenly in a median follow-up period of approximately 3 years.[14] One prospective but nonrandomized study has shown a potential survival benefit for very severe aortic stenosis with early aortic valve replacement before symptoms develop.[15]

Role of Exercise Testing in Asymptomatic Severe Aortic Stenosis

Patients with long-standing heart valve disease may become accustomed to slowly progressive functional limitation imposed by the transition to severe disease and

Table 2
Recommended follow-up intervals for aortic stenosis

Severity	Recommended Follow-up[13]
Mild	Clinic evaluation and echocardiogram every 3–5 y
Moderate	Clinic evaluation every 1 y; echocardiogram every 1–2 y
Severe	Annual clinic evaluation and echocardiogram; increase to 3–6 mo intervals if rapid progression or nearing surgical indication

Data from American College of Cardiology Foundation Appropriate Use Criteria Task Force, American Society of Echocardiography, American Heart Association, American Society of Nuclear Cardiography, Heart Failure Society of America, Heart Rhythm Society, Society for Cardiovascular Angiography and Interventions, Society of Critical Care Medicine, Society of Cardiovascular Computed Tomography, Society for Cardiovascular Magnetic Resonance, Douglas PS, Garcia MJ, Haines DE, et al. ACCF/ASE/AHA/ASNC/HFSA/HRS/SCAI/SCCM/SCCT/SCMR 2011 Appropriate Use Criteria for Echocardiography. A Report of the American College of Cardiology Foundation Appropriate Use Criteria Task Force, American Society of Echocardiography, American Heart Association, American Society of Nuclear Cardiology, Heart Failure Society of America, Heart Rhythm Society, Society for Cardiovascular Angiography and Interventions, Society of Critical Care Medicine, Society of Cardiovascular Computed Tomography, and Society for Cardiovascular Magnetic Resonance endorsed by the American College of Chest Physicians. J Am Coll Cardiol 2011;57(9):1126–66.

consequently not report symptoms despite a decline in functional status. In patients with clear evidence of severe aortic stenosis and no symptoms, there is a role for symptom-limited exercise testing, under direct cardiologist supervision, to verify that exercise capacity remains appropriate for age and that symptoms of aortic stenosis do not appear at an inappropriately low level of exercise. The role of exercise stress testing is limited to patients with asymptomatic valvular disease without a conventional indication for surgery; symptomatic aortic stenosis is a contraindication for exercise testing. Patients should be carefully monitored and the intensity of exercise protocol tailored to the functional status of each patient. Exercise testing for asymptomatic severe aortic stenosis has been demonstrated as safe if appropriately performed and of potential prognostic benefit if positive.[16,17] Although the European Society of Cardiology supports exercise testing in their diagnostic algorithm for severe asymptomatic aortic stenosis, the current ACC/AHA guidelines for valvular heart disease support only a class IIB recommendation for exercise testing.[1,18] The authors have adopted a practice of annual supervised symptom-limited exercise stress testing in patients with asymptomatic severe aortic stenosis who otherwise do not meet indications for aortic valve replacement.

Surgical Risk Assessment in Aortic Stenosis

Because of the aging population, degenerative calcific aortic stenosis is increasing in prevalence, and patients are often of advanced age with substantial comorbidities. Accurate risk assessment is important when discussing potential intervention for valve disease so that patients and families have realistic expectations. The risk of surgery, however, is often overestimated in elderly patients with valve disease and the absence of other significant comorbidities.[19] For example, an 80-year-old man with severe aortic stenosis undergoing a first-time aortic valve replacement with no other cardiac or systemic illness has an estimated perioperative risk of mortality of 1.3% and risk of combined morbidity/mortality of 11% using the Society of Thoracic Surgeons risk calculator.[20] Concomitant pulmonary disease, a combined operation, or history of prior cardiac surgery, however, markedly increases these risks. Rapid and easy-to-use online calculators (eg, www.sts.org) should be used for a starting point in discussions with patients, although the models may overlook other important variables, such as general frailty and disability in the elderly.[21]

Transcatheter Aortic Valve Replacement

The importance of careful risk assessment is further heightened by the emergence of the transcatheter aortic valve replacement (TAVR) procedure, which involves the insertion of an expandable bioprosthetic aortic valve within a stenotic aortic valve. This new procedure has gained Food and Drug Administration approval within the confines of a controlled registry at participating medical centers in operable patients. Supporting data are from the placement of aortic transcatheter valve (PARTNER) trial, which showed that the Edwards SAPIEN aortic valve resulted in improved survival and quality of life compared with standard medical therapy in severe symptomatic aortic stenosis.[22] This new therapy offers an option for the management of aortic stenosis in patients otherwise deemed high risk for traditional aortic valve replacement surgery. Currently, however, the durability of these percutaneous valves remains unknown, and the highly effective option of surgical valve replacement remains the standard of care. Intervention with TAVR earlier in the course of the disease should be avoided, given that the prognosis of asymptomatic aortic stenosis is good and that the percutaneous approach is still associated with substantial risk (stroke occurred in 5% in the PARTNER trial).[22]

MITRAL REGURGITATION
Causes

The management approach to mitral regurgitation is highly dependent on the classification of the specific valvular lesion as either organic (ie, the lesion affects the valve leaflets themselves) or functional (ie, the valve is incompetent due to structural remodeling of the LV). Also important for management, the cause should be classified as acute or chronic. The LV compensates well for long-standing, gradually progressive mitral regurgitation but quickly decompensated with acute severe regurgitation. The most common causes of mitral regurgitation are listed in **Table 3**.

Mitral Valve Prolapse

Mitral valve prolapse is a degenerative connective tissue disease of the mitral valve leaflets characterized by leaflet thickening and redundancy, with a prevalence of 2% to 3% in the population. Mitral valve prolapse is most frequently confirmed by echocardiography, either after the auscultation of a systolic murmur or as an incidental finding (see **Table 1**).[23] Redundancy of the leaflets most frequently leads to failure of coaptation with consequent mitral regurgitation. Dyspnea only develops when mitral regurgitation becomes severe; the constellation of chest pain and palpitations, previously known as a syndrome associated with mitral valve prolapse, is no longer considered a true clinical entity based on more subsequent prospective investigation.[24]

Complications of Mitral Valve Prolapse

The primary complications associated with mitral valve prolapse are

- Gradual worsening of regurgitation, typically over years
- Atrial fibrillation
- Spontaneous chordal rupture, with resultant acute severe regurgitation
- Infective endocarditis

The development of chronic severe mitral regurgitation typically is well tolerated initially, because the ventricle compensates for the volume overload state by dilation with preservation of cardiac output. There is a 7% to 10% per year incidence, however, of patients developing symptoms or cardiac decompensation requiring surgery.[25,26]

Table 3
Common causes of mitral regurgitation

Chronic Organic Mitral Regurgitation	Chronic Functional Mitral Regurgitation
Mitral valve prolapse	Dilated cardiomyopathy (either ischemic or nonischemic)
Rheumatic mitral disease	Posterior wall myocardial infarction
Endocarditis (chronic sequela)	Hypertrophic obstructive cardiomyopathy with systolic anterior motion of the mitral valve leaflets
Cleft mitral valve leaflet	

Acute Organic Mitral Regurgitation	Acute Functional Mitral Regurgitation
Mitral valve chordal rupture	Acute LV dilation from any cause
Acute infective endocarditis	Acute ischemia, particularly of the posterior wall and/or papillary muscles
	Papillary muscle rupture from acute infarction

Patients with mitral valve prolapse also have a risk of up to 8% of developing spontaneous rupture of the mitral valve chords, which may lead to acute or subacute severe regurgitation.[27] Because acute regurgitation is tolerated poorly, patients may present with pronounced dyspnea and congestive failure. A murmur may not be audible, due to the rapid equalization of pressure between the LV and left atrium, and echocardiography may be necessary to establish the diagnosis. Lastly, mitral valve prolapse is the most common underlying cause of infective endocarditis in developed countries and should always be considered in patients with mitral valve prolapse presenting with nonspecific systemic symptoms, even though the per-patient risk is not excessive.[28,29]

Functional Mitral Regurgitation

The mitral valve is integrated anatomically into the LV, with a network of chordal attachments inserting into a pair of papillary muscles that then insert into the LV myocardium. If the LV chamber becomes dilated (eg, dilated cardiomyopathy) or the posterior wall of the ventricle (where the papillary muscles attach) is dysfunctional (eg, posterior wall myocardial infarction), the mitral valve leaflets are restricted from fully closing during systole and regurgitation occurs.

Grading Mitral Valve Regurgitation Severity

The grading of mitral valve regurgitation is primarily determined with echocardiography. In routine clinical practice, the most commonly used technique relies on the ability of Doppler echocardiography to encode the regional velocity of blood flow using color flow Doppler imaging. The interpreter of the echocardiogram judges approximately what percentage of the left atrial volume is filled with regurgitant blood flow, and a grading scheme is used to determine the severity (**Fig. 2**). Although this technique is practical and clinically useful, limitations include variable machine settings that have an impact on the apparent size of the regurgitant jet and the qualitative determination that depends on the experience and expertise of the interpreter. Other echocardiographic techniques are available for the quantitative determination of regurgitant volume but also suffer from geometric assumptions and substantial interobservor variability.[30] Therefore, an integrative approach to interpretation should be

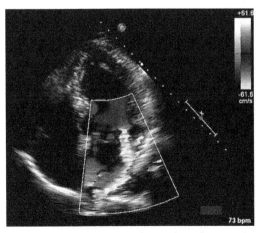

Fig. 2. Transthoracic echocardiographic image shows the color Doppler envelope of mitral regurgitation due to mitral valve prolapse. This type of eccentric Doppler jet along the left atrial wall may be underestimated qualitatively but represents severe regurgitation in this case.

used, including all available techniques when appropriate. Transesophageal echocardiography also may be helpful in more clearly defining the mitral valve anatomy and regurgitation severity.

As with the case of aortic stenosis, because of the inherent limitations and subjectivity of echocardiography, clinical correlation is always important in making management decisions. For example, a patient with mitral valve prolapse who is asymptomatic with normal LV size and function should display unequivocal severe mitral regurgitation before consideration of surgical intervention. In contrast, a symptomatic patient with reportedly moderate mitral regurgitation may warrant further testing with an exercise Doppler echocardiogram or a transesophageal echocardiogram to verify that the regurgitation is not underestimated. Exercise stress testing can also be useful in reportedly asymptomatic patients to confirm adequate functional capacity.[1] In addition, Doppler echocardiography immediately postexercise occasionally reveals more substantial regurgitation that is exercise induced and may explain the symptomatology.

Clinical Follow-up

Gradual progression of mitral regurgitation may eventually lead to severe symptomatic mitral regurgitation and cardiac decompensation. With routine clinical follow-up (**Table 4**), however, progression to severe disease generally is readily detectable, either from symptom development (dyspnea or exercise intolerance) or from structural remodeling by echocardiography.[1] Referral to a cardiologist is appropriate for moderate or severe regurgitation, although the primary care physician maintains a critical role in monitoring for symptoms.

Management of Organic Mitral Valve Regurgitation

Medical therapy with a vasodilator has not been shown beneficial in the treatment of mitral regurgitation, except for the treatment of concomitant hypertension or for stabilization in the setting of acute severe mitral regurgitation.[1] The primary focus is to determine the timing and type of surgery to be performed. As opposed to most other forms of valve disease, severe mitral regurgitation resulting from mitral valve prolapse frequently can be treated with surgical repair rather than valve replacement. Because the long-term outcomes of valve repair are believed superior to replacement, the timing of surgery is influenced by whether repair is believed feasible. The major (class I) recommendations for mitral valve surgery are as follows[1]:

- Symptomatic severe regurgitation (in the absence of severe LV dysfunction)
- Severe regurgitation with mild or moderate LV dysfunction (ejection fraction ≤60%) or with an end-systolic LV dimension ≥40 mm
- In either of the above indications, mitral valve repair is recommended over replacement with referral to a center experienced in mitral valve repair.

Table 4 Recommended follow-up for chronic mitral regurgitation	
Severity	**Recommended Follow-up[1,13]**
Mild	Clinical evaluation and echocardiogram every 3 y
Moderate	Annual clinic evaluation and echocardiogram
Severe	Annual clinic evaluation and echocardiogram; increase to every 6 mo if serial increase in LV chamber size

Class IIA (benefit likely, with less level of evidence) recommendations also include pulmonary hypertension or new-onset atrial fibrillation in the presence of severe mitral regurgitation as well as severe asymptomatic mitral regurgitation if successful mitral valve repair is probable. The latter indication is one of few in which asymptomatic valve disease, even without evidence of cardiac decompensation, is deemed enough to warrant surgical intervention. Nonetheless, intervention on asymptomatic severe mitral regurgitation, without evidence of cardiac decompensation, remains controversial, both because of subjectivity in the assessment of severity and because some prospective data support a favorable outcome without early intervention.[25] The watchful waiting approach is a reasonable alternative to early mitral valve surgery, particularly in patients with equivocally severe regurgitation, lack of access to a mitral valve repair expert (only few centers perform a high volume of this surgery), or higher surgical risk. These patients require close follow-up, however, with echocardiography at least every 12 months and at intervals of 3 to 6 months if there is evidence of significant chamber enlargement. In addition, patients should be educated about symptom development in mitral regurgitation. Once a class I indication for surgery is present, delayed intervention is associated with a worse outcome in terms of the development of heart failure and death.[31,32]

Evidence of early structural remodeling may also help in making a definitive recommendation for surgery when symptoms are not present—for example, evidence of progressive LV dilation on serial echocardiography that does not yet reach a class I indication or an elevated brain natriuretic peptide.[33] Although mitral valve repair performed by an expert surgeon should be expected to result in a durable valve with essentially normal function, complications can arise, including a suboptimal repair necessitating valve replacement, residual significant regurgitation, functional stenosis, hemolytic anemia, and death (with an operative mortality rate of 1.2%).[34]

Management of Functional Mitral Valve Regurgitation

Because the mechanism of mitral regurgitation in the presence of significant cardiomyopathy involves unfavorable geometric remodeling of the ventricle rather than inherent dysfunction of the valve leaflets, mitral valve surgery does not treat the underlying cause of the regurgitation. Intuitively, correction of mitral valve regurgitation seems to have a positive influence on the cardiomyopathy, and some retrospective or nonrandomized studies have shown a potential benefit for mitral valve repair[35–37] whereas other retrospective analysis showed no benefit.[38] Alternatively, medical therapy for the cardiomyopathy as well as biventricular pacing when a left bundle branch block is present (QRS >130 ms) also is shown to substantially improve the severity of functional mitral regurgitation.[39–42] No randomized study has compared mitral valve repair for functional regurgitation in dilated cardiomyopathy with optimal medical therapy; current ACC/AHA guidelines suggest an individualized approach in this scenario, with a class IIB recommendation for mitral valve surgery and only in the setting of refractory functional class III–IV symptoms despite optimal medical therapy for heart failure.[1] Current guidelines support concomitant mitral valve repair at the time of coronary artery bypass surgery if there is moderate or severe ischemic mitral regurgitation.[1]

OTHER VALVE DISEASE
Aortic Regurgitation

Aortic regurgitation in general can be divided into 2 underlying causes: those that involve the root of the aorta and lead to failure of coaptation of the aortic valve leaflets (eg, Marfan syndrome with aortic root dilation) and those that involve the leaflets themselves. Leaflet abnormalities can be due to an inflammatory process (eg, rheumatic heart disease) or anatomic abnormalities (eg, bicuspid aortic valve or sequelae of infective endocarditis). In addition, atherosclerotic calcification of the aortic valve that results in aortic stenosis also can cause regurgitation, albeit usually mild regurgitation. Aortic regurgitation typically is identified by a diastolic murmur, symptoms (primarily palpitations, due to the large volume of blood ejected during each contraction, or dyspnea), or as an incidental finding on echocardiography. Significant aortic regurgitation results profound volume overload of the LV, with resulting progressive dilation. In chronic regurgitation, the LV has a remarkable capability to dilate and increase its forward stroke volume, thereby compensating for the backward regurgitant flow. As a result, patients with even severe chronic regurgitation typically remain asymptomatic for years and experience no long-term cardiac sequelae despite moderate amounts of dilation. Chronic severe aortic regurgitation with marked LV chamber dilation eventually results, however, in the development of symptoms and/or LV systolic dysfunction; if this occurs, surgical intervention should proceed without delay to avoid irreversible cardiomyopathy.[1] Echocardiography is an indispensable resource for the identification of aortic regurgitation, allowing assessment of regurgitation severity and measurement of LV dimensions and ejection fraction. As with other valve lesions, the echocardiographic interpretation of regurgitation severity should be taken in context of a patient's clinical presentation and concomitant LV dilation. Cardiac MRI may have an increasing role in the future in the quantification of aortic regurgitation, because mounting evidence has shown an improved discriminatory capability for the assessment of both regurgitant volume and end-systolic volume.[43]

Mitral Stenosis

The prevalence of mitral stenosis has markedly diminished as rheumatic heart disease has become uncommon in the US population, along with that of other developed countries. Rheumatic heart disease still is responsible for the majority of patients presenting with mitral stenosis, although calcific/degenerative mitral stenosis has become more common in the aging population. In rheumatic heart disease, thickening and immobility of the mitral leaflets initially occurs along the commissural edges, with retained mobility in the remainder of the leaflets. The inflammatory process later progresses to involve more of the leaflets and the subvalvular apparatus, with the development of a diastolic pressure gradient between the left atrium and LV. In contrast, calcific/degenerative mitral stenosis results primarily from calcification at the mitral annulus with potentially progressive involvement of the leaflets themselves; the calcification can become sufficiently bulky to impede blood flow into the LV and create a substantial pressure gradient. Lastly, radiation therapy can cause stiffening and fibrosis of the mitral valve leaflets. Typically, the entire anterior leaflet becomes fibrotic and immobile, along with concomitant involvement of the aortic valve that is in the same radiation plane. Dyspnea is the most common presentation of mitral stenosis, although hemoptysis also can occasionally occur. Clinical decision making is based on the severity of symptoms, the severity of the pressure gradient across the mitral valve, and anatomic features of the mitral valve from echocardiography. Assessment of mitral gradients using cardiac catheterization requires assumptions regarding the pressure of the left atrium based on the pulmonary capillary wedge pressure or interatrial septal puncture for direct assessment. In cases of rheumatic mitral stenosis, balloon valvuloplasty is sometimes a therapeutic option that allows surgical intervention to be delayed several years. Predicting the success of balloon valvuloplasty is based on echocardiographic assessment of the anatomy of the affected mitral valve.

Pulmonic Valve Disease

Limiting pulmonic valve disease is uncommon. Pulmonic stenosis is most often caused by a congenital defect, and obstruction typically improves gradually as a child grows, as opposed to a bicuspid aortic valve, which tends to become more restricted in adulthood. Pulmonic regurgitation is most commonly related to pulmonary hypertension and may be both a clue on physical examination (early diastolic murmur at the upper sternal border, similar to aortic regurgitation) and on echocardiography to the presence of pulmonary hypertension. Pulmonic regurgitation may also be a sequela of previously corrected congenital heart disease or, rarely, due to infective endocarditis.

Tricuspid Valve Disease

Tricuspid stenosis is rare and usually due to rheumatic heart disease, in which case concomitant mitral stenosis is invariably also present. The causes of tricuspid regurgitation are analogous to those of mitral regurgitation, in that both cardiomyopathy of the right ventricle or intrinsic tricuspid valve leaflet disease can lead to significant regurgitation (**Table 5**). The most common indication for tricuspid valve surgery is at least moderate tricuspid regurgitation when cardiac surgery is performed for another reason. At least moderate tricuspid regurgitation is present in a substantial proportion of patients with severe mitral regurgitation due to mitral valve prolapse, and outcomes are better if the tricuspid valve is also repaired at the time of mitral surgery.[1] The indications for primary surgery for tricuspid valve disease are not as well validated as for left-sided valve lesions, and the decision is complicated by a prosthetic tricuspid valve that is at higher risk of thromboembolic complications. Symptoms, such as dyspnea and right-sided heart failure, that are clearly attributable to tricuspid valve regurgitation are the most well-defined surgical indication.

INFECTIVE ENDOCARDITIS
Prophylaxis

The AHA guidelines for prophylaxis against infective endocarditis in patients with predisposing cardiac lesions changed substantially in 2007.[44] These new guidelines no longer support prophylactic antibiotics in the majority of patients with valvular heart disease, reserving prophylaxis for patients with only the "highest risk of adverse outcome from infective endocarditis." The decision to change these guidelines was

Table 5	
Common causes of tricuspid regurgitation	
Chronic Organic Tricuspid Regurgitation	**Chronic Functional Tricuspid Regurgitation**
Tricuspid valve prolapse	Dilated cardiomyopathy (either ischemic or nonischemic)
Rheumatic tricuspid disease	Pulmonary hypertension
Endocarditis (chronic sequela)	
Carcinoid syndrome	
Injury from pacemaker lead implantation or cardiac biopsy	
Acute Organic Tricuspid Regurgitation	**Acute Functional Tricuspid Regurgitation**
Acute infective endocarditis	Acute right ventricular dilation from any cause

made based not on new evidence but recognition that (1) endocarditis on a per-patient basis is a rare event, (2) the majority of endocarditis cases result from daily exposure to transient bacteremia rather than from dental procedures, and (3) no randomized controlled study has been performed to test the benefit of prophylactic antibiotics. Unfortunately, a randomized controlled study of prophylactic antibiotics will never be practical because of the rarity of endocarditis on a per-patient basis. The current guidelines support prophylaxis for only the conditions listed in **Box 1**.

The new guidelines have caused some controversy regarding the implications for individual patients at risk. Because even patients without the conditions listed in **Box 1** have a high chance of morbidity and an average mortality rate of more than 20% associated with infective endocarditis, the consequences of endocarditis are great.[45] In addition, patients with predisposing cardiac lesions, as a whole, experience a substantial risk of developing endocarditis, as demonstrated by mitral valve prolapse, the most common predisposing lesion for endocarditis.[28] Furthermore, although the overall benefit of prophylaxis on a population level might be small, there is evidence in animal models that antibiotics decrease bacteremia and lower the incidence of infective endocarditis in experimental animal models.[46,47] In a case-control study performed in the Netherlands, among 438 cases of endocarditis, prophylaxis was associated with an estimated 49% efficacy at preventing endocarditis.[48] The risk of antibiotics for prophylaxis seems negligible, because there has never been a reported case of death from antibiotic-associated anaphylaxis for this condition.[44] Therefore, although the population benefit may be small, the authors' opinion is that a risk-benefit discussion should take place between physicians and individuals with predisposing cardiac lesions (eg, mitral valve prolapse with regurgitation or bicuspid aortic valve), and autonomous patients should make their own decision as to whether to take prophylactic antibiotics.[49]

Presentation and Diagnosis

The most important principle in the diagnosis of infective endocarditis is the initial consideration of the diagnosis in any patient with an unexplained fever for greater than 48 hours. Subacute endocarditis often presents with nonspecific symptoms and signs, such as chronic fevers and weight loss, that require a high degree of suspicion. Although auscultation of a murmur in this scenario should increase suspicion for the diagnosis, serial blood cultures (at least 2) are necessary in any patient with persistent fevers without a clear cause, even in the absence of a murmur (ACC/AHA class I indication).[1] The sensitivity of serial blood cultures for the diagnosis of infective

---

Box 1
AHA 2007 guidelines—conditions requiring antibiotic prophylaxis for dental procedures

Prosthetic cardiac valves or material used for valve repair

Previous endocarditis

Congenital heart disease only for the following conditions

    Uncorrected cyanotic congenital defect

    Repaired congenital defect with prosthetic material for the first 6 months postprocedure

    Repaired congenital defect with residual shunt at the site of repair with prosthetic material, indefinitely

Cardiac transplant with valvulopathy

endocarditis is 97%.[50] Furthermore, because of the importance of blood cultures in the diagnosis, antibiotics should not be initiated until after at least 2 sets of blood cultures have been drawn, because the most common cause of negative cultures is prior antibiotic use.[1] The modified Duke criteria, which rely on a combination of blood culture testing, echocardiography, and physical examination signs, establish the probability of a true diagnosis of endocarditis with good sensitivity and specificity in most cases.[1,50] Transthoracic echocardiography is recommended to investigate for the presence of endocarditis in patients with persistent bacteremia (>4 days' treatment of bacteremia) or to help identify the less common culture-negative endocarditis in patients with fever of unknown origin or other presentations compatible with endocarditis. Transthoracic echocardiography, with a sensitivity of 60% to 75%, is generally a good first-line approach, although patients with prosthetic valves generally should be evaluated with transesophageal echocardiography, with its higher sensitivity of 95%.[51] Transesophageal echocardiography should be obtained for suspected native valve endocarditis when the transthoracic study is nondiagnostic or if it is negative when the pretest probability is significant.

Treatment

After diagnosis of endocarditis is established, intravenous antibiotics should be initiated and continued for 4 to 6 weeks, per guideline recommendations.[1] Surgery for native valve endocarditis is indicated (class I) for valve stenosis or regurgitation causing heart failure; for severe aortic regurgitation or mitral regurgitation with elevated LV end-diastolic or left atrial pressures; for fungal endocarditis or other highly resistant organisms; or for complications of heart block, abscess, or destructive penetrating lesions (see ACC/AHA valve disease guidelines for details).[1] Additional indications for surgery include recurrent embolic phenomena or progressive vegetation growth despite appropriate antibiotics (class IIa) and mobile vegetation size greater than 10 mm (class IIb). A recent randomized prospective study of early surgery (within 48 hours of randomization) among patients with left-sided infective endocarditis and severe valve disease with large vegetations showed a reduction from 28% to 3% for a composite endpoint that was primarily driven by embolic events.[52] This important finding may influence future guidelines and warrants consideration in the decision making for surgery.

SUMMARY

Heart valve disease is commonly encountered in clinical practice. Primary care physicians have an important role in the initial decision to pursue echocardiography and/or cardiac referral in patients found to have murmurs and in continued follow-up for change in clinical status. A common theme for all valve disease is the need for appropriate follow-up and testing to determine the ideal timing for surgical intervention, attempting to avoid valve surgery before it is necessary yet refer for intervention before the onset of advanced and potentially irreversible cardiac remodeling and clinical decompensation. In any form of valve disease, symptoms (primarily dyspnea) remain the clearest indication for surgery, and the primary care physician maintains a critical role in both patient education and serial evaluation for these symptoms.

REFERENCES

1. American College of Cardiology/American Heart Association Task Force on Practice Guidelines, Society of Cardiovascular Anesthesiologists, Society for Cardiovascular Angiography and Interventions, Society of Thoracic Surgeons,

Bonow RO, Carabello BA, Kanu C, et al. ACC/AHA 2006 guidelines for the management of patients with valvular heart disease: a report of the American College of Cardiology/American Heart Association Task Force on Practice Guidelines (writing committee to revise the 1998 Guidelines for the Management of Patients With Valvular Heart Disease): developed in collaboration with the Society of Cardiovascular Anesthesiologists: endorsed by the Society for Cardiovascular Angiography and Interventions and the Society of Thoracic Surgeons. Circulation 2006;114(5):e84–231.

2. Cripe L, Andelfinger G, Martin LJ, et al. Bicuspid aortic valve is heritable. J Am Coll Cardiol 2004;44(1):138–43.

3. Stewart BF, Siscovick D, Lind BK, et al. Clinical factors associated with calcific aortic valve disease. Cardiovascular health study. J Am Coll Cardiol 1997; 29(3):630–4.

4. Otto CM, Pearlman AS, Gardner CL. Hemodynamic progression of aortic stenosis in adults assessed by Doppler echocardiography. J Am Coll Cardiol 1989;13(3): 545–50.

5. Davies SW, Gershlick AH, Balcon R. Progression of valvar aortic stenosis: a long-term retrospective study. Eur Heart J 1991;12(1):10–4.

6. Roger VL, Tajik AJ, Bailey KR, et al. Progression of aortic stenosis in adults: new appraisal using Doppler echocardiography. Am Heart J 1990;119(2 Pt 1):331–8.

7. Rosenhek R, Binder T, Porenta G, et al. Predictors of outcome in severe, asymptomatic aortic stenosis. N Engl J Med 2000;343(9):611–7.

8. Ross J Jr, Braunwald E. Aortic stenosis. Circulation 1968;38(Suppl 1):61–7.

9. Turina J, Hess O, Sepulcri F, et al. Spontaneous course of aortic valve disease. Eur Heart J 1987;8(5):471–83.

10. Kelly TA, Rothbart RM, Cooper CM, et al. Comparison of outcome of asymptomatic to symptomatic patients older than 20 years of age with valvular aortic stenosis. Am J Cardiol 1988;61(1):123–30.

11. Baumgartner H, Hung J, Bermejo J, et al. American Society of E, European Association of E. Echocardiographic assessment of valve stenosis: EAE/ASE recommendations for clinical practice [Erratum appears in J Am Soc Echocardiogr 2009;22(5):442]. J Am Soc Echocardiogr 2009;22(1):1–23 [quiz: 101–2].

12. Rossebo AB, Pedersen TR, Boman K, et al. Intensive lipid lowering with simvastatin and ezetimibe in aortic stenosis. N Engl J Med 2008;359(13):1343–56.

13. American College of Cardiology Foundation Appropriate Use Criteria Task Force, American Society of Echocardiography, American Heart Association, American Society of Nuclear Cardiography, Heart Failure Society of America, Heart Rhythm Society, Society for Cardiovascular Angiography and Interventions, Society of Critical Care Medicine, Society of Cardiovascular Computed Tomography, Society for Cardiovascular Magnetic Resonance, Douglas PS, Garcia MJ, Haines DE, et al. ACCF/ASE/AHA/ASNC/HFSA/HRS/SCAI/SCCM/SCCT/SCMR 2011 Appropriate Use Criteria for Echocardiography. A Report of the American College of Cardiology Foundation Appropriate Use Criteria Task Force, American Society of Echocardiography, American Heart Association, American Society of Nuclear Cardiology, Heart Failure Society of America, Heart Rhythm Society, Society for Cardiovascular Angiography and Interventions, Society of Critical Care Medicine, Society of Cardiovascular Computed Tomography, and Society for Cardiovascular Magnetic Resonance Endorsed by the American College of Chest Physicians. J Am Coll Cardiol 2011;57(9):1126–66.

14. Rosenhek R, Zilberszac R, Schemper M, et al. Natural history of very severe aortic stenosis. Circulation 2010;121(1):151–6.

15. Kang DH, Park SJ, Rim JH, et al. Early surgery versus conventional treatment in asymptomatic very severe aortic stenosis. Circulation 2010;121(13): 1502–9.
16. Amato MC, Moffa PJ, Werner KE, et al. Treatment decision in asymptomatic aortic valve stenosis: role of exercise testing. Heart 2001;86(4):381–6.
17. Das P, Rimington H, Chambers J. Exercise testing to stratify risk in aortic stenosis. Eur Heart J 2005;26(13):1309–13.
18. Vahanian A, Baumgartner H, Bax J, et al. Task force on the management of valvular hearth disease of the European Society of C, Guidelines ESCCfP. Guidelines on the management of valvular heart disease: the task force on the management of valvular heart disease of the European Society of Cardiology. Eur Heart J 2007;28(2):230–68.
19. Varadarajan P, Kapoor N, Bansal RC, et al. Survival in elderly patients with severe aortic stenosis is dramatically improved by aortic valve replacement: results from a cohort of 277 patients aged > or = 80 years. Eur J Cardiothorac Surg 2006; 30(5):722–7.
20. Risk calculator and models. The Society of Thoracic Surgeons. Available at: www.sts.org. Accessed August 8, 2012.
21. Afilalo J, Mottillo S, Eisenberg MJ, et al. Addition of frailty and disability to cardiac surgery risk scores identifies elderly patients at high risk of mortality or major morbidity. Circ Cardiovasc Qual Outcomes 2012;5(2):222–8.
22. Leon MB, Smith CR, Mack M, et al. Transcatheter aortic-valve implantation for aortic stenosis in patients who cannot undergo surgery. N Engl J Med 2010; 363(17):1597–607.
23. Freed LA, Levy D, Levine RA, et al. Prevalence and clinical outcome of mitral-valve prolapse. N Engl J Med 1999;341(1):1–7.
24. Devereux RB, Kramer-Fox R, Brown WT, et al. Relation between clinical features of the mitral prolapse syndrome and echocardiographically documented mitral valve prolapse. J Am Coll Cardiol 1986;8(4):763–72.
25. Rosenhek R, Rader F, Klaar U, et al. Outcome of watchful waiting in asymptomatic severe mitral regurgitation. Circulation 2006;113(18):2238–44.
26. Kang D-H, Kim JH, Rim JH, et al. Comparison of early surgery versus conventional treatment in asymptomatic severe mitral regurgitation. Circulation 2009; 119(6):797–804.
27. Enriquez-Sarano M, Basmadjian AJ, Rossi A, et al. Progression of mitral regurgitation: a prospective Doppler echocardiographic study. J Am Coll Cardiol 1999; 34(4):1137–44.
28. Murdoch DR, Corey GR, Hoen B, et al. International Collaboration on Endocarditis-Prospective Cohort Study I. Clinical presentation, etiology, and outcome of infective endocarditis in the 21st century: the International Collaboration on Endocarditis-Prospective Cohort Study. Arch Intern Med 2009;169(5): 463–73.
29. Clemens JD, Horwitz RI, Jaffe CC, et al. A controlled evaluation of the risk of bacterial endocarditis in persons with mitral-valve prolapse. N Engl J Med 1982;307(13):776–81.
30. Biner S, Rafique A, Rafii F, et al. Reproducibility of proximal isovelocity surface area, vena contracta, and regurgitant jet area for assessment of mitral regurgitation severity. JACC Cardiovasc Imaging 2010;3(3):235–43.
31. Ling LH, Enriquez-Sarano M, Seward JB, et al. Early surgery in patients with mitral regurgitation due to flail leaflets: a long-term outcome study. Circulation 1997;96(6):1819–25.

32. Enriquez-Sarano M, Avierinos JF, Messika-Zeitoun D, et al. Quantitative determinants of the outcome of asymptomatic mitral regurgitation. N Engl J Med 2005; 352(9):875–83.

33. Pizarro R, Bazzino OO, Oberti PF, et al. Prospective validation of the prognostic usefulness of brain natriuretic peptide in asymptomatic patients with chronic severe mitral regurgitation. J Am Coll Cardiol 2009;54(12):1099–106.

34. Gammie JS, Sheng S, Griffith BP, et al. Trends in mitral valve surgery in the United States: results from the Society of Thoracic Surgeons Adult Cardiac Surgery Database. Ann Thorac Surg 2009;87(5):1431–7 [discussion: 1437–9].

35. Bishay ES, McCarthy PM, Cosgrove DM, et al. Mitral valve surgery in patients with severe left ventricular dysfunction. Eur J Cardiothorac Surg 2000;17(3):213–21.

36. Bolling SF, Pagani FD, Deeb GM, et al. Intermediate-term outcome of mitral reconstruction in cardiomyopathy. J Thorac Cardiovasc Surg 1998;115(2):381–6 [discussion: 387–8].

37. Chen FY, Adams DH, Aranki SF, et al. Mitral valve repair in cardiomyopathy. Circulation 1998;98(Suppl 19):II124–7.

38. Wu AH, Aaronson KD, Bolling SF, et al. Impact of mitral valve annuloplasty on mortality risk in patients with mitral regurgitation and left ventricular systolic dysfunction. J Am Coll Cardiol 2005;45(3):381–7.

39. Capomolla S, Febo O, Gnemmi M, et al. Beta-blockade therapy in chronic heart failure: diastolic function and mitral regurgitation improvement by carvedilol. Am Heart J 2000;139(4):596–608.

40. Linde C, Leclercq C, Rex S, et al. Long-term benefits of biventricular pacing in congestive heart failure: results from the MUltisite STimulation in cardiomyopathy (MUSTIC) study. J Am Coll Cardiol 2002;40(1):111–8.

41. Breithardt OA, Sinha AM, Schwammenthal E, et al. Acute effects of cardiac resynchronization therapy on functional mitral regurgitation in advanced systolic heart failure [Erratum appears in J Am Coll Cardiol 2003;41(10):1852]. J Am Coll Cardiol 2003;41(5):765–70.

42. St John Sutton MG, Plappert T, Abraham WT, et al. Multicenter InSync Randomized Clinical Evaluation Study G. Effect of cardiac resynchronization therapy on left ventricular size and function in chronic heart failure. Circulation 2003; 107(15):1985–90.

43. Myerson SG, d'Arcy J, Mohiaddin R, et al. Clinical outcome in Aortic regurgitation with cardiovascular magnetic resonance. Circulation 2012;126(12):1452–60.

44. Wilson W, Taubert KA, Gewitz M, et al, American Heart Association Rheumatic Fever, Endocarditis, and Kawasaki Disease Committee, American Heart Association Council on Cardiovascular Disease in the Young, American Heart Association Council on Clinical Cardiology, American Heart Association Council on Cardiovascular Surgery and Anesthesia, Quality of Care and Outcomes Research Interdisciplinary Working Group. Prevention of infective endocarditis: guidelines from the American Heart Association: a guideline from the American Heart Association Rheumatic Fever, Endocarditis, and Kawasaki Disease Committee, Council on Cardiovascular Disease in the Young, and the Council on Clinical Cardiology, Council on Cardiovascular Surgery and Anesthesia, and the Quality of Care and Outcomes Research Interdisciplinary Working Group [Erratum appears in Circulation 2007;116(15):e376–7]. Circulation 2007;116(15):1736–54.

45. Durante-Mangoni E, Bradley S, Selton-Suty C, et al, International Collaboration on Endocarditis Prospective Cohort Study G. Current features of infective endocarditis in elderly patients: results of the International Collaboration on Endocarditis Prospective Cohort Study. Arch Intern Med 2008;168(19):2095–103.

46. Glauser MP, Francioli P. Successful prophylaxis against experimental streptococcal endocarditis with bacteriostatic antibiotics. J Infect Dis 1982;146(6):806–10.
47. Malinverni R, Overholser CD, Bille J, et al. Antibiotic prophylaxis of experimental endocarditis after dental extractions. Circulation 1988;77(1):182–7.
48. Van der Meer JT, Van Wijk W, Thompson J, et al. Efficacy of antibiotic prophylaxis for prevention of native-valve endocarditis. Lancet 1992;339(8786):135–9.
49. Bach DS. Antibiotic prophylaxis for infective endocarditis: ethical care in the era of revised guidelines. Methodist Debakey Cardiovasc J 2010;6(4):48–52.
50. Li JS, Sexton DJ, Mick N, et al. Proposed modifications to the Duke criteria for the diagnosis of infective endocarditis. Clin Infect Dis 2000;30(4):633–8.
51. Mugge A, Daniel WG, Frank G, et al. Echocardiography in infective endocarditis: reassessment of prognostic implications of vegetation size determined by the transthoracic and the transesophageal approach. J Am Coll Cardiol 1989; 14(3):631–8.
52. Kang DH, Kim YJ, Kim SH, et al. Early surgery versus conventional treatment for infective endocarditis. N Engl J Med 2012;366(26):2466–73.

The Evolution of Oral Anticoagulant Therapy

Christopher Dittus, DO, MPH*, Jack Ansell, MD

KEYWORDS

- Anticoagulation • Warfarin • Dabigatran • Rivaroxaban • Apixaban • Edoxaban
- Thromboembolism

KEY POINTS

- Develop an understanding of the coagulation cascade and the coagulation factors that are targeted by warfarin and each of the new targeted anticoagulants.
- Understand the difference in pharmacodynamics and pharmacokinetics between warfarin and the new oral anticoagulants.
- Learn the major randomized controlled trials for each indication and each new oral anticoagulant.
- Understand all the factors that influence patient compliance, anticoagulant monitoring, and reversal of the anticoagulant effect.

INTRODUCTION

Hemostasis is integral to health and survival. Ideally blood remains fluid, but rapidly clots in response to impending hemorrhage. Naturally occurring procoagulant and anticoagulant proteins exist to maintain hemostasis. Imbalance between these naturally occurring proteins may lead to clinical aberration. A general understanding of the natural physiology is helpful before mastering the therapeutic manipulation of this pathway.

The coagulation cascade is composed of 2 pathways, intrinsic and extrinsic, that combine to form a third, common, pathway (**Fig. 1**), which ultimately leads to thrombus formation. Each of these 3 pathways involves the activation of coagulation factors that circulate as proenzymes and are activated to become functional enzymes. The intrinsic pathway (factors XII, XI, IX, and VIII) is activated by contact with negatively charged surfaces, whereas the extrinsic pathway (factor VII) is activated by contact with exposed tissue factor after endothelial damage. The common pathway (factors X, V, II [prothrombin], and I [fibrinogen]) is activated by factor VIIa tissue factor or by

Conflict of interest: Dr Ansell serves as a consultant for Bristol Myers Squibb, Janssen, Boehringer Ingelheim, Pfizer, and Daiichi Sankyo Pharmaceuticals.
Department of Medicine, Lenox Hill Hospital, 100 East 77th Street, New York, NY 10075, USA
* Corresponding author.
E-mail address: cdittus@nshs.edu

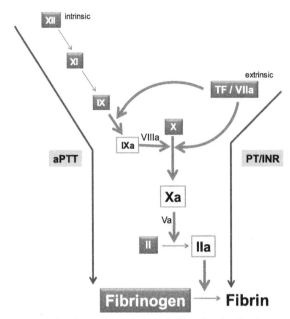

Fig. 1. Coagulation cascade. The activated partial thromboplastin time (aPTT) is a measure of the intrinsic pathway; the prothrombin time/international normalized ratio (PT/INR) is a measure of the extrinsic pathway. Xa and IIa (thrombin) are the principal targets for the new oral anticoagulants. TF, tissue factor.

factors IXa and VIIIa. Factor Xa, in conjunction with factor V, activates prothrombin to become thrombin, which in turn cleaves peptides from fibrinogen, allowing the remaining fibrin monomers to polymerize and form a fibrin clot. This fibrin clot becomes cross-linked via the action of factor XIII. Of diagnostic importance is that each pathway can be assessed by the 2 major screening assays, the activated partial thromboplastin time (aPTT) reflecting the function of the intrinsic and common pathway, and the prothrombin time (PT) reflecting the function of the extrinsic and common pathways.

Therapeutic agents involve either direct or indirect action on 1 or more of these coagulation factors. The first anticoagulant to be isolated was the parenteral agent, heparin. Heparin binds to antithrombin and accelerates its action. This complex binds to factor Xa and factor IIa (thrombin), inhibiting the action of each molecule. Low molecular weight heparin (LMWH) and fondaparinux are further refinements on heparin, with shorter chain lengths. LMWH has proportionately greater anti-Xa effect compared with its effect on thrombin, and fondaparinux has only anti-Xa action. Both of these agents have significantly less nonspecific protein binding compared with heparin, and their anticoagulant effect is predictable, thus they do not need dose monitoring. The first direct, targeted parenteral formulations were the direct thrombin inhibitors argatroban, bivalirudin, and lepirudin.[1] As the name implies, these agents directly bind to, and inhibit, thrombin; none of these agents are available in oral formulation.

The era of oral anticoagulation began with the vitamin K antagonists (VKA), the first being dicoumarol, isolated in 1940. Warfarin, a synthesized VKA, was created soon thereafter. The VKAs produce an anticoagulant effect by interfering with the synthesis of factors II, VII, IX, and X (the vitamin K–dependent factors), and reducing their concentration. Greater specificity of oral anticoagulants was achieved with the discovery of the first oral direct thrombin inhibitor, ximelagatran. Although ximelagatran was effective in numerous clinical trials, the excitement was short-lived when it was removed from the market in 2006 because of concerns over liver-function abnormalities.[2] Soon thereafter, another oral direct thrombin inhibitor, the prodrug dabigatran etexilate (Pradaxa), underwent extensive evaluation and was approved in most countries for the prevention of venous thromboembolism (VTE) in patients undergoing major joint replacement.[3] In October 2010, dabigatran etexilate was first approved in the United States for stroke prevention in nonvalvular atrial fibrillation. Simultaneously, oral direct factor Xa inhibitors have been developed and studied in various patient populations. These agents include rivaroxaban (Xarelto), apixaban (Eliquis) and, most recently, edoxaban (Lixiana). These oral inhibitors of factors IIa and Xa are the focus of this review (**Fig. 2**).

PHARMACOKINETICS AND PHARMACODYNAMICS OF ORAL ANTICOAGULANTS
Vitamin K Antagonist

Warfarin
Warfarin is rapidly absorbed after oral administration, reaching peak blood levels in 90 minutes.[4] It is highly protein bound and has a half-life of 36 to 42 hours. Warfarin is metabolized in the liver, and relies on P450 cytochrome enzymes (CYP 2C9) for this process (**Table 1**).[4] Warfarin achieves its anticoagulant effect by interfering with the synthesis of factors II, VII, IX, and X through its inhibition of vitamin K oxide reductase (VKOR). VKOR is an enzyme that reduces oxidized vitamin K, allowing it to be used again in the synthesis of the vitamin K–dependent factors (**Fig. 3**). Warfarin's pharmacokinetics are influenced by several environmental (medications, herbal remedies, diet) and genetic factors that lead to an unpredictable drug effect, which necessitates monitoring the degree of effect via the PT and its derived measure, the international normalized ratio (INR). At present, pharmacogenetic profiling (determining one's genotype for CYP2C9 or VKOR) has not shown a definitive advantage in preventing adverse drug events, and is not recommended. As mentioned previously, warfarin inhibits factors II, VII, IX, and X.[4] Of these, factors II and X (common pathway) prolong both the PT/INR and the aPTT, factor VII (extrinsic pathway) prolongs the PT/INR, and factor IX (intrinsic pathway) prolongs the aPTT. The half-life of each of these factors is important in understanding the practical concept of warfarin's delayed therapeutic effect, as well as the necessity for "bridging" therapy. Of the vitamin K–dependent factors, factor VII has the shortest half-life (6 hours) and is responsible for the initial prolongation of the PT/INR.[4] Factors II and X are responsible for the subsequent PT/INR prolongation (see **Fig. 1**). Factor II has the longest half-life of the vitamin K–dependent factors (60 hours). The long half-life of factor II is responsible for the delayed effect of warfarin.

Factor IIa Inhibition

Dabigatran etexilate
Dabigatran etexilate is a prodrug of the active anticoagulant, dabigatran. After oral administration, dabigatran etexilate is rapidly converted to dabigatran, a small, competitive, reversible, direct thrombin inhibitor.[3] Dabigatran inhibits both free and fibrin-bound thrombin. This is distinct from heparin, which only inhibits free thrombin, allowing fibrin-bound thrombin to continue to participate in thrombus formation.[1,3] Dabigatran is absorbed rapidly, reaching peak effect in approximately 2 hours, and has a short half-life of approximately 12 to 14 hours depending on renal function (see **Table 1**). It is primarily eliminated in the urine as unchanged drug, and patients

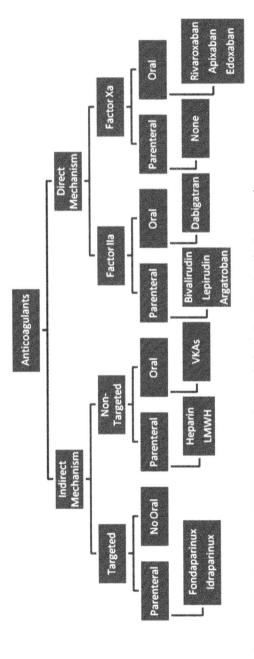

Fig. 2. Overview of anticoagulants. LMWH, low molecular weight heparin; VKA, vitamin K antagonist.

Table 1
Pharmacokinetics and pharmacodynamics of oral anticoagulants

| | VKA | Factor IIa Inhibitor | Factor Xa Inhibitors | | |
	Warfarin	Dabigatran	Rivaroxaban	Apixaban	Edoxaban
Dosing	Variable, from 2.5 to 10 mg daily	AFib: 150 mg BID (CrCl 15–30: 75 mg BID)	DVT Px: 10 mg daily AFib: 20 mg daily (CrCl <30: avoid) (C-P B or C: avoid)	DVT Px: 2.5 mg BID AFib: 5 mg BID (in Europe: CrCl <15: avoid)	30 or 60 mg daily (CrCl <30: avoid) (CrCl 30–50: reduced dose)
Oral bioavailability	High	7%	80%	66%	50%
Time to maximum plasma concentration	1.5 h (peak effect: 3–5 d)	0.5–2 h	2–4 h	1–3 h	1–2 h
Plasma protein binding	High	35%	95%	87%	40%–59%
Half-life	36–42 h	12–14 h	9–13 h	9–14 h	9–10 h
Elimination	90% liver (no renal excretion)	Renal	Two-thirds renal, one-third liver	One-quarter renal, one-half fecal (also biliary and hepatic)	One-third renal (also biliary and metabolic)
Dialysis elimination	No	65%	Unlikely owing to high protein binding	Unlikely owing to high protein binding	Likely partial
Metabolism via CYP3A4 or P-glycoprotein	CYP2C9 primarily but also CYP3A4, CYP1A2	P-Glycoprotein	Both	CYP3A4	P-Glycoprotein
Routine monitoring	Required	No	No	No	No
Reversal	Vitamin K, FFP, PCC	HD, 65%	PCC	No data	No data

Abbreviations: AFib, atrial fibrillation; BID, twice daily; C-P, Child-Pugh; CrCl, creatinine clearance; DVT Px, deep venous thrombosis; FFP, fresh frozen plasma; HD, hemodialysis; PCC, prothrombin complex concentrate; VKA, vitamin K antagonist.
Data from Refs.[3,4,6,8,9,39,40]

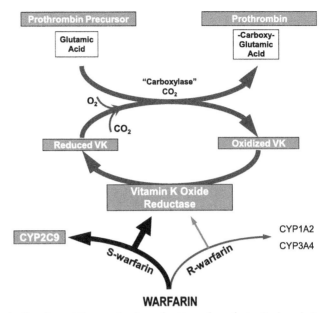

Fig. 3. Vitamin K cycle and the mechanism of action of warfarin. Reduced vitamin K partic-ipates in a carboxylation reaction, converting prothrombin precursor to functional prothrombin. In the process, vitamin K is oxidized and then recycled to reduced vitamin K by an enzyme, vitamin K oxide reductase (VKOR). Warfarin, specifically the S-isomer of the racemic preparation, inhibits VKOR, and traps vitamin K in an oxidized nonfunctional form, thus leading to impaired synthesis of the vitamin K–dependent coagulation factors. S-warfarin is also metabolized by the P450 enzyme, CYP2C9. Drugs that interfere with CYP2C9 or polymorphisms in the CYP2C9 gene or the VKOR gene lead to variations in warfarin plasma levels or the ability to inhibit the reductase enzyme. VK, vitamin K.

with renal insufficiency have higher plasma concentrations.[5] Because of renal elimina-tion and low binding of plasma protein, dabigatran is dialyzable. The anticoagulant effect of dabigatran is predictable, and thus does not require monitoring. Dabigatran does not have a specific antidote to reverse its effect, but its short half-life is advan-tageous if bleeding should occur. Because it targets the common pathway, dabigatran affects both the aPTT and the thrombin time, but has little effect on the PT/INR (**Table 2**).

Factor Xa Inhibition

Rivaroxaban

Rivaroxaban is a small molecule that directly and reversibly binds to, and inhibits, free and clot-bound factor Xa.[6] Rivaroxaban has high oral bioavailability (80%) and is rapidly absorbed, reaching a peak concentration in 2 to 4 hours (see **Table 1**). Rivarox-aban also has a short half-life of approximately 9 to 13 hours. Two-thirds of rivaroxaban is excreted through the kidney, but only one-third is unchanged drug. Additionally, rivaroxaban is partially metabolized in the liver by the cytochrome enzyme CYP3A4. Rivaroxaban affects both the aPTT and the PT/INR, although imprecisely, and neither of these laboratory measures can be used for routine monitoring (see **Table 2**).[6] A more specific laboratory test is the anti-FXa assay, which has been shown to accurately and precisely quantify rivaroxaban plasma levels.[7]

Table 2
Effect of new oral anticoagulants on standard laboratory assessments of anticoagulation

	VKA	Factor IIa Inhibitor	Factor Xa Inhibitors		
	Warfarin	Dabigatran	Rivaroxaban	Apixaban	Edoxaban
PT/INR	Yes	Minimal	Yes	Yes	Yes
aPTT	Yes	Yes	Yes	Yes	Yes
Thrombin time	No	Yes	No	No	No
Ecarin clotting time	No	Yes	No	No	No
Anti-FXa assay	No	No	Yes	Yes	Yes

Abbreviations: aPTT, activated partial thromboplastin time; PT/INR, prothrombin time/international normalized ratio; VKA, vitamin K antagonist.

Apixaban

Like rivaroxaban, apixaban directly and reversibly binds, and inhibits, factor Xa in both its free and bound forms.[8] After oral administration, roughly 66% is bioavailable and the peak plasma concentration is reached within 1 to 3 hours. The half-life of apixaban is 9 to 14 hours, and the drug is 87% protein bound. Apixaban is cleared via cytochrome P450 3A4 enzyme metabolism in the liver, as well as via renal and fecal excretion (see **Table 1**). Dosage adjustment is not required for those with mild to moderate renal impairment, but apixaban is not recommended for those with a creatinine clearance of less than 15 mL/min.[8] Like rivaroxaban, apixaban affects both the aPTT and the PT/INR with high variability. As expected, the anti-FXa assay best correlates with apixaban plasma levels, and may prove to be clinically useful in certain circumstances (see **Table 2**).[8]

Edoxaban

Edoxaban also directly and reversibly binds to, and inhibits, factor Xa.[9] Edoxaban has high specificity for both free and bound factor Xa. Compared with rivaroxaban and apixaban, edoxaban is less protein bound (40%–59%) and has less oral bioavailability (50%).[9] Peak plasma concentration of edoxaban is reached within 1 to 2 hours, and edoxaban has a half-life of approximately 9 to 11 hours (see **Table 1**). Edoxaban has predominantly renal elimination. Both the aPTT and PT/INR are affected by edoxaban, but these measures do not accurately correlate with the degree of anticoagulation (see **Table 2**).

INDICATIONS AND CLINICAL USE
Venous Thromboembolism Prophylaxis in Orthopedic Surgery Patients

Dabigatran

There have been 4 large randomized controlled trials (RCTs) evaluating the use of dabigatran for venous thromboembolism (VTE) prophylaxis in orthopedic surgery patients. RE-MODEL and RE-NOVATE evaluated the efficacy of dabigatran, 150 mg or 220 mg daily, versus enoxaparin, 40 mg daily starting the night before surgery, in the prevention of VTE after total knee replacement (TKR) and total hip replacement (THR), respectively (**Table 3**).[10,11] Dabigatran was found to be noninferior to enoxaparin in both of these studies, and won approval for the prevention of VTE in orthopedic surgery patients in Europe. In the RE-MOBILIZE study dabigatran was compared with the North American dosing of enoxaparin, 30 mg twice daily starting 12 to 24 hours after surgery, and failed to achieve noninferiority in preventing VTE and all-cause mortality.[12] These results are largely responsible for the lack of approval for this indication in the United States. In 2011, the RE-NOVATE II study found

Table 3
Randomized controlled trials (RCTs) evaluating new anticoagulants for prevention of venous thromboembolism in major orthopedic surgery

Study.Ref.	Drug, Dose	Number, Duration	Indication	Comparator	Primary Outcome Measure	Primary Safety Measure	Primary Outcome Results	Primary Safety Results
RE-MOBILIZE[12]	Dabigatran, 150 or 220 mg daily	2615, 12–15 d	TKR	Enoxaparin 30 mg BID	Total VTE and all-cause mortality	Major bleeding	150 mg: 34%, 219/649, RD: 8.4% (CI: 3.4–13.3) 220 mg: 31%, 188/604, RD: 5.8% (CI: 0.8–10.8) Enox: 25%, 163/643 Dabigatran not noninferior	150 mg: 0.6%, 5/871 220 mg: 0.6, 5/857 Enox: 1.4%, 12/868 No increase in major bleeding with either dabigatran dosing
RE-MODEL[10]	Dabigatran, 150 or 220 mg daily	2076, 6–10 d	TKR	Enoxaparin 40 mg daily	Total VTE and all-cause mortality	Major bleeding	150 mg: 40.5%, 213/526 AD: −1.3% (CI: −7.3–4.6) 220 mg: 36.4%, 183/503, AD: 2.8% (CI: −3.1–8.7) Enox: 37.7%, 193/512 Dabigatran noninferior	150 mg: 1.3%, 9/703 220 mg: 1.5%, 10/679 Enox: 1.3%, 9/694 No increase in major bleeding with either dabigatran dosing

Study	Drug, dose	N, duration	Comparator	Indication	Outcome	Results	Outcome	Results
RE-NOVATE[11]	Dabigatran, 150 or 220 mg daily	3494, 28–35 d	Enoxaparin 40 mg daily	THR	Total VTE and all-cause mortality	150 mg: 8.6%, 75/874; AD: 1.9 (CI: −0.6–4.4); 220 mg: 6%, 53/880; AD: −0.7 (CI: −2.9–1.6); Enox: 6.7%, 60/897; Dabigatran noninferior	Major bleeding	150 mg: 1.3%, 15/1163; 220 mg: 2%, 23/1146; Enox: 1.6%, 18/1154; No increase in major bleeding with either dabigatran dosing
RE-NOVATE II[13]	Dabigatran, 220 mg daily	2055, 28–35 d	Enoxaparin 40 mg daily	THR	Composite of VTE and all-cause mortality	Dab: 7.7%, 61/792; Enox: 8.8%, 69/785; RD: −1.1 (CI: −3.8–1.6); Dabigatran noninferior	Major bleeding	Dab: 1.4%, 14/1010; Enox: 0.9%, 9/1003; No increase in major bleeding with dabigatran
RECORD-1[14]	Rivaroxaban, 10 mg daily	4541, 35 d	Enoxaparin 40 mg daily	THR	Composite VTE and all-cause mortality	Riv: 1.1%, 18/1595; Enox: 3.7%, 58/1558; AR: 2.6 (CI: 1.5–3.7); Rivaroxaban superior	Major bleeding	Riv: 0.3%, 6/2209; Enox: 0.1%, 2/2224; P value: 0.18. No increase in major bleeding
RECORD-2[15]	Rivaroxaban, 10 mg daily	2509, 31–39 d	Enoxaparin 40 mg daily (10–14 d)	THR	Composite VTE and all-cause mortality	Riv: 2%, 17/864; Enox: 9.3%, 81/869; AR: 7.3 (CI: 2–9.4); Rivaroxaban superior	Major bleeding	Riv: <0.1%, 1/1228; Enox: <0.1%, 1/1229; P value: 0.25. No increase in major bleeding

(continued on next page)

Table 3
(continued)

Study[Ref.]	Drug, Dose	Number, Duration	Indication	Comparator	Primary Outcome Measure	Primary Safety Measure	Primary Outcome Results	Primary Safety Results
RECORD-3[16]	Rivaroxaban, 10 mg daily	2531, 10–14 d	TKR	Enoxaparin 40 mg daily	Composite VTE and all-cause mortality	Major bleeding	Riv: 9.6%, 79/824 Enox: 18.9%, 166/878 AR: 9.2 (CI: 5.9–12.4) Rivaroxaban superior	Riv: 0.6%, 7/1220 Enox: 0.5%, 6/1239 AR: 0.1 (P = .77), No increase in major bleeding
RECORD-4[17]	Rivaroxaban, 10 mg daily	3148, 10–14 d	TKR	Enoxaparin 30 mg BID	Composite VTE and all-cause mortality	Major bleeding	Riv: 6.9%, 67/965 Enox: 10.1%, 97/959 AR: 3.19 (CI: 0.71–5.67) Rivaroxaban superior	Riv: 0.7%, 10/1526 Enox: 0.3%, 4/1508 P value: 0.1096. No increase in major bleeding
ADVANCE-1[18]	Apixaban, 2.5 mg BID	3195, 12 d	TKR	Enoxaparin 30 mg BID	Composite VTE and all-cause mortality	Major bleeding	Apix: 9%, 104/1157 Enox: 8.8%, 100/1130 RR: 1.02 (CI: 0.78–1.32) Apixaban not noninferior	Apix: 0.7%, 11/1596 Enox: 1.4%, 22/1588 ADJ: −0.81 (CI: −1.49—0.14), No increase in major bleeding.

ADVANCE-2[19]	Apixaban, 2.5 mg BID	1973, 12 d	TKR	Enoxaparin 40 mg daily	Composite VTE and all-cause mortality	Apix: 15%, 147/976; Enox: 24%, 243/997; RR: 0.62 (CI: 0.51–0.74) Apixaban superior	Major bleeding	Apix: 0.6%, 9/1501; Enox: 0.9%, 14/1508; AD: −0.33 (CI: −0.95–0.29) No increase in major bleeding with apixaban
ADVANCE-3[20]	Apixaban, 2.5 mg BID	5407, 35 d	THR	Enoxaparin 40 mg daily	Composite VTE and all-cause mortality	Apix: 1.4%, 27/1949; Enox: 3.9%, 74/1917; RR: 0.36 (CI: 0.22–0.54) Apixaban superior	Major bleeding	Apix: 0.8%, 22/2673; Enox: 0.7%, 18/2659; AD: −0.2 (CI: −1.4–1). No increase in major bleeding with apixaban
Edoxaban trial[21]	Edoxaban, 15, 30, 60 or 90 mg	N = 776, 7–10 d	THR	Dalteparin Initial dose 2500 IU, subsequent doses 5000 IU daily	Incidence of total VTE	Incidence of VTE (P<.005): Dalt: 43.8%; Edox 15 mg: 28.2%; Edox 30 mg: 21.2%; Edox 60 mg: 15.2%; Edox 90 mg: 10.6%; Dose-response for efficacy, P<.001	Composite of major and clinically relevant nonmajor bleeding	Dalt: 0/172, 0%; Edox 15 mg: 3/192, 1.6%; Edox 30 mg: 3/170, 1.8%; Edox 60 mg: 4/185, 2.2%; Edox 90 mg: 4/177, 2.3%; P = .583

Abbreviations: AD, absolute risk difference; ADJ, adjusted risk difference; Apix, apixaban; AR, absolute risk reduction; CI, confidence interval; Dab, dabigatran; Dalt, dalteparin; Edox, edoxaban; Enox, enoxaparin; RR, relative risk; Riv, rivaroxaban; RD, risk difference; THR, total hip replacement; TKR, total knee replacement; VTE, venous thromboembolism.

dabigatran 220 mg to be noninferior to enoxaparin 40 mg daily, as in the RE-NOVATE study.[13] In each of these studies, dabigatran had a similar safety profile to enoxaparin. At present, dabigatran is not approved by the Food and Drug Administration (FDA) for VTE prophylaxis in orthopedic surgery patients.

Rivaroxaban

Four RCTs have evaluated the efficacy of a 10-mg daily dose of rivaroxaban for the prevention of VTE after THR and TKR surgery. RECORD-1 and RECORD-2 compared rivaroxaban with enoxaparin, 40 mg daily, starting the night before surgery in patients who received THR (see **Table 3**).[14,15] In RECORD-1 patients received enoxaparin for 35 days, whereas patients in RECORD-2 received enoxaparin for 10 to 14 days post-surgery. Both studies found rivaroxaban to be superior to enoxaparin, without increasing the risk of major bleeding. RECORD-3 and RECORD-4 compared rivaroxaban with enoxaparin in patients who received TKR.[16,17] Each of these studies evaluated rivaroxaban versus enoxaparin for 10 to 14 days. RECORD-4, however, used the standard North American dose of enoxaparin (30 mg twice daily), whereas RECORD-3 evaluated rivaroxaban against enoxaparin 40 mg daily (see **Table 3**). Both studies found rivaroxaban to be superior to enoxaparin without increasing the risk of major bleeding. Rivaroxaban is currently approved in the United States for VTE prophylaxis in patients undergoing total hip and knee replacement surgery.

Apixaban

Three large RCTs (ADVANCE-1, -2, and -3) evaluated apixaban as VTE prophylaxis in patients who received either a TKR or THR (see **Table 3**).[18–20] ADVANCE-1 compared apixaban, 2.5 mg twice daily with enoxaparin, 30 mg twice daily, for 12 days after TKR.[18] The primary end point was a composite of VTE and all-cause mortality. This study found that apixaban did not achieve noninferiority to 30-mg twice-daily enoxaparin. ADVANCE-2 evaluated apixaban, 2.5 mg twice daily against a lower daily dose of enoxaparin (40 mg daily) in TKR patients.[19] This trial found apixaban to be superior to enoxaparin, without an increase in major bleeding. The third trial, ADVANCE-3, compared apixaban, 2.5 mg twice daily, with enoxaparin, 40 mg daily, in THR patients.[20] This RCT also found apixaban to be superior to enoxaparin without an increase in major bleeding. At present, apixaban is not FDA-approved for this indication.

Edoxaban

Raskob and colleagues[21] evaluated the efficacy of 4 different doses (15, 30, 60, and 90 mg) of once-daily, oral edoxaban versus subcutaneous dalteparin in patients who underwent THR. In this trial, 776 patients were randomized to receive either edoxaban or dalteparin for 7 to 10 days. Results showed a statistically significant reduction in total VTE across all doses of edoxaban in a dose-response fashion, and bleeding rates were similar across all groups (see **Table 3**). At present, edoxaban is not FDA-approved for this indication.

Venous Thromboembolism Prophylaxis in Medically Ill Patients

Rivaroxaban

Recently, rivaroxaban was evaluated for efficacy in the prevention of VTE in medically ill hospitalized patients, and in patients following hospital discharge.[22] This study compared rivaroxaban, 10 mg daily for 35 days with enoxaparin, 40 mg daily for 10 days and then placebo for days 11 through 35. The study found rivaroxaban to be noninferior to enoxaparin at day 10 and superior to placebo at day 35. These encouraging results were tempered by a statistically significant increase in major bleeding in the rivaroxaban treatment group, at both day 10 and day 35 (**Table 4**).

Table 4
RCTs evaluating new anticoagulants for prevention of venous thromboembolism in medically ill patients

Study[Ref.]	Drug, Dose	Number, Duration	Indication	Comparator	Primary Outcome Measure	Primary Safety Measure	Primary Outcome Results	Primary Safety Results
MAGELLAN[22]	Rivaroxaban, 10 mg daily	8100, 35 d	VTE prophylaxis in medically ill patients	Enoxaparin 40 mg daily (10 d)	Composite of VTE-related death, PE, DVT	Major bleeding and clinically relevant nonmajor bleeding	Day 10: Riv: 2.7%, 79/2939 Enox: 2.7%, 80/2993 Day 35: Riv: 4.4%, 130/2967 Enox: 5.7%, 174/3057 Rivaroxaban noninferior at day 10, superior at day 35	Day 10: Riv: 2.8%, 111/3997 Enox: 1.2%, 48/4001 Day 35: Riv: 4.2%, 167/3997 Enox: 1.7%, 68/4001 Rivaroxaban had increased clinically significant bleeding
ADOPT[23]	Apixaban, 2.5 mg BID	6528, 30 d	VTE prophylaxis in medically ill patients	Enoxaparin 40 mg daily (6–14 d)	30-d composite of death related to VTE, PE, DVT	Major bleeding	Apix: 2.71%, 60/2211 Enox: 3.06%, 70/2284 Apixaban not superior to enoxaparin	Apix: 0.47%, 15/3184 Enox: 0.19%, 6/3217 Apixaban had increased major bleeding

Abbreviations: Apix, apixaban; CI, confidence interval; Enox, enoxaparin; HR, hazard ratio; Riv, rivaroxaban; RR, relative risk; VTE, venous thromboembolism.

Apixaban

The ADOPT trial evaluated the efficacy of apixaban in preventing VTE in medically ill hospitalized patients and following discharge.[23] This trial randomized more than 6500 patients to receive either apixaban, 2.5 mg twice daily for 30 days or enoxaparin, 40 mg daily for 6 to 14 days followed by placebo. The primary outcome found that apixaban was not superior to enoxaparin in reducing a 30-day composite of deep venous thrombosis (DVT), pulmonary embolism (PE), or death related to VTE. In addition, the apixaban group had an increase in major bleeding compared with the enoxaparin group (see **Table 4**).

Venous Thromboembolism Treatment

Dabigatran

In addition to VTE prophylaxis in orthopedic surgery patients, dabigatran has been studied for the acute and chronic treatment of VTE. Two studies, RE-COVER and RE-COVER II, evaluated the efficacy of dabigatran for the treatment of acute DVT with or without PE (**Table 5**).[24,25] Both studies compared dabigatran with the standard of care, a parenteral anticoagulant bridged to warfarin, and in each trial all patients first received a parenteral anticoagulant for a median of 9 days. Each study found dabigatran to be noninferior to the standard of care. The RE-SONATE trial evaluated dabigatran in comparison with placebo in the prevention of recurrent VTE in patients with symptomatic VTE who completed 6 to 18 months of anticoagulation with a VKA (see **Table 5**).[26] This study found a statistically significant decrease in recurrent thromboembolic events in the dabigatran arm, but no decrease in mortality. There was no increase in major bleeding in the dabigatran arm of the study. Dabigatran is not currently FDA-approved for this indication.

Rivaroxaban

Rivaroxaban has also been evaluated for use in VTE treatment. The EINSTEIN-DVT study focused on the efficacy of rivaroxaban for the treatment of DVT (see **Table 5**).[27] This trial examined rivaroxaban alone versus enoxaparin followed by a VKA. Rivaroxaban, 15 mg was given twice daily for the first 3 weeks, followed by 20 mg daily for 3, 6, or 12 months. Rivaroxaban was found to be noninferior to the standard of care, without an increase in major bleeding. The EINSTEIN-PE study had a design identical to the DVT trial except that patients had PE with, or without, DVT (see **Table 5**).[28] Rivaroxaban's efficacy was noninferior to standard therapy, with a similar rate of major and clinically relevant nonmajor bleeding, but with a significant decrease in major bleeding when evaluated alone. A related study, EINSTEIN-Extension, examined the efficacy of rivaroxaban, 20 mg daily versus placebo, for prolonged therapy (6–12 months) in patients who completed a full course of anticoagulation (6–12 months) for DVT or PE (see **Table 5**).[29] This study found rivaroxaban to be superior to placebo, with a reduced incidence of recurrent symptomatic VTE and with no statistically significant increase in major bleeding. Rivaroxaban was recently approved by the FDA for the acute and chronic treatment of VTE.

Prevention of Stroke and Systemic Embolism in Atrial Fibrillation

Dabigatran

In 2010, dabigatran was approved for the prevention of stroke and systemic embolism in patients with atrial fibrillation based on the results of the RE-LY study, a large (N = 18113) RCT evaluating dabigatran versus warfarin (INR 2–3) for the prevention of stroke in nonvalvular atrial fibrillation (**Table 6**).[30] Dabigatran was given in 2 doses, 150 mg and 110 mg, twice daily in blinded fashion, and compared with open-label

Table 5
RCTs evaluating new anticoagulants for the acute and chronic treatment of venous thromboembolism

Study Ref.	Drug, Dose	Number, Duration	Indication	Comparator	Primary Outcome Measure	Primary Safety Measure	Primary Outcome Results	Primary Safety Results
RE-COVER[24]	Dabigatran, 150 mg BID	2564, 6 mo	Treatment of acute VTE	UFH or LMWH to Warfarin (INR 2–3)	Recurrent VTE and related deaths	Major bleeding	Dab: 2.4%, 30/1274 Warf: 2.1%, 27/1265 HR: 1.10 (CI: 0.65–1.84) Dabigatran noninferior	Dab: 1.6%, 20/1274 Warf: 1.9%, 24/1265 HR: 0.82 (CI: 0.45–1.48) No increase in major bleeding with dabigatran
RE-COVER II[25]	Dabigatran 150 mg BID, after 5–11 d of LMWH or UFH	2568, 6 mo	Treatment of acute VTE	UFH or LMWH to Warfarin (INR 2–3)	Recurrent symptomatic VTE and VTE-related deaths	Major bleeding events	Dab: 2.4%, 30/1279 Warf: 2.2%, 28/1289 HR: 1.08 (CI: 0.64–1.8) Dabigatran noninferior	Dab: 15/1279 Warf: 22/1289 HR: 0.69 (CI: 0.36–1.32) No increase in major bleeding with dabigatran
RE-SONATE[26]	Dabigatran, 150 mg BID	1343, 6 mo (after 6–18 mo of treatment)	Chronic VTE Treatment	Placebo	Symptomatic, recurrent VTE	Clinically relevant bleeding, major bleeding	Dab: 0.4%, 3/681 Placebo: 5.5%, 37/662 HR: 0.08 (0.02–0.25) Dabigatran decreased VTE	Dab: 5.3% (36) Placebo: 1.8% (12) HR: 2.9, $P = .001$ Dabigatran has increase in clinically relevant bleeding, but not major bleeding

(continued on next page)

Table 5
(continued)

Study[Ref.]	Drug, Dose	Number, Duration	Indication	Comparator	Primary Outcome Measure	Primary Safety Measure	Primary Outcome Results	Primary Safety Results
EINSTEIN-DVT[27]	Rivaroxaban, 15 mg BID (3 wk), then 20 mg daily	3449, 3, 6, or 12 mo	Treatment of acute DVT (without PE)	Enoxaparin to VKA (INR 2–3)	Recurrent VTE	Major bleeding or clinically relevant nonmajor bleeding	Riv: 2.1%, 36/1731 Warf: 3%, 51/1718 HR: 0.68 (CI: 0.44–1.04) Rivaroxaban noninferior	Riv: 8.1%, 139/1718 Warf: 8.1%, 138/1711 HR: 0.97 (CI: 0.76–1.22) No increase in first major or clinically relevant nonmajor bleeding with rivaroxaban
EINSTEIN-PE[28]	Rivaroxaban, 15 mg BID (3 wk), then 20 mg daily	4832, 3, 6, or 12 mo	Acute symptomatic PE, with or without DVT	Enoxaparin to VKA (INR 2–3)	Symptomatic, recurrent VTE	Major or clinically relevant nonmajor bleeding	Riv: 2.1%, 50/2419 Warf: 1.8%, 44/2413 HR: 1.12 (CI: 0.75–1.68) Rivaroxaban noninferior	Riv: 10.3%, 249/2419 Warf: 11.4%, 274/2413 HR: 0.9 ($P = .23$) Rivaroxaban did not increase the risk of bleeding

	Rivaroxaban, 20 mg daily	1197, 6–12 mo (after full course of therapy)	Treatment of VTE	Placebo	Symptomatic, recurrent VTE	Major bleeding
EINSTEIN-Extension[29]					Riv: 1.3%, 8/602 Placebo: 7.1%, 42/594 HR: 0.18 (CI: 0.09–0.39) Rivaroxaban noninferior	Riv: 0.7%, 4/602 Placebo: 0%, 0/594 P = .11 Rivaroxaban did not increase risk of major bleeding, but did increase clinically relevant nonmajor bleeding

Abbreviations: CI, confidence interval; Dab, dabigatran; DVT, deep venous thrombosis; Enox, enoxaparin; HR, hazard ratio; LMWH, low molecular weight heparin; PE, pulmonary embolism; Riv, rivaroxaban; UFH, unfractionated heparin; VKA, vitamin K antagonist; VTE, venous thromboembolism; Warf, warfarin.

Table 6
RCTs evaluating new anticoagulants for stroke prevention in atrial fibrillation

Study[Ref.]	Drug, Dose	Number, Duration, CHADS	Indication	Comparator	Primary Outcome Measure	Primary Safety Measure	Primary Outcome Results	Primary Safety Results
RE-LY[30]	Dabigatran, 110 mg or 150 mg BID	18113, 2 y CHADS: 2	Prevention of stroke in nonvalvular atrial fibrillation	Warfarin, INR 2–3	Stroke and systemic embolism	Major bleeding	Dab (110 mg): 1.53%/y RR: 0.91 (CI: 0.74–1.11) Dab (150 mg): 1.11%/y RR: 0.66 (CI: 0.53–0.82) Warf: 1.69%/y Dabigatran 110 mg noninferior Dabigatran 150 mg superior	Dab (110 mg): 0.12%/y P value: 0.003 Dab (150 mg): 0.1%/y P value: 0.31 Warf: 0.38%/y Dabigatran 110 mg lower major bleeding and ICH Dabigatran 150 mg similar major bleeding and lower ICH
ROCKET-AF[31]	Rivaroxaban, 20 mg daily	14264, 707 d, CHADS: 3.5	Prevention of stroke in nonvalvular atrial fibrillation	Warfarin, INR 2–3	Stroke and systemic embolism	Major bleeding and clinically relevant nonmajor bleeding	Riv: 1.7%/y Warf: 2.2%/y HR: 0.79 (CI: 0.66–0.96) Rivaroxaban noninferior	Riv: 14.9%/y Warf: 14.5%/y HR: 1.03 (CI: 0.96–1.11) Rivaroxaban similar major bleeding and lower ICH
ARISTOTLE[32]	Apixaban, 5 mg BID	15000, 18 mo, CHADS: 2	Prevention of stroke in nonvalvular atrial fibrillation	Warfarin, INR 2–3	Ischemic or hemorrhagic stroke and systemic embolism	Major bleeding	Apix: 1.27%/y Warf: 1.6%/y HR: 0.79 (CI: 0.66–0.95) Apixaban superior	Apix: 2.13%/y Warf: 3.09%/y HR: 0.69 (CI: 0.6–0.8) Apixaban lower major bleeding and ICH

AVERROES[33]	Apixaban, 5 mg BID	5600, 18 mo CHADS: 2	Prevention of stroke in nonvalvular atrial fibrillation	Aspirin 81–324 mg/d	Stroke and systemic embolism	Major bleeding	Apix: 1.6%/y ASA: 3.7%/y HR: 0.45 (CI: 0.32–0.62) Apixaban superior	Apix: 1.4%/y ASA: 1.2%/y HR: 1.13 (CI: 0.74–1.75) Apixaban similar major bleeding and ICH
Edoxaban trial[34]	Edoxaban, 30 mg daily, 30 mg BID, 60 mg daily, 60 mg BID	1146, 12 wk	Safety of edoxaban in patients with nonvalvular atrial fibrillation	Warfarin (INR 2–3)	Major and/or clinically relevant bleeding	See Primary Outcome Measure	Edox 30 mg daily: 3% Edox 60 mg daily: 3.8% Edox 30 mg BID: 7.8% ($P = .029$) Edox 60 mg BID: 10.6% ($P = .002$) Warf: 3.2% Edoxaban BID increased the risk of bleeding, but daily regimens did not	See Primary Outcome Results

Abbreviations: Apix, apixaban; ASA, aspirin; CI, confidence interval; Dab, dabigatran; HR, hazard ratio; ICH, intracranial hemorrhage; Riv, rivaroxaban; RR, relative risk; Warf, warfarin.

warfarin. Enrolled patients had an average CHADS$_2$ score of 2.1, and warfarin was well managed, with an average time in therapeutic range of 64%. The trial showed that dabigatran, 110 mg twice daily, was noninferior to warfarin for the primary outcome of stroke or systemic embolism, yet was significantly safer than warfarin for major bleeding. Dabigatran, 150 mg twice daily, was found to be superior to warfarin in reducing stroke or systemic embolism, with a risk of major bleeding that was not significantly different to that with warfarin. Of note, intracranial hemorrhage was significantly reduced with both doses compared with warfarin. Dabigatran was associated with an increased incidence of dyspepsia, an increase in gastrointestinal bleeding, and a nonsignificant increase in myocardial infarction compared with warfarin.

Rivaroxaban

ROCKET-AF is the major trial comparing rivaroxaban with warfarin for the prevention of stroke and systemic embolism in patients with nonvalvular atrial fibrillation (see **Table 6**).[31] Patients enrolled in this trial had a higher mean CHADS$_2$ score of 3.5, and warfarin patients were managed with a time in therapeutic range of only 55%. Rivaroxaban, at a dose of 20 mg daily, was compared with dose-adjusted warfarin in more than 14,000 patients with atrial fibrillation. Rivaroxaban proved to be noninferior to warfarin, with a similar incidence of major bleeding. The rivaroxaban arm also experienced a significant decrease in intracranial hemorrhage and an increase in major gastrointestinal bleeding, as was seen with dabigatran.

Apixaban

Two major RCTs have evaluated apixaban for stroke prevention in patients with nonvalvular atrial fibrillation (see **Table 6**).[32,33] ARISTOTLE randomized more than 18,000 patients to receive apixaban, 5 mg twice daily, or warfarin (INR 2–3).[32] Patients had an average CHADS$_2$ score of 2.1, and warfarin-treated patients had an average time in therapeutic range of 62%. Apixaban was found to be superior to warfarin in preventing the primary outcome measure (stroke and systemic embolism), while also resulting in a significant reduction in both major bleeding and intracranial hemorrhage. The patients in the apixaban arm also experienced a significant reduction in mortality compared with warfarin. The AVERROES trial compared apixaban, 5 mg twice daily, with aspirin, 81 mg to 324 mg daily, in the prevention of stroke and systemic embolism in patients with nonvalvular atrial fibrillation who were deemed to be too risky to place on warfarin.[33] Apixaban was shown to be superior to aspirin in the prevention of stroke and systemic embolism, with a similar risk of major bleeding and intracranial hemorrhage.

Edoxaban

An RCT in 2010 evaluated the safety of edoxaban with that of warfarin in patients with atrial fibrillation (see **Table 6**).[34] More than 1000 patients were randomized to receive either edoxaban 30 mg daily, 30 mg twice daily, 60 mg daily, or 60 mg twice daily, or warfarin (goal INR 2–3). The primary outcome was major or clinically relevant nonmajor bleeding, as well as hepatic enzyme or bilirubin elevation. Daily dosing of edoxaban (30 or 60 mg) was associated with a similar safety profile to that of warfarin, but twice-daily dosing regimens were associated with an increased risk of bleeding.

Cardiovascular Outcomes in Recent Acute Coronary Syndrome

Rivaroxaban

Recently, low-dose rivaroxaban was evaluated for efficacy in improving cardiovascular outcomes in patients with recent acute coronary syndrome (ACS) (**Table 7**).[35] In this RCT, more than 15,000 patients with recent ACS were randomly assigned to receive

Table 7
RCTs evaluating cardiovascular outcomes in recent acute coronary syndrome

Study[Ref.]	Drug, Dose	Number, Duration	Indication	Comparator	Primary Outcome Measure	Primary Safety Measure	Primary Outcome Results	Primary Safety Results
ATLAS ACS2-TIMI51[35]	Rivaroxaban, 2.5 mg or 5 mg BID	15526, 13 mo	Decreasing cardiovascular events in ACS	Placebo	Composite of death from cardiovascular causes, myocardial infarction, or stroke	TIMI major bleeding not related to CABG	Riv 2.5 mg: 9.1% (P = .02) Riv: 5 mg: 8.8% (P = .03) Placebo: 10.7% Rivaroxaban 2.5 mg had a mortality benefit compared with placebo	Riv 2.5 mg: 1.8%, 65/5114 Riv 5 mg: 2.4%, 82/5115 Riv combined doses: 2.1%, 147/10229 Placebo: 0.6%, 19/5113 Rivaroxaban increased the risk of major bleeding and ICH
APPRAISE-2[36]	Apixaban, 5 mg BID	7392, 241 d	Decreasing cardiovascular events in ACS	Placebo	Cardiovascular death, myocardial infarction, or ischemic stroke	TIMI major bleeding	Apix: 7.5%, 279/3705 Placebo: 7/9%, 293/3687 HR: 0.95 (CI: 0.8–1.11, P = .51) Apixaban not superior	Apix: 1.3%, 46/3673 Placebo: 0.5%, 18/3642 HR: 2.59 (P = .001) Apixaban increased the risk of major bleeding

Abbreviations: ACS, acute coronary syndrome; Apix, apixaban; BID, twice daily; CABG, coronary artery bypass grafting; HR, hazard ratio; ICH, intracranial hemorrhage; Riv, rivaroxaban; TIMI, Thrombolysis in Myocardial Infarction.

either rivaroxaban (2.5 mg or 5 mg twice daily) or placebo for a mean of 13 months in comparison with standard treatment, which included an antiplatelet agent. The primary efficacy end point, a composite of death from cardiovascular causes, myocardial infarction, or stroke, was significantly reduced in the rivaroxaban group at both the 2.5-mg and 5-mg doses. The 2.5-mg twice-daily dose also led to a significant reduction in all-cause mortality. These positive results were tempered by the principal safety results, which revealed that rivaroxaban did not significantly increase fatal bleeding but did increase the risk of both major bleeding and intracranial hemorrhage.

Apixaban

In a similar study, the APPRAISE-2 trial evaluated the efficacy of apixaban, 5 mg twice daily, in decreasing cardiovascular events when added to standard post-ACS therapy (see **Table 7**).[36] This trial was terminated early when it was discovered that there was greater than twice the risk of major bleeding in the apixaban group compared to the placebo group. This increase in major bleeding occurred without a significant decrease in cardiovascular events in the apixaban group.

PRACTICAL MANAGEMENT
Compliance

Warfarin compliance is complicated by the necessity for both dosing and monitoring adherence. Medication compliance is improved by once-daily dosing and by warfarin's delayed offset of action. Because warfarin has a relatively long half-life, missing a dose will not lead to a total loss of anticoagulant effect. Monitoring places a burden on both the patient and the physician. Nevertheless, frequent physician visits can be beneficial because the physician is given the opportunity to provide ongoing patient education and encouragement. In addition, regular monitoring provides the physician with the opportunity to adjust the medication dose to achieve an optimal degree of anticoagulation.

Routine laboratory monitoring is not necessary with dabigatran etexilate, which removes a major source of noncompliance. Dabigatran is a twice-daily medication, which may be a source of decreased compliance when compared with the daily dosing of warfarin. The half-life of dabigatran is 12 to 14 hours, compared with a half-life of 36 to 42 hours for warfarin (see **Table 1**).[3] The shorter half-life of dabigatran makes compliance even more important, as 1 missed dose can lead to a significant loss of anticoagulant effect. A patient on warfarin can miss 1 dose and still remain fully anticoagulated until the next dose. Only patients who closely adhere to the twice-daily dosing should be candidates for the use of dabigatran.

Like dabigatran, the factor Xa inhibitors do not require monitoring, thus removing one source of noncompliance that can be found with the use of warfarin. Also, like dabigatran, the half-life of each of the factor Xa inhibitors is far shorter than that of warfarin (see **Table 1**). In fact, each of the factor Xa inhibitors have slightly shorter half-lives than dabigatran. Thus a missed dose can lead to a loss of anticoagulant effect, and compliance to the dosing regimen is extremely important. Of the 3 factor Xa inhibitors reviewed in this article, rivaroxaban and edoxaban are dosed once daily, whereas apixaban is dosed twice daily (see **Table 1**). Because once-daily dosing regimens are easier for patients to adhere to, improved compliance might be expected for rivaroxaban and edoxaban over both apixaban and the direct thrombin inhibitor, dabigatran.

Initiation and Monitoring

Warfarin can, and must be, monitored (see **Table 1**). As already mentioned, this can be a burden to the physician and patient, but once the patient has had a stable therapeutic INR this requirement becomes less frequent (every 4–6 weeks) and, consequently, less burdensome. The initial effect on the INR occurs 2 to 3 days after initiation of warfarin, and the full anticoagulant effect takes even longer.[4] During the initiation of warfarin, parenteral anticoagulation must also be administered. Parenteral anticoagulation must be maintained for at least 5 days, and until the INR has been in therapeutic range for 24 hours, for VTE treatment.[37] This delayed onset of action is a drawback of warfarin that must be corrected by administering a second, parenteral, agent.

Anticoagulant initiation is vastly simplified with dabigatran. By reaching a maximum plasma concentration in approximately 2 hours, dabigatran obviates a parenteral bridging regimen (see **Table 1**). Although dabigatran does not need to be monitored to guide therapy, when necessary, plasma drug levels can be roughly assessed with an aPTT and more specifically assessed with a thrombin time assay (see **Table 2**).

Like dabigatran, all 3 factor Xa inhibitors have a relatively rapid time to maximum plasma concentration, and parenteral bridging can be avoided when initiating therapy with any of these agents (see **Table 1**). The factor Xa inhibitors can be quantitatively monitored with a factor Xa assay, but this is not necessary for routine care, because of the predictable pharmacokinetics (see **Table 2**).

Reversal

One of the benefits of warfarin is that it can be readily reversed (see **Table 1**). This aspect is important in patients requiring urgent invasive procedures, in bleeding patients, and in patients with a significantly elevated INR.[4] The first, and simplest, reversal strategy is to hold, or discontinue, warfarin therapy. However, this strategy is viable only in stable patients, as it will take several days before normal coagulation resumes. When reversal is urgently necessary, other strategies must be implemented. Warfarin acts by inhibiting the synthesis of vitamin K–dependent coagulation factors, and by administering vitamin K, hepatic production of vitamin K–dependent clotting factors can resume.[4] This process will result in a significant impact on the INR within 12 to 24 hours. In the event of a major bleed, more rapid reversal is required. Parenteral repletion of the affected clotting factors can be achieved by giving fresh frozen plasma (FFP) or, more urgently, by giving prothrombin complex concentrate (PCC).[4] Coadministration of vitamin K is necessary whenever FFP or PCC are used to reverse the INR, as the effect of FFP, and PCC, is transient.

As with warfarin, the major adverse effect of dabigatran is bleeding. Because there is no antidote, reversal strategies target drug elimination, but also repletion of coagulation factors. By discontinuing dabigatran, 50% of the drug will be eliminated in 12 to 18 hours (in a patient with normal renal function) (see **Table 1**).[4] Dabigatran is also able to be eliminated by hemodialysis because there is low protein binding, but this method also takes time and is not practical for major, life-threatening bleeding.[3] Evidence for repletion of coagulation factor in correcting the coagulopathy induced by dabigatran, or reversing acute bleeding, is limited to a few animal studies and case reports. Recent animal studies have shown that FFP and recombinant activated factor VII may have some utility, but this has not been shown in humans.[38] A recent, small RCT evaluated the effect of PCC on the reversal of rivaroxaban and dabigatran.[39] This trial found that PCC had no effect on the anticoagulant action of dabigatran.

Reversal strategies for the factor Xa inhibitors are similar to those for dabigatran, and involve drug elimination or replacement of coagulation factors; there is no antidote for any of the factor Xa inhibitors (see **Table 1**). Like dabigatran, the shorter half-life of the factor Xa inhibitors in comparison with warfarin results in faster clearance of the drugs via normal routes of elimination. Despite 66% renal elimination, rivaroxaban cannot be removed via hemodialysis because of very high plasma protein binding (95%).[6] Apixaban has complex elimination via the kidney (25%), gastrointestinal tract (50%), and liver. Like rivaroxaban, apixaban has high protein binding (87%), and removal via hemodialysis is unlikely to be effective (see **Table 1**). Edoxaban has 33% renal elimination and is less protein bound (50%) than rivaroxaban and apixaban, therefore hemodialysis may partially remove this agent. Few studies have evaluated reversal strategies aimed at replacement of coagulation factor in the factor Xa inhibitors. FFP has not been studied for the reversal of any of these agents, and PCC has only been studied in the reversal of rivaroxaban. In this study rivaroxaban significantly prolonged the PT, which was immediately and completely reversed by administration of PCC.[39] This RCT was small (N = 12), and further studies are warranted to confirm this finding. No data exist on the reversal of apixaban and edoxaban.

SUMMARY

Before the advent of oral, targeted anticoagulants, physicians had no choice regarding the type of oral anticoagulant prescribed, as every patient received warfarin. The new oral direct thrombin and factor Xa inhibitors give the prescribing physician, as well as the patient, greater choice. Variation in dosing, half-life, elimination, monitoring, and reversal will help the clinician decide the appropriate anticoagulant for the appropriate patient. Rather than replace warfarin, each anticoagulant will now have a particular niche, and the decision of which agent to prescribe will be determined at the bedside.

REFERENCES

1. Di Nisio M, Middeldorp S, Buller HR. Direct thrombin inhibitors. N Engl J Med 2005;353:1028–40.
2. Soff GA. A new generation of oral direct anticoagulants. Arterioscler Thromb Vasc Biol 2012;32(3):569–74.
3. Blommel ML, Blommel AL. Dabigatran etexilate: a novel oral direct thrombin inhibitor. Am J Health Syst Pharm 2011;68(16):1506–19.
4. Ageno W, Gallus AS, Wittkowsky A, et al. Oral anticoagulant therapy: antithrombotic therapy and prevention of thrombosis, 9th ed: American College of Chest Physicians evidence-based clinical practice guidelines. Chest 2012;141: e44S–88S.
5. Stangier J, Rathgen K, Stahle H, et al. Influence of renal impairment on the pharmacokinetics and pharmacodynamics of oral dabigatran etexilate: an open-label, parallel-group, single-centre study. Clin Pharm 2010;49(4):259–68.
6. Kreutz R. Pharmacodynamic and pharmacokinetic basics of rivaroxaban. Fundam Clin Pharmacol 2012;26(1):27–32.
7. Asmis LM, Alberio L, Angelillo-Scherrer A, et al. Rivaroxaban: quantification by anti-Xa assay and influence on coagulation tests, a study in 9 Swiss laboratories. Thromb Res 2012;129(4):492–8.
8. Prom R, Spinler SA. The role of apixaban for venous and arterial thromboembolic disease. Ann Pharmacother 2011;45:1262–83.
9. Guigliano RP, Partida RA. Edoxaban: pharmacological principles, preclinical and early-phase clinical testing. Future Cardiol 2011;7(4):459–70.
10. Eriksson BI, Dahl OE, Rosencher N, et al. Oral dabigatran etexilate vs. subcutaneous enoxaparin for the prevention of venous thromboembolism after total knee replacement: the RE-MODEL randomized trial. J Thromb Haemost 2007;5(11): 2178–85.

11. Eriksson BI, Dahl OE, Rosencher N, et al. Dabigatran etexilate versus enoxaparin for prevention of venous thromboembolism after total hip replacement: a randomized, double-blind, non-inferiority trial. Lancet 2007;370(9591):949–56.
12. Ginsberg JS, Davidson BL, Comp PC, et al. Oral thrombin inhibitor dabigatran etexilate vs North American enoxaparin regimen for prevention of venous thrombosis after knee arthroplasty surgery. J Arthroplasty 2009;24(1):1–9.
13. Eriksson BI, Dahl OE, Huo MH, et al. Oral dabigatran versus enoxaparin for thromboprophylaxis after primary total hip arthroplasty (RE-NOVATE II): a randomised, double-blind, non-inferiority trial. Thromb Haemost 2011;105:721–9.
14. Eriksson BI, Borris LC, Friedman RJ, et al. Rivaroxaban versus enoxaparin for thromboprophylaxis after hip arthroplasty. N Engl J Med 2008;358:2765–75.
15. Kakkar AK, Brenner B, Dahl OE, et al. Extended duration rivaroxaban versus short-term enoxaparin for the prevention of venous thromboembolism after total hip arthroplasty: a double-blind, randomised controlled trial. Lancet 2008;372:31–9.
16. Lassen MR, Ageno W, Borris LC, et al. Rivaroxaban versus enoxaparin for thromboprophylaxis after total knee arthroplasty. N Engl J Med 2008;358:2776–86.
17. Turpie AG, Lassen MR, Davidson BL, et al. Rivaroxaban versus enoxaparin for thromboprophylaxis after total knee arthroplasty (RECORD4): a randomised trial. Lancet 2009;373(9676):1673–80.
18. Lassen MR, Raskob GE, Gallus A, et al. Apixaban or enoxaparin for thromboprophylaxis after knee replacement. N Engl J Med 2009;361:594–604.
19. Lassen MR, Raskob GE, Gallus A, et al. Apixaban versus enoxaparin for thromboprophylaxis after knee replacement (ADVANCE-2): a randomized double-blind trial. Lancet 2010;375:807–15.
20. Lassen MR, Gallus A, Raskob GE, et al. Apixaban versus enoxaparin for thromboprophylaxis after hip replacement. N Engl J Med 2010;363:2487–98.
21. Raskob G, Cohen AT, Eriksson BI, et al. Oral direct factor Xa inhibition with edoxaban for thromboprophylaxis after elective total hip replacement. A randomized double-blind dose-response study. Thromb Haemost 2010;104(3):642–9.
22. Cohen A, Spiro T, Buller H, et al. Rivaroxaban compared with enoxaparin for the prevention of venous thromboembolism in acutely ill medical patients. In: American College of Cardiology 60th Annual Scientific Session and Expo. New Orleans, April 5, 2011.
23. Goldhaber SZ, Leizorovicz A, Kakkar AK, et al. Apixaban versus enoxaparin for thromboprophylaxis in medically ill patients. N Engl J Med 2011;365(23):2167–77.
24. Schulman S, Kearon C, Kakkar AK, et al. Dabigatran versus warfarin in the treatment of acute venous thromboembolism. N Engl J Med 2009;361:2342–52.
25. Schulman S, Kakkar AK, Schellong SM, et al. A randomized trial of dabigatran versus warfarin in the treatment of acute venous thromboembolism (RE-COVER II). American Society of Hematology 2011 Annual Meeting (Abstract 205). San Diego, December 12, 2011.
26. Schulman S, Baanstra D, Eriksson S, et al. Dabigatran vs. placebo for extended maintenance therapy of venous thromboembolism. Abstract O-MO-037. Abstracts of the XXIII Congress of the International Society on Thrombosis and Haemostasis with the 57th Annual SSC (Scientific and Standardization Committee) Meeting. July 23-28 2011. Kyoto, Japan. J Thromb Haemost 2011;9(2):22.
27. Einstein Investigators. Oral rivaroxaban for symptomatic venous thromboembolism. N Engl J Med 2010;363:2499–510.
28. EINSTEIN-PE Investigators. Oral rivaroxaban for the treatment of symptomatic pulmonary embolism. N Engl J Med 2012;366:1287–97.

29. Romualdi E, Donadini MP, Ageno W. Oral rivaroxaban after symptomatic venous thromboembolism: the continued treatment study (EINSTEIN-extension study). Expert Rev Cardiovasc Ther 2011;9(7):841–4.
30. Connolly SJ, Ezekowitz MD, Yusuf S, et al. Dabigatran versus warfarin in patients with atrial fibrillation. N Engl J Med 2009;361:1139–51.
31. Patel MR, Mahaffey KW, Garg J, et al. Rivaroxaban versus warfarin in nonvalvular atrial fibrillation. N Engl J Med 2011;365:883–91.
32. Granger CB, Alexander JH, McMurray JV, et al. Apixaban versus warfarin in patients with atrial fibrillation. N Engl J Med 2011;365:981–92.
33. Connolly SJ, Eikelboom J, Joyner C, et al. Apixaban in patients with atrial fibrillation. N Engl J Med 2011;364:806–17.
34. Weitz JI, Connolly SJ, Patel I, et al. Randomised, parallel-group, multicentre, multinational phase 2 study comparing edoxaban, an oral factor Xa inhibitor, with warfarin for stroke prevention in patients with atrial fibrillation. Thromb Haemost 2010;104(3):633–41.
35. Mega JL, Braunwald E, Wiviott SD, et al. Rivaroxaban in patients with a recent acute coronary syndrome. N Engl J Med 2012;366:9–19.
36. Alexander JH, Lopes RD, James S, et al. Apixaban with antiplatelet therapy after acute coronary syndrome. N Engl J Med 2011;365:699–708.
37. Kearon C, Akl EA, Comerota AJ, et al. Antithrombotic therapy for VTE disease: antithrombotic therapy and prevention of thrombosis, 9th ed: American College of Chest Physicians evidence-based clinical practice guidelines. Chest 2012; 141(Suppl 2):e419S–94S.
38. Kaatz S, Kouides PA, Garcia DA, et al. Guidance on the emergent reversal of oral thrombin and factor Xa inhibitors. Am J Hematol 2012;87:S141–5.
39. Eerenberg ES, Kamphuisen PW, Sijpkens MK, et al. Reversal of rivaroxaban and dabigatran by prothrombin complex concentrate: a randomized, placebo-controlled, crossover study in healthy subjects. Circulation 2011;124(14):1573–9.
40. Garcia D, Libby E, Crowther MA. The new oral anticoagulants. Blood 2010;115: 15–20.

Carotid and Vertebral Artery Disease

Maxim Mokin, MD, PhD[a], Travis M. Dumont, MD[a],
Tareq Kass-Hout, MD[b], Elad I. Levy, MD[c],*

KEYWORDS

- Carotid artery stenosis • Vertebral artery stenosis • Stroke • Carotid endarterectomy
- Carotid artery stenting

KEY POINTS

- Extracranial carotid artery stenosis as a result of atherosclerosis can be frequently seen in patients presenting with stroke symptoms.
- Carotid ultrasound is an excellent screening test in a patient with suspected carotid artery disease, whereas conventional catheter angiography is the gold standard confirmatory test.
- Medical management is based on modification of vascular risk factors, antithrombotic therapy, and aggressive lipid-lowering therapy with statins.
- Surgical treatment (endarterectomy or stenting) is indicated in patients with symptomatic internal carotid artery stenosis of 50% or more.
- Endovascular treatment of symptomatic vertebral artery stenosis is reserved for patients with symptoms refractory to appropriate medical therapy.

Financial Relationships/Potential Conflicts of Interest: Dr Levy receives research grant support (principal investigator: Stent-Assisted Recanalization in acute Ischemic Stroke, SARIS), other research support (devices), and honoraria from Boston Scientific and research support from Codman & Shurtleff, Inc and ev3/Covidien Vascular Therapies; has ownership interests in Intratech Medical Ltd and Mynx/Access Closure; serves as a consultant on the board of Scientific Advisors to Codman & Shurtleff, Inc; serves as a consultant per project and/or per hour for Codman & Shurtleff, Inc, ev3/Covidien Vascular Therapies, and TheraSyn Sensors, Inc; and receives fees for carotid stent training from Abbott Vascular and ev3/Covidien Vascular Therapies. Dr Levy receives no consulting salary arrangements. All consulting is per project and/or per hour. Dr Mokin has received an educational grant from Toshiba. Dr Kass-Hout has received research funding from the Genentech Medical Educational and Research Department. Dr Dumont reports no financial relationships.

[a] Department of Neurosurgery, Gates Vascular Institute, Kaleida Health, School of Medicine and Biomedical Sciences, University at Buffalo, State University of New York, 100 High Street, Suite B4, Buffalo, NY 14203, USA; [b] Department of Neurology, Emory University, 49 Jesse Hill Jr Drive Southeast, Suite 126, Atlanta, GA 30303, USA; [c] Departments of Neurosurgery and Radiology, Gates Vascular Institute, Kaleida Health, Toshiba Stroke Research Center, School of Medicine and Biomedical Sciences, University at Buffalo, State University of New York, 100 High Street, Suite B4, Buffalo, NY 14203, USA
* Corresponding author.
E-mail address: elevy@ubns.com

INTRODUCTION

Extracranial carotid artery disease is commonly seen in patients presenting with stroke symptoms. Carotid stenosis as a cause of stroke (so-called "symptomatic" stenosis) can be seen in as many as 10% to 30% of such patients, depending on the percentage of stenosis used to define the presence of symptomatic carotid artery lesions.[1,2] Atherosclerotic lesions causing focal carotid stenosis are typically found at the bifurcation area. The severity of stenosis, estimated by the diameter, as of the most narrow segment in comparison with the diameter of the normal (nondiseased) carotid artery,[3] defines the magnitude of hemodynamic changes and the risk of developing a future cerebrovascular ischemic event (ie, stroke or transient ischemic attack [TIA]). This relationship was demonstrated in patients with both symptomatic and asymptomatic stenosis. The management of patients with vertebral artery disease is less understood. Both diseases, however, share several common features relative to diagnostic evaluation and medical and surgical treatment, largely because the development of focal atherosclerotic lesions is the main underlying mechanism in patients with extracranial carotid and vertebral artery stenosis. Carotid and vertebral artery dissections are more frequent in younger people and their mechanism and management have some unique features, distinguishing this entity from atherosclerotic lesions.

PRESENTING SYMPTOMS AND DIAGNOSTIC TESTS
Atherosclerosis

Atherosclerosis is a systemic disease and the presence of carotid artery plaques is frequently encountered in patients with coronary artery or peripheral vascular disease.[4,5] Similar to the degree of stenosis, plaque composition and morphology are important determinants when estimating the risk of stroke and thus should be carefully evaluated in patients with carotid disease. Ulcerative plaques with irregular edges, presence of intraplaque hemorrhages, and lipid-rich plaques are considered features of "unstable" plaques that have shown a strong association with a higher risk of subsequent cerebrovascular ischemic events.[6,7] **Box 1** summarizes the characteristics suggestive of high-risk plaques. In contrast, plaques with smooth walls and a homogeneous appearance are more stable.

Clinical Presentation

Clinical symptoms in patients with carotid artery disease can occur via 2 distinct pathways. First is inadequate cerebral blood perfusion as a result of hemodynamic stenosis, which is more commonly observed in patients with poorly developed collateral circulation. The circle of Willis allows cross-filling of intracranial vessels through

---

Box 1
Morphologic features suggestive of unstable plaques indicating high risk for rupture and ischemic events

- Intraplaque hemorrhage
- Lipid-rich plaque composition
- Irregular/ulcerated surface
- Thin or ruptured fibrous caps
- Presence of necrotic lipid cores

communication between the anterior and posterior circulation, as well as communication between the right and the left hemispheres. Patients with poor collateral supply (either because of anatomic variations or intracranial atherosclerosis) are not able to adequately redistribute blood flow to the affected brain regions. This commonly occurs in the setting of a sudden drop in blood pressure secondary to dehydration or impaired cardiac output, such as in patients with myocardial infarction, or in patients undergoing surgeries, such as coronary-artery bypass graft.

The second mechanism is plaque rupture and obstruction of smaller, more distally located blood vessels with plaque material causing embolic strokes. Depending on the size and number of the emboli originating from the carotid artery plaque, the symptoms can vary from benign transient events to more severe permanent neurologic deficits.

Clinical symptoms can range from brief neurologic findings (ie, TIAs, which are defined as transient neurologic deficits that resolved within 24 hours) to devastating permanent deficits, depending on the availability of collateral blood flow, comorbid conditions that affect cerebral vasculature (hypertension, diabetes, previous substance abuse), and concurrent treatment (eg, antiplatelet agents, antihyperlipidemic agents [statins]).

As a general rule, patients with strokes secondary to carotid artery disease tend to present with asymmetric neurologic symptoms. These commonly include numbness or weakness of the contralateral (to the lesion) face, arm, or leg. Speech deficits, such as word-finding difficulty (expressive aphasia), or inability to follow commands (receptive aphasia) typically occur as a result of strokes located in the dominant (usually left) hemisphere. Nondominant (usually right) hemispheric symptoms manifest with more subtle deficits, such as neglect, and these deficits are more difficult to recognize. In fact, patients sometimes are not aware of their deficits. Transient loss of vision in one eye (amaurosis fugax) is seen in patients with ophthalmic artery embolism. Clinical symptoms that should prompt a physician to initiate a carotid stenosis diagnostic evaluation are provided in **Box 2**.

It should be noted that similar symptoms can be observed due to other etiologies of TIAs or stroke, such as intracranial atherosclerosis, small vessel disease, or cardioembolic strokes; however, there is one syndrome that is rather unique to patients with severe carotid artery stenosis. It is called a "shaking TIA" and is thought to occur because of hemodynamic insufficiency causing global ischemia of one hemisphere. Clinically, this syndrome presents with transient episodes of limb shaking or flapping and can be mistaken for a focal seizure.[8,9]

Establishing the diagnosis of vertebral artery stenosis or occlusion based on clinical presentation is more challenging. Symptoms are often vague or have an anatomic distribution that can be localized to multiple brain territories. Syncope, dizziness,

---

Box 2
Clinical symptoms and physical findings suggestive of carotid stenosis

- Carotid bruit on physical examination
- Transient monocular blindness (amaurosis fugax)
- Inattention (neglect)
- Aphasia (expressive, receptive, mixed)
- Slurred speech (dysarthria), often as a result of facial droop
- Unilateral face, arm, leg numbness or weakness (paresis)

and unsteady gait can be mistakenly attributed to vestibular system disorders or cardiac dysfunction. Patients can present with weakness or numbness affecting both the right and left sides of the face and/or extremities. Cranial nerve palsies (as a result of brainstem strokes) are common and detailed examination of extraocular movements and facial muscle strength should be performed as part of the diagnostic evaluation. Unilateral visual field deficits (homonymous hemianopia) are sometimes described by patients as vision loss in one eye but should be distinguished from monocular blindness by performing visual field testing in each eye.

Diagnostic Tests

A variety of diagnostic testing modalities are currently available for clinicians, and the choice depends on multiple factors, including the goal of the test (screening vs confirmatory diagnosis), comorbid conditions (renal function tests, history of iodine contrast allergy), and index of suspicion. As a general rule, noninvasive imaging tests should be obtained initially in patients with neurologic symptoms of possible ischemic origin. According to the most recent guidelines on the management of patients with carotid artery disease, carotid ultrasonography should be the first diagnostic test in those patients.[10] In patients with acute ischemic symptoms attributable to carotid artery disease, however, either magnetic resonance angiography (MRA) or computed tomographic angiography (CTA) is also indicated.

Carotid ultrasound

This relatively low-cost, noninvasive test can be easily performed at bedside or in the outpatient office setting and has become the most commonly used initial tool in the arsenal of many primary care physicians, neurologists, and endovascular or vascular interventionists. It allows visual inspection of vessel diameter, tortuosity, and plaque composition. Intraplaque hemorrhages and plaques with hypoechoic lesions are associated with higher risk of stroke, and can be diagnosed using carotid ultrasound (**Fig. 1**A).[11,12] The degree of carotid artery stenosis is calculated based on peak systolic velocity measurements (**Fig. 2**B, **Table 1**).[13] Reliability of findings can be influenced by operator experience and variations in specific techniques used when acquiring the study. Other limitations of carotid ultrasound include dependence of velocity measurements on cardiac output (especially in patients with poor ejection fraction) in cases with concurrent intracranial stenosis (tandem lesions).

Magnetic resonance and computed tomographic angiography

Magnetic resonance angiography (MRA) and computed tomographic angiography (CTA) provide excellent spatial resolution of the extracranial and intracranial portions of the carotid and vertebral arteries. CTA uses iodine contrast media, which can be a limiting factor in patients with a previous history of an allergy to this agent. MRA can be performed without contrast media (called time-of-flight MRA); unfortunately, the quality of images can potentially be suboptimal because of significant motion artifacts. Also, MRA can sometimes overestimate the true degree of carotid or vertebral stenosis (called flow void artifacts), especially at the carotid bifurcation. These limitations can be overcome with gadolinium contrast-enhanced MRA.[14] One of the most important advantages of using MRA in evaluating carotid disease is its ability to characterize carotid plaque morphology. This helps identify carotid plaques with high-risk features for rupture and distal cerebral embolization, such as detection of necrotic lipid cores, intraplaque hemorrhages, and thin fibrous plaques (see **Fig. 1**B).[15,16]

CTA is another excellent noninvasive imaging modality that provides high-quality resolution of both extracranial and intracranial vasculature. It is often used in cases

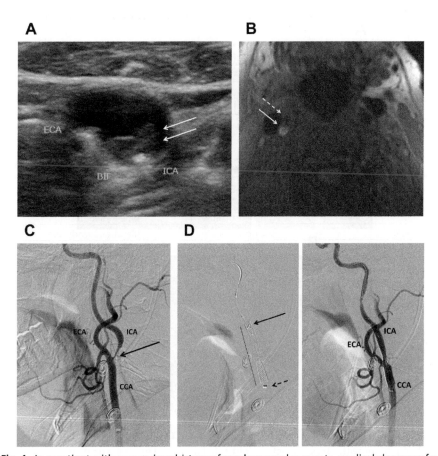

Fig. 1. In a patient with no previous history of cerebrovascular events, medical clearance for a planned major surgical procedure was requested by the surgeon. (*A*) Ultrasound of the carotid arteries showed a moderate plaque in the right internal carotid artery (ICA) with a hemorrhagic component (*arrows*). Because the plaque was an incidental discovery during a routine medical clearance evaluation, this right ICA stenosis should be considered asymptomatic. Measurement of velocities showed ≥70% stenosis. BIF, carotid bifurcation; ECA, external carotid artery. (*B*) MRA confirmed the presence of intraplaque hemorrhage within the ICA plaque (*arrows*). For comparison, the normal appearance of the ECA lumen is shown (*dotted arrow*). (*C*) Diagnostic digital subtraction angiogram confirmed the presence of critical right ICA stenosis at the origin of the right ICA (*arrow*). CCA, common carotid artery. (*D*) The presence of intraplaque hemorrhages indicates high-risk features for plaque rupture and distal cerebral embolization. Both medical and surgical treatment options were discussed with the patient. Carotid endarterectomy could be safely performed given the rather focal appearance of the lesion; however, the patient preferred carotid artery stenting. Left image (intraoperative digital subtraction angiogram, unsubtracted view) allows better visualization of the devices used during the procedure. Right image (*same view*) shows contrast injection within the vessel lumen. A stent (*long line*) can be seen within the distal end of the CCA and extending into the proximal portion of the ICA. A filter basket designed to capture embolic debris (distal protection device) is being removed after successful deployment of the stent (*arrow*). A guide catheter within the CCA that was used to deliver the stent and the filter can be seen at the bottom of the image (*dotted arrow*).

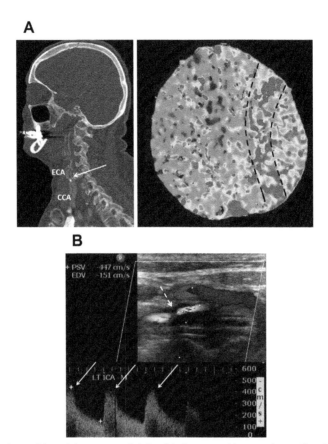

Fig. 2. A patient with sudden onset of right-sided arm and leg weakness (hemiparesis) presented to the emergency room. (*A*) An emergent CTA revealed evidence of critical stenosis of the left ICA (*arrow, left image*). Computed tomographic perfusion study (*right image*) showed a perfusion deficit in the so-called "watershed" territory: an area localized between the territories of 2 arteries, in this case, the left anterior cerebral and middle cerebral arteries (indicated by *dotted lines*). This pattern of ischemia is indicative of hemodynamic ICA stenosis. (*B*) Carotid ultrasound showed significantly elevated peak systolic velocities within the left ICA (*arrows*; maximal peak velocity of 447 cm/s), indicating presence of critical stenosis. Color-flow analysis shows a flow jet through the stenotic area (*dotted arrow*). Red color over the arterial lumen shows blood flow toward the probe and blue indicates flow away from the probe. EDT, end diastolic velocity; LT ICA, left internal carotid artery; PSV, peak systolic velocity. (*C*) The presence of an extensive ulcerative plaque with irregular borders (*arrows*) was confirmed by conventional diagnostic angiography. (*D*) Because of the extensive length of the plaque, extending high into the neck, and anticipated difficulty with an open surgical approach (carotid endarterectomy), carotid stenting was performed. Flow cessation with occlusive balloons (indicated by *arrows*), known as "proximal protection," was chosen instead of "distal protection" with filters because of concerns for possible plaque disruption and distal embolization.

in which MRA cannot be performed because of imaging-incompatible implanted devices, such as defibrillators or pacemakers, or when a reliable history cannot be obtained for medical clearance, which becomes especially important when evaluating patients in an acute setting, such as in the emergency room (see **Fig. 2**A). Radiation

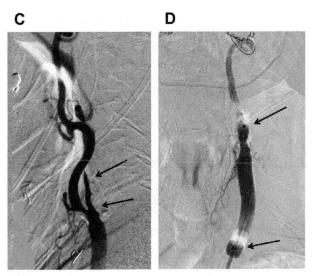

Fig. 2. (*continued*)

exposure and risk of acute kidney injury associated with administration of iodine contrast media are the 2 main limiting factors of this imaging modality. CTA is less susceptible to motion or flow artifacts than MRA.

Digital subtraction angiography
Conventional catheter angiography remains the gold standard for diagnosing carotid and vertebral artery disease (see **Figs.** 1C and 2C). With widespread use of noninvasive imaging technology, digital subtraction angiography is now mainly used as a confirmatory test when equivocal results are obtained during the imaging evaluation process. Its technical ability to provide multiple vessel views from virtually any angle

Table 1
Estimation of internal carotid artery stenosis

Estimation of Carotid Stenosis	Ultrasound Findings
"Normal" ICA	ICA PSV <125 cm/s and no plaque or intimal thickening is visualized
<50% ICA stenosis	ICA PSV <125 cm/s and plaque or intimal thickening is visualized
50%–69% ICA stenosis	ICA PSV of 125–230 cm/s and plaque is visualized
>70% ICA stenosis	ICA PSV >230 cm/s and visible plaque and lumen narrowing are seen
Near-occlusion of ICA	ICA PSV may be high, low, or undetectable. A markedly narrowed lumen is visualized.
Total ICA occlusion	No detectable patent lumen and no flow are seen

Abbreviations: ICA, internal carotid artery; PSV, peak systolic velocity.
Adapted from Grant EG, Benson CB, Moneta GL, et al. Carotid artery stenosis: grayscale and Doppler ultrasound diagnosis—Society of Radiologists in Ultrasound Consensus Conference. Ultrasound Q 2003;19:190–8.

under different magnifications allow excellent visualization of a stenotic area in question and calculation of the degree of stenosis. Selective catheterization of cervical vessels also provides valuable information about the extent of collateral blood supply. Neurologic complications following cerebral angiography are rare. According to recent studies, the risk of TIA or stroke is less than 1%.[17,18]

Table 2 provides a summary comparison of the technical advances and limitations of carotid ultrasonography and magnetic resonance, computed tomographic, and digital subtraction angiography.

Table 2
Comparison of advantages and limitations among carotid ultrasonography and magnetic resonance, computed tomographic, and digital subtraction angiography techniques

Imaging Modality	Advantages	Disadvantages
Ultrasonography	Inexpensive Can be performed at bedside Noninvasive Excellent screening tool Allows plaque composition analysis	Less accurate than CTA or MRA for measuring degree of stenosis. False results in patients with tandem stenosis (multiple stenotic lesions), with poor cardiac function. May overestimate severity of stenosis if contralateral carotid occlusion is present. Technique is highly operator-dependent.
CTA	Noninvasive Higher specificity than ultrasound Easy to use in emergency situations (eg, acute stroke)	Beam artifact from calcified lesions. Caution in patients with iodine allergy. Concern for radiation exposure. Risk of contrast-induced nephropathy.
MRA	Noninvasive Excellent ability to characterize plaque morphology Noninvasive test of choice to detect arterial dissection (carotid or vertebral?) No radiation exposure	Multiple devices are not MR-compatible (pacemakers, defibrillators, old surgical hardware)
Conventional catheter angiography (digital subtraction angiography)	Gold standard in determining degree of stenosis Diagnostic and interventional portions can be performed during same session.	Invasive Expensive Risk of contrast-induced nephropathy Concern for radiation exposure

Abbreviations: CTA, computed tomographic angiography; MR, magnetic resonance; MRA, magnetic resonance angiography.

MANAGEMENT OF CAROTID AND VERTEBRAL ARTERY DISEASES

We have witnessed tremendous advances in both medical and surgical management of patients with extracranial vertebral and especially carotid artery disease over the past decade. Medical management is based on several principles, including elimination or modification of vascular risk factors (such as hypertension, diabetes, obesity, and smoking), antithrombotic therapy, and aggressive lipid-lowering therapy with statins.

Guidelines for surgical treatment of carotid stenosis (either by means of endarterectomy or stenting) differ depending on whether a patient is considered to have symptomatic or asymptomatic stenosis. Patients are considered to be symptomatic if they have had a TIA or stroke involving the particular carotid artery within the previous 6 months.[10] If neurologic symptoms occurred beyond 6 months or the finding of carotid stenosis was incidental, such stenosis is considered asymptomatic.

Medical Management

The first step in the management of patients with newly diagnosed disease of the carotid or vertebral artery should be addressing risk factor modifications. The American Heart Association/American Stroke Association guidelines strongly recommend that all patients with a previous history of stroke or TIA or with a history of high-grade carotid artery stenosis follow a "cardiosmart" lifestyle.[19] Risk-factor modification should be aggressive, with the goal to target blood pressure to be lower than 130/80, low-density lipoprotein level to be less than 100 mg/dL in low-risk patients and less than 70 mg/dL in high-risk patients, hemoglobin A1C less than 7%, and a body mass index between 18.5 and 24.9. This should be achieved rigorously by increased physical activity; using alcohol in moderation if consumed; decreased sodium intake; and a daily healthy diet that is rich in whole grains, fresh fruits, vegetables, and low-fat dairy products. Trans fats should be specifically avoided.

Data on secondary prevention of stroke or TIA in patients with carotid or vertebral artery stenosis are extensive and aim at targeting the risk factors from multiple angles. Antiplatelet medication, such as aspirin, clopidogrel, or Aggrenox (combination of aspirin and extended-release dipyridamole; Boehringer Ingelheim Pharmaceuticals, Ridgefield, CT, USA) is proven to reduce the risk of secondary stroke; however, studies failed to show any clinical significance of using one antiplatelet medication over the other.[20–22] Evidence to support the clinical benefit of dual antiplatelet therapy is currently lacking. Because of higher risk for hemorrhagic complications (mainly gastrointestinal bleeding), a combination of 2 antiplatelet agents is not recommended[23]; however, under certain circumstances, such as in patients with a recent stenting procedure, 2 agents are required to prevent in-stent thrombosis (typically a combination of aspirin and clopidogrel for a period of 3 months).

Cholesterol-lowering drugs, especially statins, decrease stroke risk in patients with vascular disease,[24] although the benefits may be due to other actions of these drugs (anti-inflammatory effect on the plaque lesion) and not just their ability to reduce cholesterol levels. **Table 3** summarizes landmark studies evaluating medical therapies for primary and secondary stroke prevention applicable to patients with carotid and vertebral artery disease.

Carotid Artery Stenosis: Surgical Approaches, Techniques, and Risks

According to the American Heart Association/American Stroke Association guidelines for the primary prevention of stroke, prophylactic carotid endarterectomy or stenting is recommended in highly selected patients with carotid stenosis of 60% or more.[25] The

Table 3
Landmark randomized trials evaluating medical management of cerebrovascular diseases applicable to patients with carotid and vertebral artery stenosis

Trial	Design	Findings
MATCH,[21] 2004	Aspirin + clopidogrel compared with clopidogrel alone after recent stroke or TIA	No value of adding aspirin to clopidogrel
CHARISMA,[20] 2006	Clopidogrel and aspirin vs aspirin alone in patients at high risk for atherothrombotic events	No significant difference between the 2 regimens
SPARCL,[24] 2006	Atorvastatin vs placebo in patients with recent stroke or TIA	Atorvastatin reduced the incidence of strokes and other cardiovascular events
PRoFESS,[22] 2008	Aspirin and extended-release dipyridamole (Aggrenox) vs clopidogrel for recurrent stroke	Similar rates of recurrent stroke between the 2 groups

Abbreviations: CHARISMA, Clopidogrel for High Atherothrombotic Risk and Ischemic Stabilization, Management, and Avoidance; MATCH, Management of Atherothrombosis with Clopidogrel in High-risk Patients with Recent Transient Ischaemic Attack or Ischaemic Stroke; PRoFESS, Prevention Regimen for Effectively Avoiding Second Strokes; SPARCL, Stroke Prevention by Aggressive Reduction in Cholesterol Levels; TIA, transient ischemic attack.

benefit of surgery, however, is most significant in asymptomatic patients with degree of stenosis of 80% or more.

In patients with symptomatic carotid artery stenosis, surgical revascularization is recommended in patients with 50% or more stenosis.[10] Carotid revascularization is not recommended in patients with complete (100%) occlusion of the carotid artery.

Carotid Endarterectomy

Carotid endarterectomy is probably the most rigorously studied surgical procedure and has proven clinical benefit over medical treatment of carotid stenosis.[26–29] The procedure involves removing the offending carotid plaque and reconstructing the carotid artery. The artery is directly approached through a linear incision on the neck and requires minimal but meticulous dissection of the surrounding tissues. A typical procedure requires approximately 20 to 40 minutes of carotid artery manipulation and invariably involves temporary occlusion of the carotid artery. The most frequent risks of carotid endarterectomy include stroke and myocardial infarction. The estimated risk of major complications from carotid endarterectomy from the most recently completed randomized trial, the Carotid Revascularization Endarterectomy versus Stenting Trial (CREST),[30,31] is on the order of 5% (2.3% stroke and 2.3% myocardial infarction).

Carotid endarterectomy may be performed with local anesthetics or general anesthesia. The choice of anesthesia does not appear to affect surgical outcome and is typically directed by surgeon preference. Endarterectomy with a local anesthetic requires a cooperative patient, and, when possible, allows the surgeon the advantage of performing neurologic examinations throughout the procedure. General anesthesia allows the surgeon to control hemodynamic factors more easily and ensures minimal movement of the operative field during dissection and arterial closure. The use of neurophysiologic monitoring with electroencephalography and sometimes somatosensory-evoked potentials generally accompanies general anesthesia to ensure adequate blood flow during the procedure, although it is not requisite.[32,33]

The surgical technique of carotid endarterectomy has been well refined, although varied techniques may be used based on surgeon preference or vascular anastomotic reserve. Before the procedure, an understanding of the vascular anatomy of the circle of Willis and contralateral carotid artery may be helpful in determining the optimal surgical technique. For example, a patient with no contralateral occlusion and a complete circle of Willis is theoretically more likely to tolerate prolonged clamping of the carotid artery during endarterectomy.

Once the endarterectomy is completed, reconstruction of the carotid artery is performed. This requires closing the incision of the common and internal carotid artery and is generally performed with a simple closure of the incision. For cases in which the internal carotid artery is small, a patch may be sewn into place to widen the intraluminal area.

Carotid Stenting

Carotid stenting was initially introduced as an alternative treatment for carotid stenosis for patients considered at high risk of experiencing perioperative complications with carotid endarterectomy. With improvements in techniques and outcomes, carotid stenting is now more frequently used.[34–37] Simply described, in this procedure, a meshlike tubular device is placed within the lumen of the afflicted vessel to force open the artery at its narrowed segment and to reconstruct the artery from the inside. The approach is typically performed through a needle-puncture wound over the femoral artery. A typical procedure requires approximately 5 to 15 minutes of carotid artery manipulation. Estimated risks of major complications from carotid stenting from the most recently completed randomized trial (CREST) is on the order of 5% (4.1% stroke and 1.1% myocardial infarction).[30,31]

New devices for carotid stenting

The basic technical component of carotid stenting requires an exchange (or switching out) of a series of devices, including embolic protection filters, stents, and angioplasty balloons. Most common stent devices were tested thoroughly for safety with a series of trials and registries after Food and Drug Administration approval throughout the past decade.[38] Stent devices for use in internal carotid artery stenosis are self-expanding and delivered on a wire through a catheter-based system. Individual stents have characteristics that make them more useful in certain clinical and anatomic circumstances.[39,40] For instance, some stents are designed with a finer mesh (smaller open-cell area) that may limit distal embolization of a high-risk plaque with intraplaque hemorrhage or necrosis. Other stents are designed with built-in flexibility (open-cell stents), which may be favorable for cases in which the diseased carotid artery has a distinctive curve. No significant difference in the incidence of perioperative stroke has been appreciated with the use of different stents.[41,42]

Embolic protection devices may be used to prevent thromboembolism during stenting procedures. The earliest experiences with carotid stenting did not include embolic protection devices, and the resultant rate of intraprocedural embolic stroke was unacceptably high. Thromboembolism associated with passage of the stent through the area of stenosis or with expansion of the stent (particularly in cases with hemorrhage or necrosis within the plaque) is averted with embolic protection devices. Devices used to prevent thromboembolism during carotid stenting include filter devices, flow cessation or reversal catheters, and distal aspiration catheters. All these devices are designed to prevent plaque that is dislodged during stent placement from traveling into the brain and causing a stroke.

Distal embolic protection devices are small filters (porous umbrellalike devices) that are expanded within the internal carotid artery past the area of stenosis and just before its entry to the intracranial vault (see **Fig. 1**D). Distal embolic protection devices are placed before passage of the stent through the area of carotid stenosis and are designed to capture small particles of plaque dislodged during placement of the stent. Filter devices are widely used in the most recent and ongoing carotid stenting trials.[30,31,43–45] Their use is now well established, and such devices are used for most carotid-stenting procedures. The principal downside to distal embolic protection devices is that such devices must be passed through the area of stenosis before their deployment distal to the area of stenosis, which may produce unwanted thromboembolic debris with placement. This problem may be encountered in particular in patients with "high risk" carotid plaques with critical stenosis ($\geq$95%) or dangerous features (intraplaque hemorrhage or necrosis).

Flow cessation or reversal catheters are devices placed proximal to the area of stenosis with occlusive balloons that are inflated within the common and external carotid arteries to stop or reverse flow through the area of stenosis during placement of a stent (see **Fig. 2**D). These so-called "proximal protection" catheters prevent plaque dislodged during placement of the stent from entering the intracranial vault, and thus prevent perioperative stroke. Two prospective carotid stenting registries testing the safety of flow cessation[46] and reversal[47] have yielded the lowest incidence of perioperative stroke for any prospective carotid stenting study to date. The downside to proximal protection is that stasis or reversal of flow is requisite. This may not be tolerated by patients with contralateral carotid stenosis or occlusion.

Vertebral Artery Stenosis: Surgical Approaches, Techniques, and Risks

Stenosis of the vertebral artery tends to occur at the origin (or ostium). Because of the deep location of this artery within the inferior triangle of the neck, endarterectomy is rarely performed; and surgical techniques may require arterial bypass. Endovascular stenting is more easily accomplished.

Vertebral artery stenosis is much less common and studied than carotid artery stenosis. Treatment is reserved for patients with stenosis in a dominant vertebral artery with symptomatology refractory to appropriate medical therapy. In part because of the clinical rarity of vertebral artery stenosis, devices used for treatment of this disease were not specifically designed for such an application. The anatomic features of vertebral artery stenosis (including the typical location at the ostium and small diameter) make use of distal embolic protection filters difficult; thus, stenting without distal embolic protection devices is routine. In addition, small stents are more likely to develop restenosis or cracking because of positioning within the ostium of the vessel. Use of drug-eluting stents and open-cell stents with angioplasty balloons designed to form-fit the stent to the vessel opening may reduce the risk of complications after stenting.[48–50]

CAROTID AND VERTEBRAL ARTERY DISSECTION

Even though arterial dissection accounts for approximately 2% of all ischemic strokes, it is considered to be the second leading cause of stroke in patients younger than 45 years, accounting for 10% to 25% of ischemic strokes in this population.[51,52] However, estimating the real incidence of arterial dissection is difficult because many of these patients are asymptomatic and likely underdiagnosed. It is worth mentioning that spontaneous cervicocerebral dissections are more common in men.

Pathogenesis

Although some dissections are iatrogenic or secondary to severe trauma, most occur spontaneously. Arterial dissections are usually a direct cause of an intimal tear with a subsequent intramural hematoma, referred to as a false lumen. The intramural hematoma could be primarily in the tunica media layer (the muscular middle layer of the blood vessel), which results in no communication between the true and the false lumens. Dissections of the extracranial carotid and vertebral arteries account for most of the cervicocerebral dissections, likely because of the greater mobility of these segments (as compared with intracranial segments) over bony structures. Underlying arteriopathy, such as fibromuscular dysplasia or heritable connective tissue disorder, has been postulated to lead to arterial dissection.[53,54] Ischemic strokes that are caused by arterial dissection are mostly attributable to distal thromboembolism, luminal stenosis, or occlusion.

Clinical Presentation

The most common symptom associated with carotid artery dissection is pain on the ipsilateral side of the head, face, or neck. Onset of the pain is usually gradual and could radiate to the face, jaw, ear, or even the pharynx. Involvement of the sympathetic fibers of the internal carotid plexus is common in extracranial carotid artery dissection and results in partial Horner syndrome (ipsilateral ptosis and miosis). Cranial nerve palsies have also been reported. Most ischemic stroke manifestations occur within 1 week of the onset of the pain.[55] These manifestations are usually associated with occlusions and stenosis greater than 80% and they are mostly territorial, supporting an embolic etiology.[56]

Headache and neck pain are also common in vertebral artery dissection.[57] Ischemic stroke and TIAs occur shortly after the headache onset.[58] Subarachnoid hemorrhage is also a common presentation of intracranial vertebral artery dissection.

Diagnosis

Once a clinical diagnosis of cervicocerebral dissection is suspected, MRA of the extracranial vessels is the most specific noninvasive modality to confirm the diagnosis. In particular, fat-suppression techniques are important to differentiate small intramural hematomas from surrounding soft tissues.[59,60] For situations in which MRA is not feasible, other noninvasive studies, such as CTA, might be helpful. Conventional angiography remains the gold standard in accurately defining the exact level and arterial territory of the dissection.[61] If endovascular therapy is necessary, it can be performed in tandem with diagnostic conventional angiography.

Treatment

With appropriate management, the prognosis is usually excellent, with a high chance of complete recovery.[62,63] Clinical trials to definitively support different types of medical therapy in patients with arterial dissection are still lacking. The most acceptable therapy for extracranial cervicocerebral arterial dissection is anticoagulation with heparin as an immediate therapy and warfarin as a subsequent therapy for 3 to 6 months until the dissection is healed, which is usually assessed by either multimodal ultrasound studies, CTA, or MRA.[62] The value of anticoagulation over antiplatelet therapy is questionable and still under study.[64]

Endovascular therapy is typically indicated for patients with persistent ischemic symptoms while receiving medical therapy or those who have contraindications to systemic anticoagulation. Catheter-directed intervention allows reestablishment of the true lumen by means of balloon angioplasty and stenting, which in turn will help to restore normal hemodynamic flow and reduce the risk of stroke.[63,65] Surgical treatment (such as carotid reconstruction or bypass surgery) is usually reserved for patients in whom optimal medical therapy is a failure and who are not candidates for endovascular therapy.

SUMMARY

Extracranial carotid and vertebral artery stenosis can present with a variety of clinical symptoms. Depending on the clinical scenario (emergent evaluation of a patient with stroke vs a routine outpatient visit) different imaging modalities should be applied as a part of the diagnostic evaluation. Medical treatment should involve management of cerebrovascular risk factors and antiplatelet and cholesterol-lowering agents. The degree of carotid artery stenosis and relevance to clinical symptoms (symptomatic vs asymptomatic stenosis) should be taken into account when considering surgical treatment. Carotid artery stenting has become a commonly used alternative to carotid endarterectomy, largely because of advances in techniques and development of new devices. Surgical treatment of patients with vertebral artery stenosis is typically reserved in cases refractory to appropriate medical therapy. Carotid and vertebral artery dissections can present with unique symptoms, and their mechanisms are different from formation of extracranial atherosclerotic lesions.

ACKNOWLEDGMENTS

We thank Paul H. Dressel, BFA, for preparation of the illustrations and Debra J. Zimmer for editorial assistance.

REFERENCES

1. Jeng JS, Sacco RL, Kargman DE, et al. Apolipoproteins and carotid artery atherosclerosis in an elderly multiethnic population: the Northern Manhattan stroke study. Atherosclerosis 2002;165:317–25.
2. Kolominsky-Rabas PL, Weber M, Gefeller O, et al. Epidemiology of ischemic stroke subtypes according to TOAST criteria: incidence, recurrence, and long-term survival in ischemic stroke subtypes: a population-based study. Stroke 2001;32:2735–40.
3. Fox AJ. How to measure carotid stenosis. Radiology 1993;186:316–8.
4. Brevetti G, Sirico G, Giugliano G, et al. Prevalence of hypoechoic carotid plaques in coronary artery disease: relationship with coexistent peripheral arterial disease and leukocyte number. Vasc Med 2009;14:13–9.
5. Brevetti G, Sirico G, Lanero S, et al. The prevalence of hypoechoic carotid plaques is greater in peripheral than in coronary artery disease and is related to the neutrophil count. J Vasc Surg 2008;47:523–9.
6. Sadat U, Weerakkody RA, Bowden DJ, et al. Utility of high resolution MR imaging to assess carotid plaque morphology: a comparison of acute symptomatic, recently symptomatic and asymptomatic patients with carotid artery disease. Atherosclerosis 2009;207:434–9.
7. Takaya N, Yuan C, Chu B, et al. Association between carotid plaque characteristics and subsequent ischemic cerebrovascular events: a prospective assessment with MRI—initial results. Stroke 2006;37:818–23.
8. Ali S, Khan MA, Khealani B. Limb-shaking transient ischemic attacks: case report and review of literature. BMC Neurol 2006;6:5.

9. Baquis GD, Pessin MS, Scott RM. Limb shaking—a carotid TIA. Stroke 1985;16: 444–8.
10. Brott TG, Halperin JL, Abbara S, et al. 2011 ASA/ACCF/AHA/AANN/AANS/ACR/ ASNR/CNS/SAIP/SCAI/SIR/SNIS/SVM/SVS guideline on the management of patients with extracranial carotid and vertebral artery disease. A report of the American College of Cardiology Foundation/American Heart Association Task Force on Practice Guidelines, and the American Stroke Association, American Association of Neuroscience Nurses, American Association of Neurological Surgeons, American College of Radiology, American Society of Neuroradiology, Congress of Neurological Surgeons, Society of Atherosclerosis Imaging and Prevention, Society for Cardiovascular Angiography and Interventions, Society of Interventional Radiology, Society of NeuroInterventional Surgery, Society for Vascular Medicine, and Society for Vascular Surgery. Circulation 2011;124:e54–130.
11. Sabetai MM, Tegos TJ, Nicolaides AN, et al. Hemispheric symptoms and carotid plaque echomorphology. J Vasc Surg 2000;31:39–49.
12. Tegos TJ, Sohail M, Sabetai MM, et al. Echomorphologic and histopathologic characteristics of unstable carotid plaques. AJNR Am J Neuroradiol 2000;21:1937–44.
13. Grant EG, Benson CB, Moneta GL, et al. Carotid artery stenosis: grayscale and Doppler ultrasound diagnosis—Society of Radiologists in Ultrasound Consensus Conference. Ultrasound Q 2003;19:190–8.
14. Nederkoorn PJ, van der Graaf Y, Eikelboom BC, et al. Time-of-flight MR angiography of carotid artery stenosis: does a flow void represent severe stenosis? AJNR Am J Neuroradiol 2002;23:1779–84.
15. Oppenheim C, Touze E, Leclerc X, et al. High resolution MRI of carotid atherosclerosis: looking beyond the arterial lumen. J Radiol 2008;89:293–301 [in French].
16. Takaya N, Yuan C, Chu B, et al. Presence of intraplaque hemorrhage stimulates progression of carotid atherosclerotic plaques: a high-resolution magnetic resonance imaging study. Circulation 2005;111:2768–75.
17. Dawkins AA, Evans AL, Wattam J, et al. Complications of cerebral angiography: a prospective analysis of 2,924 consecutive procedures. Neuroradiology 2007; 49:753–9.
18. Fifi JT, Meyers PM, Lavine SD, et al. Complications of modern diagnostic cerebral angiography in an academic medical center. J Vasc Interv Radiol 2009;20:442–7.
19. Furie KL, Kasner SE, Adams RJ, et al. Guidelines for the prevention of stroke in patients with stroke or transient ischemic attack: a guideline for healthcare professionals from the American Heart Association/American Stroke Association. Stroke 2011;42:227–76.
20. Bhatt DL, Fox KA, Hacke W, et al. Clopidogrel and aspirin versus aspirin alone for the prevention of atherothrombotic events. N Engl J Med 2006;354:1706–17.
21. Diener HC, Bogousslavsky J, Brass LM, et al. Aspirin and clopidogrel compared with clopidogrel alone after recent ischaemic stroke or transient ischaemic attack in high-risk patients (MATCH): randomised, double-blind, placebo-controlled trial. Lancet 2004;364:331–7.
22. Sacco RL, Diener HC, Yusuf S, et al. Aspirin and extended-release dipyridamole versus clopidogrel for recurrent stroke. N Engl J Med 2008;359:1238–51.
23. Adams RJ, Albers G, Alberts MJ, et al. Update to the AHA/ASA recommendations for the prevention of stroke in patients with stroke and transient ischemic attack. Stroke 2008;39:1647–52.
24. Amarenco P, Bogousslavsky J, Callahan A 3rd, et al. High-dose atorvastatin after stroke or transient ischemic attack. N Engl J Med 2006;355:549–59.

25. Goldstein LB, Bushnell CD, Adams RJ, et al. Guidelines for the primary prevention of stroke: a guideline for healthcare professionals from the American Heart Association/American Stroke Association. Stroke 2011;42:517–84.
26. North American Symptomatic Carotid Endarterectomy Trial Collaborators. Beneficial effect of carotid endarterectomy in symptomatic patients with high-grade carotid stenosis. N Engl J Med 1991;325:445–53.
27. Executive Committee for the Asymptomatic Carotid Atherosclerosis Study. Endarterectomy for asymptomatic carotid artery stenosis. JAMA 1995;273:1421–8.
28. Halliday A, Mansfield A, Marro J, et al. Prevention of disabling and fatal strokes by successful carotid endarterectomy in patients without recent neurological symptoms: randomised controlled trial. Lancet 2004;363:1491–502.
29. Mayberg MR, Wilson SE, Yatsu F, et al. Carotid endarterectomy and prevention of cerebral ischemia in symptomatic carotid stenosis. Veterans Affairs Cooperative Studies Program 309 Trialist Group. JAMA 1991;266:3289–94.
30. Brott TG, Hobson RW 2nd, Howard G, et al. Stenting versus endarterectomy for treatment of carotid-artery stenosis. N Engl J Med 2010;363:11–23.
31. Mantese VA, Timaran CH, Chiu D, et al. The Carotid Revascularization Endarterectomy versus Stenting Trial (CREST): stenting versus carotid endarterectomy for carotid disease. Stroke 2010;41:S31–4.
32. Hamdan AD, Pomposelli FB Jr, Gibbons GW, et al. Perioperative strokes after 1001 consecutive carotid endarterectomy procedures without an electroencephalogram: incidence, mechanism, and recovery. Arch Surg 1999;134:412–5.
33. Kalkman CJ. Con: routine shunting is not the optimal management of the patient undergoing carotid endarterectomy, but neither is neuromonitoring. J Cardiothorac Vasc Anesth 2004;18:381–3.
34. Bladin C, Chambers B, New G, et al. Guidelines for patient selection and performance of carotid artery stenting. ANZ J Surg 2010;80:398–405.
35. Dumont TM, Rughani AI. National trends in carotid artery revascularization surgery. J Neurosurg 2012;116:1251–7.
36. Ricotta JJ, Aburahma A, Ascher E, et al. Updated Society for Vascular Surgery guidelines for management of extracranial carotid disease. J Vasc Surg 2011;54:e1–31.
37. Siddiqui AH, Natarajan SK, Hopkins LN, et al. Carotid artery stenting for primary and secondary stroke prevention. World Neurosurg 2011;76:S40–59.
38. Kan P, Mokin M, Dumont TM, et al. Cervical carotid artery stenosis: latest update on diagnosis and management. Curr Probl Cardiol 2012;37:127–69.
39. Hart JP, Bosiers M, Deloose K, et al. Impact of stent design on the outcome of intervention for carotid bifurcation stenosis. J Cardiovasc Surg (Torino) 2010; 51:799–806.
40. Muller-Hulsbeck S, Preuss H, Elhoft H. CAS: which stent for which lesion. J Cardiovasc Surg (Torino) 2009;50:767–72.
41. Tadros RO, Spyris CT, Vouyouka AG, et al. Comparing the embolic potential of open and closed cell stents during carotid angioplasty and stenting. J Vasc Surg 2012;56(1):89–95.
42. Timaran CH, Rosero EB, Higuera A, et al. Randomized clinical trial of open-cell vs closed-cell stents for carotid stenting and effects of stent design on cerebral embolization. J Vasc Surg 2011;54:1310–1316.e1 [discussion: 1316].
43. Carotid stenting vs. surgery of severe carotid artery disease and stroke prevention in asymptomatic patients (ACT 1). Available at: http://clinicaltrials.gov/ct2/show/NCT00106938. Accessed August 24, 2012.
44. Ederle J, Dobson J, Featherstone RL, et al. Carotid artery stenting compared with endarterectomy in patients with symptomatic carotid stenosis (International

Carotid Stenting Study): an interim analysis of a randomised controlled trial. Lancet 2010;375:985–97.

45. Reiff T, Stingele R, Eckstein HH, et al. Stent-protected angioplasty in asymptomatic carotid artery stenosis vs. endarterectomy: SPACE2—a three-arm randomised-controlled clinical trial. Int J Stroke 2009;4:294–9.

46. Ansel GM, Hopkins LN, Jaff MR, et al. Safety and effectiveness of the INVATEC MO.MA proximal cerebral protection device during carotid artery stenting: results from the ARMOUR pivotal trial. Catheter Cardiovasc Interv 2010;76:1–8.

47. Clair DG, Hopkins LN, Mehta M, et al. Neuroprotection during carotid artery stenting using the GORE flow reversal system: 30-day outcomes in the EMPiRE Clinical Study. Catheter Cardiovasc Interv 2011;77:420–9.

48. Dumont TM, Kan P, Snyder KV, et al. Stenting of the vertebral artery origin with ostium dilatation: technical note. J Neurointerv Surg 2012. [Epub ahead of print].

49. Ogilvy CS, Yang X, Natarajan SK, et al. Restenosis rates following vertebral artery origin stenting: does stent type make a difference? J Invasive Cardiol 2010;22: 119–24.

50. Stayman AN, Nogueira RG, Gupta R. A systematic review of stenting and angioplasty of symptomatic extracranial vertebral artery stenosis. Stroke 2011;42:2212–6.

51. Bogousslavsky J, Pierre P. Ischemic stroke in patients under age 45. Neurol Clin 1992;10:113–24.

52. Giroud M, Fayolle H, Andre N, et al. Incidence of internal carotid artery dissection in the community of Dijon. J Neurol Neurosurg Psychiatry 1994;57:1443.

53. Schievink WI, Wijdicks EF, Michels VV, et al. Heritable connective tissue disorders in cervical artery dissections: a prospective study. Neurology 1998;50:1166–9.

54. Stanley JC, Fry WJ, Seeger JF, et al. Extracranial internal carotid and vertebral artery fibrodysplasia. Arch Surg 1974;109:215–22.

55. Baumgartner RW, Bogousslavsky J. Clinical manifestations of carotid dissection. Front Neurol Neurosci 2005;20:70–6.

56. Baumgartner RW, Arnold M, Baumgartner I, et al. Carotid dissection with and without ischemic events: local symptoms and cerebral artery findings. Neurology 2001;57:827–32.

57. Silbert PL, Mokri B, Schievink WI. Headache and neck pain in spontaneous internal carotid and vertebral artery dissections. Neurology 1995;45:1517–22.

58. Arnold M, Bousser MG, Fahrni G, et al. Vertebral artery dissection: presenting findings and predictors of outcome. Stroke 2006;37:2499–503.

59. Jacobs A, Lanfermann H, Neveling M, et al. MRI- and MRA-guided therapy of carotid and vertebral artery dissections. J Neurol Sci 1997;147:27–34.

60. Schievink WI. Spontaneous dissection of the carotid and vertebral arteries. N Engl J Med 2001;344:898–906.

61. Provenzale JM. Dissection of the internal carotid and vertebral arteries: imaging features. AJR Am J Roentgenol 1995;165:1099–104.

62. Desfontaines P, Despland PA. Dissection of the internal carotid artery: aetiology, symptomatology, clinical and neurosonological follow-up, and treatment in 60 consecutive cases. Acta Neurol Belg 1995;95:226–34.

63. Pham MH, Rahme RJ, Arnaout O, et al. Endovascular stenting of extracranial carotid and vertebral artery dissections: a systematic review of the literature. Neurosurgery 2011;68:856–66.

64. Menon R, Kerry S, Norris JW, et al. Treatment of cervical artery dissection: a systematic review and meta-analysis. J Neurol Neurosurg Psychiatry 2008;79:1122–7.

65. DeOcampo J, Brillman J, Levy DI. Stenting: a new approach to carotid dissection. J Neuroimaging 1997;7:187–90.

Ischemic Bowel Syndromes

Jose A. Silva, MD, Christopher J. White, MD*

KEYWORDS

- Ischemic bowel disease • Acute mesenteric ischemia • Chronic mesenteric ischemia
- Atherosclerotic vascular disease

KEY POINTS

- Atherosclerotic vascular disease involving the mesenteric arteries occurs frequently in the elderly population.
- Although the prevalence of ischemic bowel disease is difficult to determine, acute mesenteric ischemia has been reported to cause in 1 in 1000 hospital admissions, whereas chronic mesenteric ischemia is estimated to affect 1 in 100,000 individuals.
- Mesenteric ischemia generally manifests in its chronic form as postprandial abdominal pain resulting in significant weight loss, and in its acute form as an abrupt development of abdominal pain, lower gastrointestinal bleeding, and subsequent intestinal necrosis.

INTRODUCTION

Atherosclerotic vascular disease involving the mesenteric arteries (**Fig. 1**) occurs frequently in the elderly population. Although the prevalence of ischemic bowel disease is difficult to determine, acute mesenteric ischemia (AMI) has been reported to cause in 1 in 1000 hospital admissions, whereas chronic mesenteric ischemia (CMI) is estimated to affect 1 in 100,000 individuals.[1,2]

Mesenteric ischemia generally manifests in its chronic form as postprandial abdominal pain resulting in significant weight loss, and in its acute form as an abrupt development of abdominal pain, lower gastrointestinal bleeding, and subsequent intestinal necrosis. This article discusses the cause, clinical manifestations, diagnosis, and management of AMI and CMI.

AMI
Etiology and Pathophysiology

AMI occurs as a result of hypoxemia, which leads to intestinal infarction. It is not unusual for patients to have a history of atherosclerotic vascular disease (eg, previous myocardial infarction and/or angina pectoris, congestive heart failure, stroke, or

Department of Cardiology, John Ochsner Heart and Vascular Institute, Ochsner Clinic Foundation, 1514 Jefferson Highway, New Orleans, LA 70118, USA
* Corresponding author.
E-mail address: drcjwhite@gmail.com

Prim Care Clin Office Pract 40 (2013) 153–167
http://dx.doi.org/10.1016/j.pop.2012.11.007
0095-4543/13/$ – see front matter © 2013 Elsevier Inc. All rights reserved.

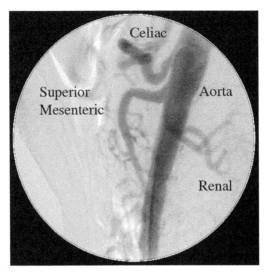

Fig. 1. Angiography of the celiac trunk and superior mesenteric artery showing a mild amount of atherosclerotic plaque.

peripheral vascular disease).[3,4] AMI may be caused by embolism, thrombosis, or occlusive vascular disease, or may be iatrogenic (**Fig. 2**). Arterial thrombosis accounts for approximately 12% and venous thrombosis for 8% of the cases of AMI.[1,5–7]

Arterial embolism is the most common cause of AMI, accounting for approximately half of all cases (**Fig. 3**).[1,5] The heart is by far the most common source ($\approx$80%) of embolization, with atrial fibrillation the most frequent cause ($\approx$75%), followed by thrombi from the left ventricle after a recent myocardial infarction ($\approx$25%).[8] Deficiencies of protein C and S, antithrombin III deficiency, antiphospholipid antibodies, heparin-induced thrombocytopenia, factor V Leiden mutation, the use of contraceptives and other estrogen-containing medications, and malignancy may induce a hypercoagulable state that may lead to arterial or venous thrombosis of the mesenteric circulation.[1,5–7,9,10]

Nonocclusive AMI refers to intestinal ischemia without arterial or venous obstruction, occurring in approximately 20% of patients who ultimately develop AMI.[1] This condition is usually the result of low cardiac output states, leading to decreased mesenteric perfusion. Nonocclusive AMI has been described in patients with congestive heart failure, sepsis, profound hypotension, and hypovolemia. These conditions induce splanchnic vasoconstriction,[11,12] which may lead to intestinal infarction. In

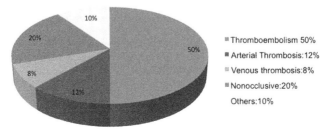

Fig. 2. Most frequent causes of AMI.

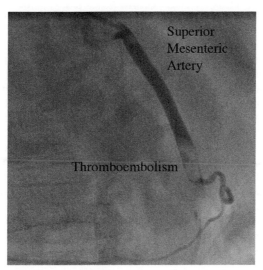

Fig. 3. Angiography of a thromboembolic event causing AMI. The angiogram shows large filling defect (thrombus) causing total occlusion of the superior mesenteric artery.

addition, drugs such as ergot alkaloids, cocaine, and digitalis have been implicated in the development of splanchnic vasoconstriction.[9,10,12,13]

Assessment of AMI

AMI mostly affects elderly individuals, who often have other comorbid conditions. Because of their age and multiple ailments, these patients have a decreased physiologic reserve, which renders them vulnerable. Consequently, a high degree of suspicion and early diagnosis of this condition are critical to decrease morbidity and mortality. Clinicians must have a high index of suspicion when assessing patients with abdominal pain and risk factors for mesenteric atherosclerotic disease and bowel ischemia.

Clinical Presentation

The presentation of AMI may be subtle and nonspecific before florid symptoms appear. Symptoms will depend on the location and extent of arterial obstruction and the degree of vascular collateral development.[14] Abdominal pain is the dominant symptom, occurring in nearly 85% of patients.[4,8,15] A change in mental status is present in almost 30% of elderly patients.[16] The abdominal pain is often severe and typically disproportionate to the physical findings.[17] Localized pain is often periumbilical and is usually related to small bowel ischemia. In patients with a history of CMI before the development of acute abdominal pain, acute arterial thrombosis superimposed on severe mesenteric atherosclerotic disease is often the underlying pathologic event.[18–20] Nonocclusive arterial disease must be suspected in patients with or without abdominal pain who develop diarrhea and bacteremia after cardiopulmonary resuscitation.[21,22]

Other symptoms of AMI include diarrhea, nausea, and vomiting, which occur in approximately 50% of patients.[23] The diarrhea is frequently bloody, particularly with intestinal infarction.[24] Gastrointestinal emptying with vomiting and diarrhea occurs as a result of intense muscular spasm and hyperperistalsis during early intestinal ischemia.[25]

Mesenteric venous thrombosis has a variable and often more subtle and less severe clinical presentation. The progression toward more severe symptoms is also slower than when the arterial circulation is compromised. Abdominal pain ($\approx$85%), anorexia ($\approx$50%), nausea and vomiting ($\approx$45%), upper and lower gastrointestinal bleeding ($\approx$35% and $\approx$20%, respectively), and constipation ($\approx$10%) are the typical symptoms. Typically, patients endure pain for several days (mean duration, 5 days) before seeking medical attention.[5,26]

The abdomen may be soft with minimal tenderness on direct deep palpation, and bowel sounds are usually normal. With increasing bowel ischemia, patients may develop abdominal distention and decreased bowel sounds as a result of hypoperistalsis from intestinal ischemia. Nearly 75% of patients will have fecal occult blood,[24] and if ischemia progresses toward bowel infarction, they develop peritoneal signs, such as abdominal rigidity and abdominal pain on palpation, with rebound tenderness, fever, and tachycardia.[12] If surgical intervention is not performed early in the course of the disease, patients will develop sepsis, hypotension, and renal failure, and will die.

Diagnosis of AMI

Acute intestinal ischemia causes several laboratory abnormalities, which are usually nonspecific. Leukocytosis with a left shift is common.[4,14,19,22,25,27] The serum amylase concentration may be elevated.[25,28] Metabolic acidosis as a result of lactic acid accumulation develops in most patients.[19,22,29] In addition, intestinal necrosis is associated with elevated serum lactate, phosphate, and alkaline phosphatase levels, and with prerenal azotemia, hypoxemia, bacteremia, and sepsis.[27–33]

Plain abdominal radiographs may show no abnormalities until late in the clinical course. They are, however, useful in identifying other serious intra-abdominal conditions, such as small bowel obstruction, adynamic ileus, colonic pseudo-obstruction, and mechanical obstruction, which usually show nonspecific radiographic patterns of intestinal dilation, focal gas-filled bowel loops, thickened bowel loops, and air-fluid levels.

Specific radiographic findings include thumbprinting from intestinal edema, hemorrhage, and muscle necrosis, resulting in rigid aperistaltic bowel loops in approximately 25% of patients.[34] Ominous roentgenographic findings include pneumoperitoneum as a result of intestinal perforation; pneumatosis intestinalis; or portal vein pneumatosis (gas-forming bacteria in the bowel wall or extending into the portal vein).[35] Duplex ultrasonography of the mesenteric arteries may be useful to diagnose acute mesenteric occlusion but is dependent on adequate preparation, such as fasting and technologist experience.

Computed tomographic angiography (CTA) is a sensitive and specific imaging modality to assess vascular patency of the mesenteric arterial and venous system. In addition, pneumatosis of the intestinal wall can be quickly diagnosed, and 3-dimensional reconstructions allow visualization of complex anatomy.[35,36]

Invasive angiography remains the gold standard diagnostic test for confirming or excluding the diagnosis of mesenteric occlusive disease (see **Fig. 3**). Angiography is also important for the definitive diagnosis of nonocclusive mesenteric ischemia. Angiography is important to determine the anatomy before performing either surgical or endovascular revascularization. The decision to proceed with mesenteric angiography before exploratory laparotomy may be difficult in some circumstances and must be individualized according to the patient's clinical condition.[5,32]

Management of AMI

General measures

Patients with AMI require aggressive fluid resuscitation and hydration. In addition, their metabolic acidosis and electrolyte imbalances must be corrected and they should be given antibiotic coverage for gram-negative and anaerobic bacteria. Intestinal decompression with a nasogastric tube is important, and discontinuation of medications that promote splanchnic vasoconstriction, such as vasopressin and digoxin, is also recommended.[19,22,23]

Surgical therapy

The traditional treatment of AMI has been surgical revascularization with exploratory laparotomy for assessment of intestinal viability and resection of the infarcted bowel.[8] The initial steps after laparotomy are to determine or confirm the cause and extent of the mesenteric occlusive disease and to assess bowel viability.[19,20,37,38] The surgical treatment of AMI includes mesenteric arterial embolectomy and mesenteric artery bypass, in addition to removal of necrotic bowel during the surgical procedure. Early diagnosis and treatment are critical to decrease the incidence of intestinal infarction and the need for bowel resection, and have a dramatic impact on procedural mortality.[19,20,38]

Pooled data from 24 studies describing the surgical outcome of 1234 patients with AMI between 1967 and 2000 showed a mortality rate of 69% (range, 24%–92%).[38] Determination of bowel viability and removal of necrotic bowel are critical, because infarcted intestine causes bowel perforation, peritonitis, and sepsis. In some instances, when questionably viable bowel is not removed at initial laparotomy, patients are returned to the operating room for a "second-look" laparotomy 12 to 36 weeks after the initial surgical procedure.[19,20,39]

Endovascular therapy

Percutaneous catheter–based endovascular revascularization procedures may be performed at invasive angiography.[38,40–43] The success of endovascular strategies for treating AMI ultimately depends on the promptness of diagnosis and early initiation of therapy. Several small series have also shown the successful use of local infusions of fibrinolytic therapy for thrombotic occlusions.[44–49] A drawback of catheter-directed fibrinolysis is that reperfusion may take several hours, potentially jeopardizing intestinal viability or worsening intestinal ischemia/infarction. Therefore, these patients require close surveillance.

Whether every patient with AMI should undergo laparoscopic assessment or exploratory laparotomy to rule out bowel infarction is debatable. Many experts advocate the use of routine surgical exploration to assess intestinal viability and removal of necrotic bowel.[38] Investigators have suggested that patients who have undergone an angiographically successful endovascular procedure can be managed with minimally invasive laparoscopic assessment for intestinal viability or no surgical exploration at all.[42,43]

CMI
Prevalence

Mesenteric arterial stenoses occur commonly, particularly in the elderly population with established atherosclerotic disease. An angiographic study found asymptomatic mesenteric stenosis in 40% of patients with abdominal aortic aneurysm, 29% with aortoiliac obstructive disease, and 25% with peripheral arterial disease of the lower extremities.[50] Ultrasound surveillance in a healthy group of elderly individuals (age >65 years) found a 17.5% prevalence of asymptomatic (>70%) stenosis in at least one mesenteric artery.[50,51] Although occlusive mesenteric artery stenosis is common, the development of symptoms of CMI is unusual, probably because of the rich communication among the 3 mesenteric vessels and the development of collaterals from other arteries.

Etiology

Atherosclerotic disease is the predominant (>95%) cause of mesenteric arterial stenoses.[14] Other causes of CMI include vascular conditions, such as fibromuscular dysplasia, Takayasu disease, Buerger disease, and radiation-induced and autoimmune arteritis.[52,53]

The origin of the celiac trunk from the aorta can be extrinsically compressed by the arcuate ligament of the diaphragm, causing significant, sometimes critical, stenosis of this vessel.[54] Whether isolated extrinsic compression of the celiac trunk can lead to the development of symptomatic chronic mesenteric ischemia or the so-called celiac axis compression syndrome or median arcuate compression syndrome has been debated.[55,56]

Natural History

Few data address the progression of mesenteric arterial disease, and consequently the natural history of this condition is incompletely understood.[57,58] In asymptomatic patients with established mesenteric atherosclerotic disease, development of AMI or CMI occurs only in patients with multivessel involvement. A prospective study using invasive abdominal angiography in 980 patients showed significant (>50%) stenosis of at least 1 mesenteric artery in 82 patients. At a mean follow-up of 2.6 years, CMI only developed in 4 (4.9%) of the 82 patients, and these had involvement of all 3 mesenteric arteries.[59]

The natural history of patients with symptomatic CMI is the opposite. Some investigators have suggested that between 20% and 50% of patients with symptomatic CMI will develop AMI.[1] The remaining patients continue to experience symptomatic chronic postprandial abdominal pain, weight loss, and emaciation.[60]

Pathophysiology of CMI

Symptoms of CMI usually develop when at least 2 mesenteric arteries are affected by hemodynamically significant stenoses.[57,59] Single-vessel stenosis rarely causes CMI, except when mesenteric arterial interconnections are congenitally poorly developed; in acute or subacute stenoses in which little time is available for the development of collaterals; or in patients in whom it was previously interrupted because of previous abdominal surgery or intestinal resection.

Clinical Presentation

The typical symptoms of CMI include abdominal pain, usually triggered by food ingestion, and weight loss (**Table 1**).[18] The abdominal pain is usually described as dull aching and sometimes as "crampy" in the periumbilical area. It begins within 1 hour after food ingestion and subsides 1 to 2 hours later. Because of the postprandial abdominal pain, many patients develop a so-called fear of food and decrease their caloric intake, resulting in weight loss. Patients with typical CMI commonly have a 20- to 40-lb weight loss by the time of diagnosis.[57] Significant weight loss may help differentiate patients with functional bowel symptoms from those with CMI. Patients with CMI may have an abdominal bruit localized in the epigastrium that may be heard.

Table 1
Most frequent symptoms of CMI

Typical symptoms	78%
• Postprandial abdominal pain	
• Fear for food	
• Weight loss	
Ischemic gastropathy	14%
• Nausea, vomiting	
• Fullness	
• Abdominal pain	
• Right upper quadrant discomfort	
• Weight loss	
Ischemic colitis	8%
• Abdominal pain	
• Gastrointestinal bleeding	
• Hematochezia	

Data from Silva JA, White CJ, Collins TJ, et al. Endovascular therapy for chronic mesenteric ischemia. J Am Coll Cardiol 2006;47:944–50.

Ischemic gastropathy, ischemic colitis, and malabsorption are manifestations of CMI (see **Table 1**). Ischemic gastropathy usually manifests as nausea, vomiting, fullness, right upper quadrant discomfort, abdominal pain, and weight loss.[61–63] Ischemic colitis usually manifests as abdominal pain, gastrointestinal bleeding, and/or hematochezia.[27,57,64,65]

Diagnosis of CMI

The diagnosis of CMI is often challenging. Some investigators have reported that only 50% of patients with CMI present with typical symptoms.[66] The authors recently reported on a series of 59 patients with CMI, and found a typical presentation in 78%, and ischemic gastropathy or ischemic colitis in the remaining 22%.[67]

Table 2						
Results of CMI with surgical revascularization						
	N	Procedural Mortality	Procedural Morbidity	Symptoms Relief	Symptoms Recurrence	Follow-Up (y)
Hollier et al,[74] 1981	56	8.9%	—	96%	26.5%	3
Cunningham et al,[75] 1991	85	12%	47%	97%	14%	5
Cormier et al,[76] 1991	103	4%	—	—	4%	5.5
McAfee et al,[77] 1992	58	10%	49%	96%	10%	3.3
Christensen et al,[78] 1994	53	0%	—	—	30%	
Gentile et al,[79] 1994	23	0%	—	100%	10%	3.3
Johnston et al,[80] 1995	21	0%	19%	—	14%	
Taylor and Porter,[81] 1995	58	0%	9%	—	4%	4.5
Mateo et al,[82] 1999	85	8%	33%	81%	24%	4.8
Foley et al,[83] 2000	49	12%	35%	—	21%	3.5
Cho et al,[84] 2002	25	4%	60%	—	21%	5.3
English et al,[85] 2004	58	29%	62%	94%	43%	3

Table 3
Results of CMI treated with stent placement

	N	Procedural Success	Symptom Relief	In-Hospital Mortality	Procedural Complications	Symptom Recurrence	Primary Patency Rate	Follow-Up (mo)
Sheeran et al,[87] 1999	12	92%	83%	8%	0%	18%	83%	15.7
Sharafuddin et al,[88] 2003	25	96%	88%	0%	12%	17%	92%	15
Silva et al,[67] 2006	59	96%	88%	1.7%	2.5%	17%	71%	38
AbuRahma et al,[89] 2003	22	96%	95%	0%	0%	34%	30%	26
Resch et al,[90] 2005	17	94%	82%	5.8%	5.8%	17%	69%	14
Brown et al,[91] 2005	14	100%	100%	0%	0%	50%	43%	13
Schaefer et al,[92] 2006	19	96%	78%	10%	0%	22%	82%	17

The diagnosis of CMI is based on symptoms of bowel ischemia in the presence of hemodynamically significant stenoses in more than 1 mesenteric artery. Because of the difficulty in establishing this diagnosis, a multidisciplinary team approach is encouraged.[68] Duplex ultrasonography, cross-sectional imaging with CTA, and magnetic resonance angiography are all adequate to establish the presence of mesenteric arterial stenosis.[69–72] Invasive angiography is used less frequently for screening but is recommended for patients with an inconclusive noninvasive imaging study or in whom revascularization therapy is being considered.

Management of CMI

Medical therapy

Patients with CMI, like others with atherosclerotic vascular disease, should be treated with aggressive lipid-lowering therapy, smoking cessation, optimization of blood pressure, diabetes control, and antiplatelet therapy with aspirin. In addition, because of the detrimental actions of digoxin in the splanchnic circulation, which cause vasoconstriction and ischemia, it should be avoided in these individuals.[9]

Although some patients with CMI may experience improvement or relief of symptoms with medical therapy, they usually experience disease progression and development of AMI, inanition, and death unless revascularization is performed. Therefore, the current recommendation is for all patients with symptomatic CMI to be referred for either endovascular or surgical revascularization therapy.[73]

Surgical therapy

Open surgery for CMI includes a variety of surgical techniques, with reported early success rates of 91% to 96% and late success rates between 80% and 90%.[37,57] **Table 2** summarizes the outcomes of 12 surgical studies, showing mortality rates ranging from 0% to 29% and morbidity rates ranging from 9% to 62%.[74–85] These results have been confirmed by a recent surgical study of 336 patients from the Nationwide Inpatient Sample as part of the Healthcare Cost and Utilization Project, showing an in-hospital mortality rate of 14.7% for surgical revascularization for CMI, a complication rate of 44.6%, and a median hospital stay of 14 days.[86]

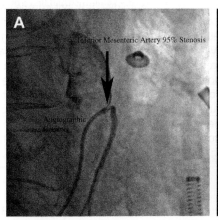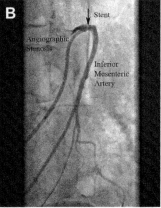

Fig. 4. (A) Angiogram of a critical 95% stenosis of the ostium of the inferior mesenteric artery (IMA) in a patient with CMI. (B) Angiogram after treatment of the IMA with a stent (arrow) placement showing an excellent angiographic result.

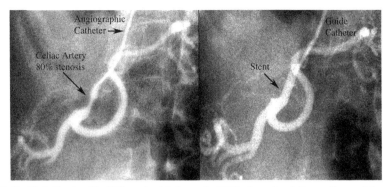

Fig. 5. (*Left*) Patient with CMI and a high-grade 80% stenosis at the ostium of the celiac artery. (*Right*) After endovascular stent (*arrow*) placement.

Endovascular therapy

Catheter-based endovascular revascularization techniques are generally preferred alternatives to open surgery because of the lower morbidity. Endovascular therapies may be repeated if necessary, generally without increased patient risk compared with the first procedure, and prior angioplasty does not preclude surgery if required at a later date.

Aorto-ostial stenoses are common causes of CMI and are difficult to treat with balloon angioplasty alone because of elastic recoil. Stent placement defeats this recoil, resulting in larger lumen diameter and a higher procedural success rate than for balloon dilation alone. Data in the literature are still limited addressing the role of endoluminal stents for the treatment of CMI (**Table 3**).[67,87–93]

The authors reported favorable results of primary stent placement for CMI in 59 patients (79 vessels).[67] The procedural success rate was 96%, with symptom relief in 88%. At a mean follow-up of 38 ± 15 months, 17% had a recurrence of symptoms, but none developed AMI and all underwent successful repeat revascularization without complications (**Figs. 4** and **5**).

No comparative clinical trials exist of surgical versus percutaneous revascularization strategies. Because patients with CMI are severely malnourished and frequently experience significant cardiac and neurovascular morbidity, it is not surprising that surgical revascularization is associated with high rates of procedural morbidity ($\approx 45\%$) and mortality ($\approx 15\%$).[94] Whether patients who survive surgery have higher patency rates and symptom-free survival than those treated with stent revascularization remains controversial.[66,94,95] The results of percutaneous revascularization have prompted several investigators to advocate this strategy as the preferred treatment for patients with CMI,[91] or as a bridging procedure for further surgical revascularization in patients who experience symptom recurrence after percutaneous treatment once the surgical risk has been decreased. The complications of endovascular therapy are usually related to vascular access and include hematomas, pseudoaneurysms, abrupt occlusion, and retroperitoneal bleeding.[67,91,94,95]

REFERENCES

1. Stoney RJ, Cunningham CG. Acute mesenteric ischemia. Surgery 1993;114: 372–80.
2. Marston A. Diagnosis and management of intestinal ischemia. Ann R Coll Surg Engl 1972;50:29–41.

3. Reiner PM, Jimenez FA, Rodriguez FL. Atherosclerosis in the mesenteric circulation: observations and correlations with aortic and coronary atherosclerosis. Am Heart J 1963;66:200–9.
4. Reinus JF, Brandt LJ, Boley SJ. Ischemic diseases of the bowel. Gastroenterol Clin North Am 1990;19:319–43.
5. Rhee RY, Gloviczki P, Medoza CT, et al. Mesenteric venous thrombosis: still a lethal disease in the 1990s. J Vasc Surg 1994;20:688–97.
6. Greengard JS, Eichinger S, Griffin JH, et al. Brief report: variability of thrombosis among siblings with resistance to activated protein C due to an Arg to Gln mutation in the gene for factor 5. N Engl J Med 1994;331:1559–62.
7. Greene FL, Ariyan S, Stausel HC Jr. Mesenteric and peripheral vascular ischemia secondary to ergotism. Surgery 1977;81:176–9.
8. Svensson PJ, Dahlback B. Resistance to activated protein C as a basis for venous thrombosis. N Engl J Med 1994;330:517–22.
9. Kim EH, Gewertz BL. Chronic digitalis administration alters mesenteric vascular reactivity. J Vasc Surg 1987;5(2):382–9.
10. Nalbandian H, Sheth N, Dietrich R, et al. Intestinal ischemia caused by cocaine ingestion: report of two cases. Surgery 1985;97:374–6.
11. Granger DN, Richardson PD, Kvietys PR, et al. Intestinal blood flow. Gastroenterology 1980;78:837–63.
12. Reilly PM, Bulkley GB. Vasoactive mediators and splanchnic perfusion. Crit Care Med 1993;21(Suppl 2):S55–68.
13. Levinsky RA, Lewis RM, Bynum TE, et al. Digoxin induced intestinal vasoconstriction. The effects of proximal arterial stenosis and glucagon administration. Circulation 1975;52(1):130–6.
14. Capell M. Intestinal (mesenteric) vasculopathy I. Gastroenterol Clin North Am 1998;27:783–825.
15. Howard TJ, Plaskon LA, Wiebke EA, et al. Nonocclusive mesenteric ischemia remains a diagnostic dilemma. Am J Surg 1996;171:405–8.
16. Finucane PM, Arunachalam T, O'Dowd J, et al. Acute mesenteric infarction in elderly patients. J Am Geriatr Soc 1989;37:355–8.
17. Eldrup-Jorgensen J, Hawkins RE, Bredenberg CE. Abdominal vascular catastrophes. Surg Clin North Am 1997;77:1305–20.
18. Dunphy JE. Abdominal pain of vascular origin. Am J Med Sci 1936;192:109–12.
19. Kaleya RN, Boley SJ. Acute mesenteric ischemia. An aggressive diagnostic and therapeutic approach. Can J Surg 1992;35:613–23.
20. Endean ED, Barnes S, Kwolek CJ, et al. Surgical management of thrombotic acute intestinal ischemia. Ann Surg 2001;6:801–8.
21. Gaussorges P, Guergniant PY, Vedrinne JM, et al. Bacteremia following cardiac arrest and cardiopulmonary resuscitation. Intensive Care Med 1988;14:575–7.
22. Kaleya RN, Boley SJ. Acute mesenteric ischemia. Crit Care Clin 1995;11:479–512.
23. Ottinger LW, Austen WG. A study of 136 patients with mesenteric infarction. Surg Gynecol Obstet 1967;124:251–61.
24. Ottinger LW. The surgical management of acute occlusion of the superior mesenteric artery. Ann Surg 1978;188:721–31.
25. Marston A, Taylor M. Acute mesenteric ischemia. In: Taylor MB, Gollan JL, Steer ML, et al, editors. Gastrointestinal emergencies. 2nd edition. Baltimore (MD): Williams & Wilkins; 1997. p. 555–70.
26. Boley SJ, Kaleya RN, Brandt LJ. Mesenteric venous thrombosis. Surg Clin North Am 1992;72:183–201.

27. Boley SJ, Brandt LJ, Veith FJ. Ischemic disorders of the intestines. Curr Probl Surg 1978;15:1–85.
28. Tsai CJ, Kuo YC, Chen PC, et al. The spectrum of acute intestinal vascular failure: a collective review of 43 cases in Taiwan. Br J Clin Pract 1990;44:603–8.
29. Boley SJ, Feinstein FR, Sammartano R, et al. New concepts in the management of emboli of the superior mesenteric artery. Surg Gynecol Obstet 1981;153: 561–9.
30. Lange H, Jackel R. Usefulness of plasma lactate concentration in the diagnosis of acute abdominal disease. Eur J Surg 1994;160:381–4.
31. Koborozos B, Vyssoulis G, Manouras A, et al. Serum phosphate levels in acute bowel ischemia. Ann Surg 1985;10:242–4.
32. Barnett S, Davison E, Bradley E. Intestinal alkaline phosphatase and base deficit in mesenteric occlusion. J Surg Res 1976;20:243–6.
33. Brandt LJ, Smithline AE. Ischemic lesions of the bowel. In: Feldman M, Sleisenger MH, Scharschmidt BF, editors. Sleisenger and Fordtran's gastrointestinal and liver disease: pathophysiology, diagnosis, management. 6th edition. Philadelphia: WB Saunders; 1998. p. 2009–24.
34. Klein HM, Lensing R, Klosterhalfen B, et al. Diagnostic imaging of mesenteric infarction. Radiology 1995;197:79–82.
35. Wolf EL, Sprayregen S, Bakal CW. Radiology in intestinal ischemia: plain film, contrast, and other imaging studies. Surg Clin North Am 1992;72:107–24.
36. Perez C, Llauger J, Puig J, et al. Computed a findings in bowel ischemia. Gastrointest Radiol 1989;14:241–5.
37. Cleveland TJ, Nawaz S, Gaines PA. Mesenteric arterial ischemia: diagnosis and therapeutic options. Vasc Med 2002;7:311–21.
38. Park WM, Gloviczki P, Cherry KJ Jr, et al. Contemporary management of acute mesenteric ischemia: factors associated with survival. J Vasc Surg 2002;35: 445–52.
39. Kaleya RN, Sammartano RJ, Boley SJ. Aggressive approach to acute mesenteric ischemia. Surg Clin North Am 1992;72:157–82.
40. VanDeinse WH, Zawacki JK, Phillips D. Treatment of acute mesenteric ischemia by percutaneous transluminal angioplasty. Gastroenterology 1986;91:475–8.
41. Loomer DC, Johnson SP, Diffin DC, et al. Superior mesenteric artery stent placement in a patient with acute mesenteric ischaemia. J Vasc Interv Radiol 1999;10: 29–32.
42. Leduc FJ, Pestieau SR, Detry O, et al. Acute mesenteric ischemia: minimal invasive management by combined laparoscopy and percutaneous transluminal angioplasty. Eur J Surg 2000;166:345–7.
43. Demirpolat G, Oran I, Tamsel S, et al. Acute mesenteric ischemia: endovascular therapy. Abdom Imaging 2007;32(3):299–303.
44. Calin GA, Calin S, Ionescu R, et al. Successful local fibrinolytic treatment and balloon angioplasty in superior mesenteric arterial embolism: a case report and literature review. Hepatogastroenterology 2003;50:732–4.
45. Simo G, Echenagusia AJ, Camunez F, et al. Superior mesenteric arterial embolism: local fibrinolytic treatment with urokinase. Radiology 1997;204:775–9.
46. Turegano Fuentes F, Simo Muerza G, Echenagusia Belda A, et al. Successful intraarterial fragmentation and urokinase therapy in superior mesenteric artery embolism. Surgery 1995;117:712–4.
47. McBride KD, Gaines PA. Thrombolysis of a potentially occluding superior mesenteric artery thromboembolus by infusion of streptokinase. Cardiovasc Intervent Radiol 1994;17:164–6.

48. Boyer L, Delorme JM, Alexandre M, et al. Local fibrinolysis for superior mesenteric artery thromboembolism. Cardiovasc Intervent Radiol 1994;17:214–6.
49. Gallego AM, Ramirez P, Rodriguez JM, et al. Role of urokinase in the superior mesenteric artery embolism. Surgery 1996;120:111–3.
50. Valentine RJ, Martin JD, Myers SI, et al. Asymptomatic celiac and superior mesenteric artery stenoses are more prevalent among patients with unsuspected renal artery stenoses. J Vasc Surg 1991;14:195–9.
51. Hansen KJ, Wilson DB, Craven TE, et al. Mesenteric artery disease in the elderly. J Vasc Surg 2004;40:45–52.
52. Palubinskas AJ, Ripley HR. Fibromuscular hyperplasia in extra-renal arteries. Radiology 1964;82:451–4.
53. Harris MT, Lewis BS. Systemic diseases affecting the mesenteric circulation. Surg Clin North Am 1992;72:245–59.
54. Stanley JC, Fry WJ. Median arcuate ligament syndrome. Arch Surg 1971;103:252–8.
55. Bech FR. Celiac artery compression syndromes. Surg Clin North Am 1997;77: 409–24.
56. Reilly LM, Ammar AD, Stoney RJ, et al. Late results following operative repair for celiac artery compression syndrome. J Vasc Surg 1985;2:79–91.
57. van Bockel JH, Geelkerken RH, Wasser MN. Chronic splanchnic ischemia. Best Pract Res Clin Gastroenterol 2001;15:99–119.
58. Zierler RE, Bergelin RO, Isaacson JS, et al. Natural history of atherotic renal artery stenosis: a prospective study with duplex ultrasonography. J Vasc Surg 1994;19: 250–7.
59. Thomas JH, Blake K, Pierce GE, et al. The clinical course of asymptomatic mesenteric arterial stenosis. J Vasc Surg 1998;27:840–4.
60. Kwaan JH, Connolly JE. Prevention of intestinal infarction resulting from mesenteric arterial occlusive disease. Surg Gynecol Obstet 1983;157:321–4.
61. Liberski SM, Koch KL, Atnip RG, et al. Ischemic gastroparesis: resolution after revascularization. Gastroenterology 1990;99:252–7.
62. Babu SC, Shah PM. Celiac territory ischemic syndrome in visceral artery occlusion. Am J Surg 1993;166:227–30.
63. Kathleen MC, Quigley TM, Kozarek RA, et al. Lethal nature of ischemic gastropathy. Am J Surg 1993;165:646–9.
64. Geelkerken RH, Schulze Kool LJ, Breslau PJ, et al. Transient colonic ischemia: consequence of a rare anatomical variation of the mesenteric arteries. Eur J Surg 1996;162:827–9.
65. Cappell MS. Intestinal (mesenteric) vasculopathy. II. Ischemic colitis and chronic mesenteric ischemia. Gatroenterol Clin North Am 1998;27:827–60, vi.
66. Geelkerken RH, Van Bockel JH, De Roos WK, et al. Chronic mesenteric vascular syndrome. Results of reconstructive surgery. Arch Surg 1991;126:1101–6.
67. Silva JA, White CJ, Collins TJ, et al. Endovascular therapy for chronic mesenteric ischemia. J Am Coll Cardiol 2006;47:944–50.
68. Bradbury AW, Brittenden J, McBride K, et al. Mesenteric ischaemia: a multidisciplinary approach. Br J Surg 1995;82:1446–59.
69. Geelkerken RH, Van Bockel JH. Duplex ultrasound examination of splachnic vessels in the assessment of splachnic ischemic symptoms. Eur J Vasc Endovasc Surg 1999;18:371–4.
70. Moneta GL, Lee RW, Yeager RA, et al. Mesenteric duplex scanning: a blinded prospective study. J Vasc Surg 1993;17:79–86.
71. Behar JV, Nelson RC, Zidar JP, et al. Thin-section multidetector CT angiography of renal artery stents. AJR Am J Roentgenol 2002;178:1155–9.

72. Maintz D, Tombach B, Juergens KU, et al. Revealing in-stent restenoses of the iliac arteries: comparison of multidetector CT with MR angiography and digital radiographic angiography in a phantom model. Am J Roentgenol 2002;179: 1319–22.

73. Hirsh AT, Haskal ZJ, Hertzer NR, et al. ACC/AHA 2005 Guidelines for the management of patients with peripheral arterial disease (lower extremity, renal, mesenteric, and abdominal aortic): executive summary. J Am Coll Cardiol 2006;47: 1239–312.

74. Hollier LH, Bernatz PE, Pairolero PC, et al. Surgical management of chronic intestinal ischemia: a reappraisal. Surgery 1981;90:940–6.

75. Cunningham CG, Reilly LM, Rapp JH, et al. Chronic visceral ischemia. Three decades of progress. Ann Surg 1991;214:276–88.

76. Cormier JM, Fichelle JM, Vennin J, et al. Atherosclerotic occlusive disease of the superior mesenteric artery: late results of reconstructive surgery. Ann Vasc Surg 1991;5:510–8.

77. McAfee MK, Cherry KJ, Naessens JM, et al. Influence of complete revascularization on chronic mesenteric ischemia. Am J Surg 1992;164:220–4.

78. Christensen MG, Lorentzen JE, Schroeder TV. Revascularization of atherosclerotic mesenteric arteries: experience in 90 consecutive patients. Eur J Vasc Surg 1994;8:297–302.

79. Gentile AT, Moneta GL, Taylor LM, et al. Isolated bypass to the superior mesenteric artery for intestinal ischemia. Arch Surg 1994;129:926–31.

80. Johnston KW, Lindsay TF, Walker PM, et al. Mesenteric arterial bypass grafts: early and late results and suggested surgical approach for chronic and acute mesenteric ischemia. Surgery 1995;118:1–7.

81. Taylor LM, Porter JM. Treatment of chronic visceral ischemia. In: Rutherford RB, editor. Vascular surgery. Philadelphia: WB Saunders; 1995. p. 1301–11.

82. Mateo RB, O'Hara PJ, Hertzer NR, et al. Elective surgical treatment of symptomatic chronic mesenteric occlusive disease: early results and late outcomes. J Vasc Surg 1999;29:821–32.

83. Foley MI, Moneta GL, Abou-Zamzam AM, et al. Revascularization of the superior mesenteric artery alone for the treatment of intestinal ischemia. J Vasc Surg 2000; 32:37–47.

84. Cho JS, Carr JA, Jacobsen G, et al. Long-term outcome after mesenteric artery reconstruction: a 37-year experience. J Vasc Surg 2002;35:453–60.

85. English WP, Pearce JD, Craven TE, et al. Chronic visceral ischemia: symptom-free survival after open surgical repair. Vasc Endovascular Surg 2004;38:493–503.

86. Derrow AE, Seeger JM, Dame DA, et al. The outcome in the United States after thoracoabdominal aortic aneurysm repair, renal artery bypass, and mesenteric revascularization. J Vasc Surg 2001;34:54–61.

87. Sheeran SR, Murphy TP, Khwaja A, et al. Stent placement for the treatment of mesenteric artery stenosis or occlusions. J Vasc Interv Radiol 1999;10:861–7.

88. Sharafuddin MJ, Olson CH, Sun S, et al. Endovascular treatment of celiac and mesenteric arteries stenoses: applications and results. J Vasc Surg 2003;38: 692–8.

89. AbuRahma AF, Stone PA, Bates MC, et al. Angioplasty/stenting of the superior mesenteric artery and celiac trunk: early and late outcomes. J Endovasc Ther 2003;10:1046–53.

90. Resch T, Lindh M, Dias N, et al. Endovascular recanalisation in occlusive mesenteric ischemia—feasibility and early results. Eur J Vasc Endovasc Surg 2005;29: 199–203.

91. Brown DJ, Schermerhorn ML, Powell RJ, et al. Mesenteric stenting for chronic mesenteric ischemia. J Vasc Surg 2005;42:268–74.
92. Schaefer PJ, Schaefer FK, Hinrichsen H, et al. Stent placement with the monorail technique for treatment of mesenteric artery stenosis. J Vasc Interv Radiol 2006; 17(4):637–43.
93. Rose SC, Quigley TM, Raker EJ. Revascularization for chronic mesenteric ischemia: comparison of operative bypass grafting and percutaneous translumi-nal angioplasty. J Vasc Interv Radiol 1995;6:339–49.
94. Kasirajan K, O'Hara PJ, Gray BH, et al. Chronic mesenteric ischemia. Open surgery versus percutaneous angioplasty and stenting. J Vasc Surg 2001;33: 63–71.
95. Sivamurthy N, Rhodes JM, Lee D, et al. Endovascular versus open mesenteric revascularization: immediate benefits do not equate with short term functional outcomes. J Am Coll Surg 2006;202:859–67.

Vascular Medicine
Aortic and Peripheral Arterial Disease

Fadi Elias Shamoun, MD[a], Grant T. Fankhauser, MD[b],
Martina Mookadam, MD[c],*

KEYWORDS

- Abdominal aortic aneurysm • Aortic dissection • Medical therapy
- Peripheral vascular disease

KEY POINTS

- The medical management of patients with an abdominal aortic aneurysm (AAA) includes modification of risk factors, smoking cessation, cardiovascular risk treatment, and hypertensive therapy. One small study showed that mild exercise could decrease the rate of progression; however, no specific therapy has been shown to alter disease outcome.
- Many AAA and thoracic aortic aneurysms are now amenable to endovascular treatment. Endovascular repair offers the benefit of shorter hospital stays and lower perioperative morbidity and mortality.
- Most patients with peripheral arterial disease (PAD) are asymptomatic or have atypical symptoms; only a few present with classic intermittent claudication or critical limb ischemia. Smoking and diabetes mellitus are the most important risk factors for developing PAD.

INTRODUCTION

Vascular diseases are among the most challenging problems in primary care. Patients with aortic and peripheral vascular diseases are at higher risk of morbidity and mortality from a cardiovascular stand point. The complexity of these cases and new advances in medical and interventional procedures will increase treatment options. This review discusses the management of patients with aortic aneurysmal diseases, acute aortic syndrome, peripheral vascular disease screening, and medical therapy.

The authors have nothing to disclose.
[a] Department of Carviovascular Medicine, Mayo Clinic, 13400 East Shea Boulevard, Scottsdale, AZ 85259, USA; [b] Department of Vascular Surgery, Mayo Clinic, 13400 East Shea Boulevard, Scottsdale, AZ 85259, USA; [c] Department of Family Medicine, Mayo Clinic, 13400 East Shea Boulevard, Scottsdale, AZ 85259, USA
* Corresponding author.
E-mail address: mookadam.martina@mayo.edu

Prim Care Clin Office Pract 40 (2013) 169–177
http://dx.doi.org/10.1016/j.pop.2012.11.001
0095-4543/13/$ – see front matter © 2013 Elsevier Inc. All rights reserved.

ANEURYSMS OF THE AORTA
Epidemiology of AAAs

Abdominal aortic aneurysms (AAAs) are the thirteenth leading cause of death in the United States. They are the tenth leading cause of death in men older than 65 years. AAAs occur in 2% to 6.5% of men older than 60 years, with 10% to 15% of these cases being familial. Most of the persons who have an AAA (80%) are asymptomatic and are diagnosed incidentally.[1] In a few, the AAA can cause pain in the abdomen, the back, or the flank. Physical examination may reveal a pulsatile abdominal mass or livedo of the extremities, which indicates atheroembolism (**Fig. 1**). The atheroembolisms result in blue or gangrenous toes, livedo reticularis, accelerating hypertension, increased serum creatinine level, and eosinophilia. Other aneurysms such as a popliteal aneurysm may also be present in patients who have an AAA. Popliteal artery aneurysms tend to lead to arterial ischemia rather than rupture.

The prevalence of AAAs and their risk factors was studied in the ADAM (Aneurysm Detection and Management) trial, which enrolled 73,451 US veterans aged 50 to 79 years. The prevalence was found to be 4.6% in the general population versus 5.9% in white male smokers and 1.9% in white female smokers. Risk factors associated with AAAs included smoking (odds ratio [OR], 5.57), family history of AAA (OR, 1.95), age (OR, 1.65), coronary artery disease (OR, 1.62), hyperlipidemia (OR, 1.54), and chronic obstructive pulmonary disease (OR, 1.28).[2]

AAA screening is typically based on physical examination; however, the physical examination alone lacks sensitivity.[3] Screening as recommended by the US Preventive Services Task Force involves 1-time screening ultrasonography for men aged 65 to 75 years who have a history of smoking.[1] Kim and colleagues[4] conducted a cost-saving analysis for AAA screening. Estimated savings during a 7-year follow-up were 19,500 per year per life saved.

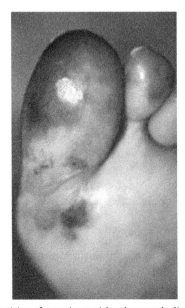

Fig. 1. Livedo on the extremities of a patient with atheroembolism. Classic skin discoloration on the left leg of a patient with an ascending aortic atheroma indicates atheroemboli secondary to an AAA.

Medical Management of AAAs

The medical management of patients with an AAA includes risk factor modification, smoking cessation, cardiovascular risk treatment, and hypertensive therapy. One small study showed that mild exercise could decrease the rate of progression,[5] however, no specific therapy has been shown to alter disease outcome.

Screening for AAA Size and Growth Rate

According to several investigators,[6–8] the clinical indications for AAA repair include 1 of the following criteria:

1. Diameter greater than 5.0 cm
2. Expansion rate of more than 0.5 cm/year
3. Inflammatory or infectious cause
4. Concomitant recurrent atheroaneurysms
5. Symptomatic or ruptured AAA

AAA Repair Outcomes

The EVAR[9] (Endovascular Aneurysm Repair) trial was a randomized trial of open surgical AAA repair in 626 patients compared with endovascular AAA repair in 626 patients. The EVAR researchers found comparable AAA-related mortality within 6 years of AAA repair and comparable all-cause mortality within 2 years (**Fig. 2**).[9] In a large population-based study of US Medicare recipients undergoing AAA repair, Schermerhorn and colleagues[10] found that patients undergoing endovascular procedures suffered fewer medical complications after repair compared with patients having

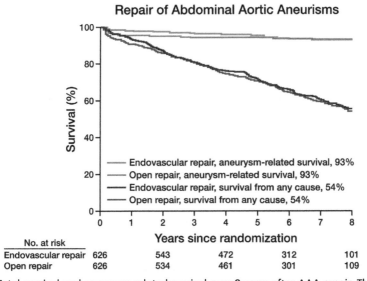

Fig. 2. Total survival and aneurysm-related survival over 8 years after AAA repair. The early benefit of lower aneurysm-related mortality after endovascular repair was lost over time, partly because of fatal endograft ruptures, until by year 8 there was no significant difference in the risk of death from any cause between the 2 groups. (*Modified from* Greenhalgh RM, Brown LC, Powell JT, et al; United Kingdom EVAR Trial Investigators. Endovascular versus open repair of abdominal aortic aneurysm. N Engl J Med 2010;362:1869; with permission.)

open repair (n = 22,830 in the matched cohorts), regardless of age. However, late survival was similar for the 2 groups, converging after 3 years (**Fig. 3**).[10]

As a result of these and other findings, AAA treatment recommendations were recently updated by a consortium of professional medical groups, including the American College of Cardiology Foundation, the American Heart Association Task Force on Practice, the American Stroke Association, and representatives from thoracic surgery, radiology, cardiovascular anesthesiology, cardiovascular angiography, and vascular medicine.[11] In particular, the group agreed that no firm recommendation could be made on the optimal treatment approach to AAAs. The available evidence regarding open versus endovascular procedures is inadequate to make firm recommendations regarding the optimal method of treatment. The early mortality advantage of endovascular procedures may be lost during follow-up.[11]

Thoracic Aortic Aneurysms

The prevalence of thoracic aortic aneurysms in the general population may be as high as 10.4 per 100,000 person-years, with men and women equally affected, as found in the 1998 population-based epidemiologic study conducted by Clouse and colleagues[12] of the population of Olmsted County, Minnesota, for 1980 to 1994. The overall 5-year survival in 133 patients with degenerative thoracic aortic aneurysms was 56% for the 15-year period studied. However, female sex was associated with an increased risk of rupture (risk ratio, 6.8; 95% confidence interval, 2.3–19.9; $P = .01$).[12]

Risk factors include hypertension, history of familial aneurysms, congenital bicuspid aortic valve, connective tissue disease, and the syndromes Ehlers-Danlos, Marfan, Loeys-Dietz, and Turner. Infectious and inflammatory causes include syphilis, giant cell arteritis, Takayasu arteritis, Behçet syndrome, ankylosing spondylitis, and deceleration trauma. Thoracic aortic aneurysms have a 5-year cumulative risk of rupture of about 16% if they measure 4 to 5.9 cm and almost double that (31%) if they are greater than 6 cm.[12]

The indications for surgery in thoracic abdominal aneurysms are: (1) diameter greater than 5.5 cm; (2) symptomatic; (3) rapid enlargement; (4) traumatic origin;

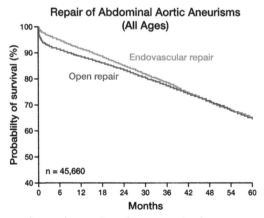

Fig. 3. Survival after endovascular repair and open repair of AAAs. By postoperative year 3, survival of patients treated surgically for AAAs differed little by type of procedure (endovascular repair or open repair). (*Modified from* Schermerhorn ML, O'Malley AJ, Jhaveri A, et al. Endovascular vs. open repair of abdominal aortic aneurysms in the Medicare population. N Engl J Med 2008;358:470; with permission.)

(5) infections caused by syphilis and rarely from mycotic aneurysms from bacterial endocarditis; (6) bicuspid aortic valve; and (7) Marfan or Turner syndromes.[11,13]

The natural history of thoracic abdominal aneurysms, as studied in the Yale database, showed a progressive enlargement of 0.1 to 0.25 cm per year.[13] Factors that worsen prognosis include diastolic hypertension, size greater than 6 cm of the ascending aorta, traumatic aneurysm, and association with coronary artery disease and carotid disease.

Medical management includes β-blockers to control changes in blood pressure and a vasodilator. Patients should discontinue tobacco use and should undergo treatment of any associated coronary and carotid disease. Follow-up clinical and noninvasive imaging tests should be conducted at 3 months, then at 6 months, and then yearly, depending on the case.[14] Most AAA and many thoracic aortic aneurysms are now amenable to endovascular treatment. Endovascular repair offers the benefit of shorter hospital stays and lower perioperative morbidity and mortality. These advantages come at the expense of higher costs and more frequent reintervention. In most cases, anatomy determines the eligibility for endovascular treatment. Aneurysms around the renal or visceral arteries (celiac or superior mesenteric) precluded endovascular treatment in the past; however, new advances in endografts with branches or fenestrations for the renal and visceral arteries open the possibility for endovascular treatment of aneurysms previously deemed unsuitable. Patients unfit for large, open surgeries may soon be able to undergo less invasive treatment of thoracic aortic aneurysms and AAAs.[15]

Acute Aortic Dissection

Most patients with acute aortic dissection (98%) present with severe chest or back pain. Acute aortic dissections are associated with hypertension (49%), aortic regurgitation (28%), pulse deficit, deferential blood pressure (31%), and focal neurologic deficit (17%).[16,17] Chest pain with congestive heart failure, shock, cerebrovascular accidents, syncope, paraplegia, and acute arterial occlusion should raise the suspicion of acute aortic dissection. Chest radiographs usually reveal a widened mediastinum and an increased aortic diameter, tracheal deviation to the right, and left pleural effusion; however, a normal chest radiograph does not exclude aortic dissection. Involvement of the ascending thoracic aorta (Stanford type A) is a surgical emergency, with mortality near 11%, and surgery requiring complete circulatory arrest. Type B aortic dissections are treated medically (and overall have the best prognosis among all aortic dissections). Medical therapy includes intravenous β-blockers and pain control in the acute phase and long-term blood pressure control. Surgical treatment of type B aortic dissections is indicated in cases of end-organ ischemia or refractory pain.[11,18]

Peripheral Arterial Disease

Most patients with peripheral arterial disease (PAD) are asymptomatic or have atypical symptoms; only a few present with classic intermittent claudication or critical limb ischemia. Smoking and diabetes mellitus are the most important risk factors for developing PAD.[6] In a primary care population defined by age and common risk factors, the prevalence of PAD was approximately 1 in 3 patients.[19] The prevalence of PAD increases with age, ranging from less than 10% for persons aged 55 to 59 years to almost 60% for persons aged 85 to 89 years.[20,21]

PAD is a coronary artery disease risk equivalent, and patients with both coronary artery disease and PAD have a 4.6% increase in all-cause mortality and a 23.1% risk of cardiovascular death, myocardial infarction, stroke, or hospitalization for atheroembolic events.[22,23] Cardiovascular and all-cause mortality correlate with ankle brachial index (**Fig. 4**).[24] A good reference on PAD for patient education can be found at the Web site of the Vascular Disease Foundation (http://www.vdf.org/). On physical examination, patients with PAD may have elevation pallor and dependent rubor (**Fig. 5**). Ankle brachial index (ABI) is more than 95% sensitive and specific for patients with PAD (ABI >1.30 is noncompressible; 1.0–1.29 is normal; 0.91–0.99 is borderline or equivocal; 0.41–0.9 is mild to moderate; and 0.0–0.4 reflects severe PAD, with patients likely to have rest pain).

The most effective therapy for PAD and claudication is exercise (PAD rehabilitation program), with more than 100% improvement in pain-free walking time and distance. This treatment approach is limited by availability of programs and motivation of the patient. Medication options are limited as well. Only 2 medications are approved in the United States for claudication: cliostazol and pentoxiphyllin. The more effective is cliostazol, which can improve pain-free walking time by as much as 50%. Cliostazol is contraindicated in patients with congestive heart failure. Pentoxiphyllin is less effective, needs to be dose-adjusted in renal insufficiency, and is mostly used in patients with small vessel disease.

Angioplasty is performed in approximately 15% of patients with PAD and provides relief of symptoms. Its use may be limited by availability and cost. Lower extremity bypass surgery is also effective, often resulting in complete symptom relief. Limitations include graft failure and high morbidity and mortality in the perioperative period, and it is therefore performed in less than 5% of patients. In some studies, aspirin has been shown to be equivalent to placebo,[24] and statins have been found to have an uncertain effect on claudication.[25] Standard of care for all PAD patients must include aspirin and risk factor modification for vascular disease with statins and angiotensin-converting enzyme inhibitors.[26] Participation in an exercise training program has been associated with improvement in pain-free walking time.[27]

The indications for revascularization in patients with PAD are rest pain, nonhealing ulceration, and life-style–limiting symptoms. The 5-year primary patency rate for angioplasty with or without stenting in peripheral vessels compared with bypass grafting is shown in **Fig. 6**.[28] When comparing bypass grafting, vein grafting was superior

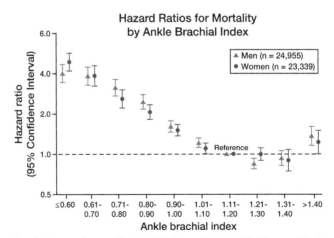

Fig. 4. Hazard ratio for total mortality by ABI. (*From* Fowkes FG, Murray GD, Butcher I, et al. Ankle brachial index combined with Framingham Risk Score to predict cardiovascular events and mortality: a meta-analysis. JAMA 2008;300(2):201; with permission.)

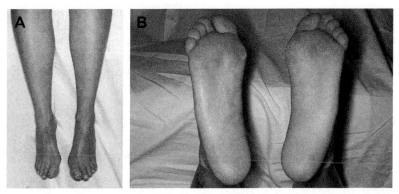

Fig. 5. Dependent rubor. A 47-year-old woman presented for an evaluation of a painful leg. Examination showed several cyanotic and mottled toes. In the dependent position, the right foot was erythematous and cool to touch (*A*). Pallor developed rapidly with foot elevation (*B*). Dependant rubor is a sign of severe PAD. This patient had an ABI of 0.4 in the right leg and 0.7 in the left.

to synthetic conduit rates of patency, although all forms of revascularization are modest in the smaller vessels. For many patients with high perioperative risk, angioplasty with and without stenting can still provide satisfactory results.

Acute arterial occlusion is manifested by 5 Ps: pain, pulselessness, pallor, paresthesias, and paralysis. These manifestations may be embolic, thrombus in situ (eg, popliteal aneurysms), or trauma and dissection (eg, those related to fibromuscular dysplasia or the vascular type of Ehler-Danlos syndrome). Treatment in these patients includes starting anticoagulation therapy, protecting the tissue of the limb with a vascular boot, pharmacologic or surgical thromboembolectomy, and bypass grafting or percutaneous transluminal angioplasty.

Symptomatic patients can benefit from endovascular intervention. Stenotic lesions from the iliac arteries to the tibial arteries are amenable to angioplasty with optional stent placement. Endovascular intervention can frequently be performed as an

5-Year Primary Patency Rates

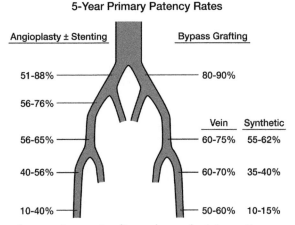

Fig. 6. Five-year primary patency rate after endovascular intervention.

outpatient procedure. Endovascular intervention is not as durable as peripheral arterial bypass, but interventions can be repeated and surgical bypass is always a later possibility. Endovascular therapy may be offered for mild to moderate claudication, whereas surgical bypass is likely not offered until rest pain or tissue loss develops. Advances in technology will make more lesions amenable to endovascular treatment and extend the patency after intervention.[6]

REFERENCES

1. Fleming C, Whitlock EP, Beil TL, et al. Screening for abdominal aortic aneurysm: a best-evidence systematic review for the U.S. Preventive Services Task Force. Ann Intern Med 2005;142:203–11.
2. Lederle FA, Johnson GR, Wilson SE, et al. Prevalence and associations of abdominal aortic aneurysm detected through screening. Aneurysm Detection and Management (ADAM) Veterans Affairs Cooperative Study Group. Ann Intern Med 1997;126:441–9.
3. Fink HA, Lederle FA, Roth CS, et al. The accuracy of physical examination to detect abdominal aortic aneurysm. Arch Intern Med 2000;160:833–6.
4. Kim LG, P Scott RA, Ashton HA, et al. A sustained mortality benefit from screening for abdominal aortic aneurysm. Ann Intern Med 2007;146:699–706.
5. Tew GA, Moss J, Crank H, et al. Endurance exercise training in patients with small abdominal aortic aneurysm: a randomised controlled pilot study. Arch Phys Med Rehabil 2012;93(12):2148–53.
6. Hirsch AT, Haskal ZJ, Hertzer NR, et al. ACC/AHA 2005 guidelines for the management of patients with peripheral arterial disease (lower extremity, renal, mesenteric, and abdominal aortic): executive summary a collaborative report from the American Association for Vascular Surgery/Society for Vascular Surgery, Society for Cardiovascular Angiography and Interventions, Society for Vascular Medicine and Biology, Society of Interventional Radiology, and the ACC/AHA Task Force on Practice Guidelines (Writing Committee to Develop Guidelines for the Management of Patients With Peripheral Arterial Disease) endorsed by the American Association of Cardiovascular and Pulmonary Rehabilitation; National Heart, Lung, and Blood Institute; Society for Vascular Nursing; TransAtlantic Inter-Society Consensus; and Vascular Disease Foundation. J Am Coll Cardiol 2006;47:1239–312.
7. Lederle FA, Johnson GR, Wilson SE, et al. Rupture rate of large abdominal aortic aneurysms in patients refusing or unfit for elective repair. JAMA 2002;287:2968–72.
8. Ashton HA, Buxton MJ, Day NE, et al, Multicentre Aneurysm Screening Study Group. The Multicentre Aneurysm Screening Study (MASS) into the effect of abdominal aortic aneurysm screening on mortality in men: a randomised controlled trial. Lancet 2002;360:1531–9.
9. United Kingdom EVAR Trial Investigators, Greenhalgh RM, Brown LC, Powell JT, et al. Endovascular versus open repair of abdominal aortic aneurysm. N Engl J Med 2010;362:1863–71.
10. Schermerhorn ML, O'Malley AJ, Jhaveri A, et al. Endovascular vs. open repair of abdominal aortic aneurysms in the Medicare population. N Engl J Med 2008;358:464–74.
11. Hiratzka LF, Bakris GL, Beckman JA, et al. 2010 ACCF/AHA/AATS/ACR/ASA/SCA/SCAI/SIR/STS/SVM guidelines for the diagnosis and management of patients with thoracic aortic disease: a report of the American College of

Cardiology Foundation/American Heart Association Task Force on Practice Guidelines, American Association for Thoracic Surgery, American College of Radiology, American Stroke Association, Society of Cardiovascular Anesthesiologists, Society for Cardiovascular Angiography and Interventions, Society of Interventional Radiology, Society of Thoracic Surgeons, and Society for Vascular Medicine. Circulation 2010;121:e266–369.

12. Clouse WD, Hallett JW Jr, Schaff HV, et al. Improved prognosis of thoracic aortic aneurysms: a population-based study. JAMA 1998;280:1926–9.

13. Elefteriades JA. Natural history of thoracic aortic aneurysms: indications for surgery, and surgical versus nonsurgical risks. Ann Thorac Surg 2002;74: S1877–80 [discussion: S1892–8].

14. Pape LA, Tsai TT, Isselbacher EM, et al. Aortic diameter >or = 5.5 cm is not a good predictor of type A aortic dissection: observations from the International Registry of Acute Aortic Dissection (IRAD). Circulation 2007;116:1120–7.

15. Dillavou ED, Muluk SC, Makaroun MS. Improving aneurysm-related outcomes: nationwide benefits of endovascular repair. J Vasc Surg 2006;43:446–51.

16. Klompas M. Does this patient have an acute thoracic aortic dissection? JAMA 2002;287:2262–72.

17. Park SW, Hutchison S, Mehta RH, et al. Association of painless acute aortic dissection with increased mortality. Mayo Clin Proc 2004;79:1252–7.

18. Hagan PG, Nienaber CA, Isselbacher EM, et al. The International Registry of Acute Aortic Dissection (IRAD): new insights into an old disease. JAMA 2000; 283:897–903.

19. Hirsch AT, Criqui MH, Treat-Jacobson D, et al. Peripheral arterial disease detection, awareness, and treatment in primary care. JAMA 2001;286:1317–24.

20. Meijer WT, Hoes AW, Rutgers D, et al. Peripheral arterial disease in the elderly: The Rotterdam Study. Arterioscler Thromb Vasc Biol 1998;18:185–92.

21. Criqui MH, Fronek A, Barrett-Connor E, et al. The prevalence of peripheral arterial disease in a defined population. Circulation 1985;71:510–5.

22. Steg PG, Bhatt DL, Wilson PW, et al. One-year cardiovascular event rates in outpatients with atherothrombosis. JAMA 2007;297:1197–206.

23. Grundy SM, Cleeman JI, Merz CN, et al. Implications of recent clinical trials for the National Cholesterol Education Program Adult Treatment Panel III guidelines. Circulation 2004;110:227–39.

24. Fowkes FG, Murray GD, Butcher I, et al. Ankle brachial index combined with Framingham Risk Score to predict cardiovascular events and mortality: a meta-analysis. JAMA 2008;300:197–208.

25. Mondillo S, Ballo P, Barbati R, et al. Effects of simvastatin on walking performance and symptoms of intermittent claudication in hypercholesterolemic patients with peripheral vascular disease. Am J Med 2003;114:359–64.

26. 2011 Writing Group Members, 2005 Writing Committee Members, ACCF/AHA Task Force Members. 2011 ACCF/AHA focused update of the guideline for the management of patients with peripheral artery disease (updating the 2005 guideline): a report of the American College of Cardiology Foundation/American Heart Association Task Force on practice guidelines. Circulation 2011;124:2020–45.

27. Hiatt WR, Wolfel EE, Meier RH, et al. Superiority of treadmill walking exercise versus strength training for patients with peripheral arterial disease. Implications for the mechanism of the training response. Circulation 1994;90:1866–74.

28. Norgren L, Hiatt WR, Dormandy JA, et al. Inter-Society Consensus for the Management of Peripheral Arterial Disease (TASC II). Eur J Vasc Endovasc Surg 2007;33:S1–35.

Hypertension

Katherine H. Winter, MD, MPH, Laura A. Tuttle, MA,
Anthony J. Viera, MD, MPH*

KEYWORDS

- Hypertension • Blood pressure • Antihypertensive therapy • Diabetes • Diuretics
- Angiotensin-converting enzyme inhibitors • Angiotensin receptor blockers
- Calcium channel blockers

KEY POINTS

- Antihypertensive treatment substantially reduces the risk of heart failure, stroke, and myocardial infarction.
- A thiazide-type diuretic such as chlorthalidone should usually be part of the therapeutic regimen, with additional agents based on comorbidities.
- Secondary causes of hypertension should be considered in all children with hypertension as well as adults with early onset hypertension or resistant hypertension.

EPIDEMIOLOGY

Hypertension is the most common modifiable risk factor for cardiovascular disease (CVD), affecting 1 in 3 American adults.[1] The risk of having hypertension increases with age (**Box 1**), with a 90% lifetime risk of developing hypertension for people living in the United States.[2] The prevalence of hypertension also varies by race/ethnicity, with non-Hispanic Blacks having the highest prevalence (38.6%).[1]

Hypertension contributes to nearly 50% of all adverse CVD outcomes in developed nations such as the United States, including myocardial infarction (MI), heart failure, stroke, and kidney disease.[1,2] In addition, CVD morbidity and mortality are positively correlated with the degree of elevation of blood pressure (BP), without any evidence of a threshold down to at least 115/75 mm Hg.[3] Control of BP can reduce heart failure, stroke, and MI risks by 50%, 40%, and 25%, respectively.[2] Recent data suggest that even among "normotensive" patients, BP-lowering drugs reduce adverse CVD outcomes in patients with risk factors for atherosclerotic disease.[4]

Data from the most recent National Health and Nutrition Examination Survey showed that although the proportion of hypertensive patients receiving pharmacologic

Disclosure: Dr Viera serves on the Medical Advisory Board for Suntech Medical, manufacturer of a brand of ambulatory blood pressure monitor.
Department of Family Medicine, University of North Carolina at Chapel Hill, 590 Manning Drive, CB 7595, Chapel Hill, NC 27599-7595, USA
* Corresponding author.
E-mail address: anthony_viera@med.unc.edu

Prim Care Clin Office Pract 40 (2013) 179–194
http://dx.doi.org/10.1016/j.pop.2012.11.008
0095-4543/13/$ – see front matter © 2013 Elsevier Inc. All rights reserved.

Box 1	
Prevalence of hypertension by age group	
Age Group	**Prevalence of Hypertension**
18–39 y	7.4%
40–64 y	35.6%
65+ y	69.7%

treatment has risen (from 60.3% to 69.9%) over the past decade, only about 46% are considered controlled (defined as systolic/diastolic BP <140/90 mm Hg).[1]

SCREENING FOR HYPERTENSION

The US Preventive Services Task Force (USPSTF) in 2007 issued a grade "A" recommendation to screen all adults aged 18 years and older for high BP.[5] The guideline recommends averaging 2 or more BPs in 2 separate office visits over a period of 1 to several weeks. The exception to this rule are those patients with a single greatly elevated BP reading in the office setting (systolic BP >200 mm Hg and/or diastolic BP >120 mm Hg) in the absence of a recognized cause of secondary elevation.[6] Although the USPSTF guideline did not specify a screening interval, the authors cite the seventh report of Joint National Committee on Prevention, Detection, Evaluation, and Treatment of High Blood Pressure (JNC7)'s guidelines of screening every 2 years in those with BP less than 120/80 mm Hg and every year in prehypertensive patients.[2,5]

CURRENT DIAGNOSIS AND MANAGEMENT GUIDELINES

The JNC developed the most widely accepted guideline for managing hypertension in the United States.[2] The most recent JNC report was published in 2003 (known as JNC7). The JNC7 report classifies hypertension into prehypertension, Stage I, and Stage II according to the degree of BP elevation (**Table 1**).[2]

Recommendations for the approach to management depend in part on whether patients have comorbidities. Major CVD comorbidities include heart failure, history of MI or stroke, coronary artery disease, diabetes, and chronic kidney disease

Table 1			
Classification of hypertension initial BP management			
BP Classification	**Systolic (mm Hg)**	**Diastolic (mm Hg)**	**Management[a]**
Prehypertension	120–139 or	80–89	Screen every year; pharmacotherapy not indicated
Stage I hypertension	140–159 or	90–99	Thiazide-type diuretic (eg, chlorthalidone) for most; consider ACEI (or ARB), BB, CCB, or combination of these depending on comorbidities
Stage II hypertension	≥160 or	≥100	Initial therapy with 2-drug combination (usually thiazide-type diuretic and ACEI or ARB, CCB, or BB)

Abbreviations: ACEI, angiotensin-converting enzyme inhibitor; ARB, angiotensin II receptor blocker; BB, beta-blocker; CCB, calcium channel blocker.
[a] For all categories, lifestyle modifications, as described in the next section, should be encouraged.

(CKD). The goal for these patients is a BP less than 130/80 mm Hg. For those without these comorbidities, the goal BP is usually less than 140/90 mm Hg. A goal of BP less than 150/90 mm Hg is reasonable for patients aged 80 years and older.[7] As a general rule, in patients with BP significantly above target level (>20/10 mm Hg), 2 BP agents should be initiated.[2] The JNC8 guideline is forthcoming at the time of this writing.

The 2007 Canadian Hypertension Education Program (CHEP) also stratifies individuals by the presence of target end-organ damage or other CVD risk factors. However, the CHEP threshold for initiating therapy among those without compelling indications is greater than or equal to 160 mm Hg systolic or greater than or equal to 100 mm Hg diastolic, or the equivalent of the JNC7's Stage II hypertension.[2,8] Otherwise the goals of therapy and recommended pharmacologic agents are similar between JNC and CHEP.

LIFESTYLE MODIFICATIONS FOR HYPERTENSION

All patients should be advised about lifestyle modifications for lowering BP. In those with mild hypertension, a 3 to 6-month trial of lifestyle modifications may be warranted before any drug therapy is prescribed. Even when drug therapy is prescribed, however, patients should be reminded that lifestyle modifications remain an important part of managing high BP. The 5 key lifestyle recommendations for managing high BP are: weight loss, exercise, the Dietary Approaches to Stopping Hypertension (DASH) eating plan, reduced sodium intake, and moderation of alcohol drinking (**Table 2**).[2]

The DASH eating plan along with limited sodium intake of 1600 mg per day can decrease BP as well as single drug therapy.[9] In some cases, lifestyle modifications may allow an individual previously taking antihypertensive drugs to decrease or even cease drug treatment.[10] Although lifestyle modifications have been shown to have a significant effect on BP, the success depends on the motivation and commitment of the patient to adhere to the modifications, as well as the physician's commitment to counsel patients on the recommendations and potential benefits.

Many patients choose to pursue natural dietary supplements to decrease BP in conjunction with or instead of lifestyle modifications or drug therapy recommended by their physician. However, quality research regarding dietary supplements continues to be limited.

Table 2
Lifestyle modifications for reducing blood pressure

Recommendation	Description	Approximate Systolic BP Reduction
Weight loss	Achieve/maintain body mass index of 18.5–24.9 kg/m²	5–20 mm Hg
DASH eating plan	Diet rich in fruits, vegetables, and low-fat dairy with reduced fat intake	8–14 mm Hg
Exercise	Regular aerobic activity at least 30 min/d	4–9 mm Hg
Reduced dietary sodium intake	Maximum 2400 mg of sodium daily (ideally 1600 mg or less)	2–8 mm Hg
Moderate alcohol drinking	Maximum 2 drinks[a] per day for men; maximum 1 drink per day for women	2–4 mm Hg

[a] A "drink" is 1 oz or 30 mL ethanol; eg, 24 oz beer, 10 oz wine, or 3 oz 80-proof whiskey.

EVALUATION

Patients with newly diagnosed hypertension should have an evaluation that consists of 3 major goals: (1) assessing concomitant cardiovascular risk factors, (2) considering secondary causes of hypertension, and (3) assessing the presence or absence of end-organ damage.[2]

Identification of other cardiovascular risk factors and comorbid conditions is essential as the presence of these risk factors (**Box 2**) substantially increase a patient's overall morbidity and mortality.[2,5] These risk factors are identified both in the patient's history and physical examination.[6] Suggested laboratory tests include an electrocardiogram, urinalysis, fasting blood glucose, hematocrit, serum potassium, creatinine, calcium, and fasting lipid profile.[2]

TARGET ORGAN DAMAGE

Chronic hypertension demonstrates a wide range of systemic effects, most prominently in the brain, heart, kidneys, and microvasculature. Damage to these organs contributes to high rates of morbidity and mortality among hypertensive patients. Examples include vascular and hemorrhagic stroke, retinopathy, left ventricular hypertrophy, proteinuria, and renal failure.

With regard to primary and secondary stroke prevention, studies estimate that BP control reduces the risk of first stroke by 32% and recurrent strokes by up to 30%.[11] Several meta-analyses have demonstrated that all classes of BP medications are similarly effective in preventing stroke; however, calcium channel blockers (CCBs) appear to be the most effective for primary prevention of stroke.[2,11–13] In addition, hypertension is the most important modifiable risk factor in vascular dementia, defined as cognitive decline secondary to destruction of brain tissue by cardiovascular insults.[14] Although the data are limited with regards to the effect that controlling BP would have on slowing the progression or preventing dementia, a recent study suggests that hypertension increases the odds of vascular dementia before stroke by 40%.[4] Target organ damage visible on the retina is associated with increased risk of stroke.[15]

SECONDARY HYPERTENSION

Secondary hypertension refers to hypertension that is attributable to an underlying identifiable cause. Approximately 10% of people with hypertension have a secondary

---

Box 2
Cardiovascular risk factors

Cigarette smoking

Obesity (body mass index $\geq$30 kg/m^2)

Physical inactivity

Dyslipidemia

Diabetes mellitus

Microalbuminuria or glomerular filtration rate <60 mL/min

Age (>55 men, >65 women)

Family history of premature CVD (men <55 years, women <65 years)

form.[16] Identification of an underlying cause is important if the underlying cause is correctable. Remember to consider exogenous agents that may be contributing to elevated BP. Commonly used medications such as oral contraceptives and antidepressants (eg, serotonin-norepinephrine reuptake inhibitors) can raise BP and a trial off these agents, if possible, may be all that is needed to reduce BP. Secondary causes should especially be considered in patients with resistant hypertension (RHTN) or those who develop hypertension early (<18 years) or late in life.[17,18] **Table 3** lists the most important causes (excluding the risk factor of obesity and elevated BP due to exogenous agents) by age group. Please note there is some overlap in causes among the categories.

Renal Artery Stenosis

In youth, renal artery stenosis (RAS) is predominantly caused by fibromuscular dysplasia (FMD), whereas in the elderly RAS is typically a result of atherosclerosis.[18,22] Although these entities differ in pathophysiology, the hemodynamic effects are similar and ultimately can lead to RHTN and impairment in renal function.[22]

FMD occurs in 4% of all adult women aged 20 to 60 years.[23] Little is known about the pathophysiology, but it is described as a noninflammatory, nonatherosclerotic arterial disease. Renal and carotid arteries are affected most, and hyperplasia of arterial lumens leads to stenotic "webs." These webs lead to aberrant flow patterns including poststenotic dilation and aneurysms. Catheter-based angiography, in conjunction with intravascular ultrasound (IVUS), is considered the gold standard for the diagnosis of FMD. IVUS detects stenosis that cannot be seen on imaging by measurement of pressure gradients. Computed tomography angiography and magnetic resonance angiography can also be used to diagnose FMD but are less sensitive in detecting stenosis (however, they can accurately identify aneurysms). Angioplasty is the treatment of choice.[23]

RAS secondary to atherosclerosis is suspected in patients with known atherosclerotic disease (coronary artery, cerebrovascular disease, or peripheral vascular disease), late onset (>55 years), severe hypertension, difficult to control hypertension, new or worsening renal dysfunction, or sudden "flash" pulmonary edema.[24] Bilateral RAS should be considered in patients with a rise in serum creatinine value of greater than or equal to 0.5 to 1 mg/dL, when started on an angiotensin-converting enzyme (ACE) inhibitor or angiotensin receptor blocker (ARB).[2,18]

In many cases, atherosclerotic RAS appears to be an incidental finding with few discernable physiologic effects.[25] Antihypertensives such as ACEs and ARBs, statins, and aspirin are used in medical management of RAS.[24,25] In patients with worsening renal function, refractory hypertension, or recurrent episodes of "flash," pulmonary edema renal artery revascularization is advocated.[24] However, a recent trial demonstrated that revascularization did not improve outcomes (including control of hypertension and preservation of renal function) compared with medical therapy alone.[26] Thus, diagnosing atherosclerotic RAS may be of little utility in most cases.

Endocrinologic Disorders

Triiodothyronine (T3), the active form of thyroid hormone after conversion from T4, increases heart rate and cardiac output (through the renin-angiotensin-aldosterone system. Not surprisingly, hyperthyroidism correlates with a rise in systolic BP. In contrast, patients with hypothyroidism have decreased cardiac output, which over time leads to a rise in diastolic BP.[27] Thyroid function testing and thyroid antibodies, if necessary, are used to establish the diagnosis.

Table 3
Most important secondary causes of hypertension by age group

Age Group & Causes	Signs or Symptoms	Laboratory Tests	Imaging or Other Studies
Children			
Renal parenchymal disease	Dysuria, recurrent urinary tract infection, hematuria May be asymptomatic	BUN/creatinine Urinalysis Urine culture	Renal ultrasound
Coarctation of the aorta	Difference in systolic BP between arms Delayed or absent femoral pulses Murmur	N/A	Echocardiogram
Young Adults			
Coarctation of the aorta	Same as mentioned earlier		
Renal artery stenosis from fibromuscular dysplasia	Mostly young women	N/A	Angiography IVUS MRA/CTA
Middle-aged Adults			
Obstructive sleep apnea	Snoring, witnessed apnea spells, daytime somnolence		Polysomnography (sleep study)
Hypo or hyperthyroidism	Bradycardia/ tachycardia Cold/ heat intolerance Constipation/diarrhea Irregular menses Thyromegaly	TSH, free T4	In hyperthyroid patients, consider radioactive iodine uptake scan
Hyperaldosteronism	Classic hypokalemia not seen in many	PAC/PRA ratio If ratio >25, refer for saline loading test	CT abdomen
Chronic kidney disease	Fatigue Edema	BUN/creatinine Anemia of chronic disease	Ultrasound showing small hyperechoic kidneys
Cushing syndrome	Central obesity Rapid weight gain Moon facies Buffalo hump	24-h urinary-free cortisol (2/3 tests must be positive) LDST	HDST MRI brain CT adrenals
Pheochromocytoma	Headaches Palpitations Flushing Syncope Labile blood pressures Orthostatic hypotension	24-h urinary fractionated metanephrines Plasma free metanephrines	CT adrenals
Older Adults			
Chronic kidney disease	Same as mentioned earlier		

(continued on next page)

Table 3 *(continued)*			
Age Group & Causes	Signs or Symptoms	Laboratory Tests	Imaging or Other Studies
Renal artery stenosis from atherosclerosis	Known risk factors or atherosclerotic disease	Rise in creatinine of >30% after ACEI/ARB	MRA/CTA renal artery doppler

Abbreviations: ACEI, angiotensin-converting enzyme inhibitor; ARB, angiotensin II receptor blocker; BUN, blood urea nitrogen; CTA, computed tomography angiography; CT, computed tomography; DMSA, dimercaptosuccinic acid scan; FT4, free thyroxine; HDST, high-dose dexamethasone suppression test; IVUS, intravascular ultrasound; LDST, low-dose dexamethasone suppression test; MRA, magnetic resonance angiography; MRI, magnetic resonance imaging; PAC, plasma aldosterone concentration; PRA, plasma renin activity; TSH, thyroid stimulating hormone; UTI, urinary tract infection; VCUG, voiding cystourethrogram.
Data from Refs.[17–21]

Cushing syndrome and primary hyperaldosteronism are other secondary causes of hypertension. Cushing syndrome can have 3 causes: (1) increased secretion of adrenocorticotropic hormone (ACTH) by the pituitary (ie, Cushing disease), (2) increased secretion of cortisol from the adrenal gland (without stimulation by ACTH), or (3) ectopic ACTH production. A 24-hour urinary free cortisol or salivary cortisol is a first-line test. Second line tests include low-dose and high-dose dexamethasone suppression tests, brain magnetic resonance imaging to rule out pituitary adenoma, or computed tomography of the adrenals to rule out hyperplasia or adenomas to further elucidate the cause.

Primary hyperaldosteronism (PH) results from oversecretion of aldosterone from the adrenal glands. About two-thirds of patients with PH have bilateral adrenal hyperplasia, whereas about one-third have an aldosterone-secreting adenoma.[18] Prospective studies of patients with RHTN have found the prevalence of primary aldosteronism ranging from 14% to 21%.[28] Testing for primary hyperaldosteronism requires measurement of plasma aldosterone concentration and renin activity. A ratio below 20 (when plasma aldosterone is reported in ng/dL and plasma renin activity in ng/ml/hr) effectively rules out PH. A ratio of 20 or higher with a serum aldosterone level greater than 15 ng/dL suggests PH, but the diagnosis must be confirmed by specialized testing. Further testing includes a saline loading test and radiographic studies of the adrenals.[18,29]

Secondary hyperaldosteronism occurs when juxtaglomerular cells of the kidneys sense decreased renal perfusion and secrete renin (resulting in increased aldosterone). A variety of disease states contribute to poor renal perfusion including congestive heart failure and liver cirrhosis.

OUT-OF-OFFICE BP MEASUREMENT

BP assessments for diagnosis of hypertension and monitoring response to treatment have traditionally been based on office BP measurement (OBPM) using a small number of auscultatory or oscillometric readings. However, office measurements only give a "snapshot" of BP and often provide a poor estimate of true BP because of the inherent variability of BP.[30] BP average outside the office setting may be lower than that measured in the office setting (ie, white coat effect). On the other hand, BP average outside the office may actually be higher than that measured in the office setting (ie, masking effect). The only way to detect white coat hypertension (elevated office BP with normal out-of-office BP) or masked hypertension (normal office BP with elevated out-of-office BP) is to use out-of-office measurements.[31,32]

The 2 main methods available for out-of-office BP measurements are home BP monitoring (HBPM) (also called "self-BP monitoring") and ambulatory BP monitoring (ABPM). Both methods have been shown to predict target organ damage and CVD risk better than office BP.[33,34] HBPM and ABPM provide multiple measurements of BP outside the office setting, allowing opportunity to possibly detect white coat or masked hypertension. HBPM and ABPM are not interchangeable techniques, however. They both are valuable in diagnosing and managing hypertension, but each has its own set of strengths and limitations (**Table 4**).

Home BP Monitoring

HBPM is typically an inexpensive and widely accepted method of assessment. A clinician should ensure that patients obtain a validated model with appropriate cuff size and are trained in proper technique. A list of validated models is available online at www.dableducational.org. Unfortunately, many hypertensive patients pursue purchasing and using a home monitor on their own, with little or no guidance from a clinician.[35] Outside of some initial training and occasional verification of valid readings, HBPM requires little intervention from the clinician.

HBPM measurements can assist in clarifying a patient's BP status, but any average should be based on a systematic method of obtaining readings. One such protocol is to have patients take 3 readings in the morning and evening for 5 consecutive days. These measurements should be recorded (ideally stored in the monitor's memory) and brought to the office. To obtain the average, the first 2 days' readings and the first reading of each remaining triplicate are dropped and the remaining 12 readings are averaged.[34] This average is used to help clarify diagnosis or current level of BP control. When such readings are highly discordant from office readings, however, we recommend pursuing ABPM if possible.

HBPM has also been shown to improve patients' compliance with treatment and hypertension control and is used as an educational tool to increase patients' awareness and understanding of BP control. Studies have shown that self-BP monitoring at home may improve awareness and understanding of concordance, leading to better compliance and BP management.[36]

HBPM is, however, dependent on the willingness and ability of the patient and his/her continued efforts to obtain readings. In addition, HBPM does not effectively capture BP measurements outside the home or during sleep.

Table 4
Comparison of out-of-office BP techniques

	HBPM	ABPM
Benefit		
Provides BP measures outside the office	●	●
Provides BP measures outside the office and home		●
Predicts cardiovascular risk better than OBPM	●	●
Assesses nocturnal BP patterns		●
Reinforces BP control	●	
Limitation		
Requires continued, consistent efforts by the patient	●	
Requires more intervention by the provider		●
Not widely available		●

Ambulatory BP Monitoring

ABPM not only offers many of the same benefits of HBPM, but also provides other unique information. With ABPM, patients wear a monitor that automatically records BP at preprogrammed intervals throughout the course of 24 (sometimes 48) hours. This method allows for measurements to be obtained during individuals' daily activities that would not be feasible with HBPM, such as during work and social interactions.

ABPM also captures the diurnal rhythm of BP (**Fig. 1**). Measurement of nighttime BP is valuable because lack of a nocturnal fall in BP ("nondipping") conveys additional cardiovascular risk.[37] Many studies have used the overall 24 hour BP average as the cardiovascular risk predictor, but others have reported that the best prediction of risk comes from the nighttime BP.[38] Studies have also shown that an excessive morning surge of BP may be related to increased cardiovascular risk.[39]

Contrary to the economic and practical benefits of HBPM, ABPM is typically less available, more costly, and not as well tolerated by patients, thereby limiting its use for repeated monitoring sessions. Use of ABPM also requires it to be arranged by the medical provider and an appointment for the patient to be fitted with the monitor and instructed on its wear. Currently, reimbursement for ABPM is limited, with most insurance providers only reimbursing for suspected white coat hypertension. Based largely on cost-effectiveness analysis demonstrating that ABPM can reduce the number of patients labeled as hypertensive, the current UK guideline recommends that ABPM should be performed on any patients with suspected hypertension with an OBPM of 140/90 mm Hg or higher.

AUTOMATED OFFICE MEASUREMENT TECHNIQUES

In an effort to improve assessment of BP in the clinical setting, oscillometric devices have been introduced that can take multiple consecutive readings without repeated intervention from the provider. These automated office devices are intended to be used while the patient is allowed to rest alone in a quiet and private area. Typically, 6 measurements are automatically taken 1 minute apart. The first is automatically discarded and the remaining 5 readings are automatically averaged.[40] Studies have suggested that automated office BP measurement eliminates white coat effect and provides an estimate of BP similar to daytime ABPM.[41,42]

SPECIAL POPULATIONS AND COMORBIDITIES
Children

In children, hypertension is defined as average systolic BP or diastolic BP that is greater than or equal to the 95th percentile for sex, age, and height on 3 or more occasions. BP charts are available at http://www.nhlbi.nih.gov/guidelines/hypertension/child_tbl.pdf. The National Institutes of Health recommends that children older than 3 years seen in medical care settings should have their BP measured at each encounter.[17]

Secondary hypertension is more common among children compared with adults. In this age group, intrinsic renal disease and aortic coarctation are the most common secondary causes of hypertension. Glomerulonephritis, congenital abnormalities, and reflux nephropathy can all contribute to renal parenchymal disease in children.[18] A urinalysis, urine culture, and renal ultrasound are recommended as part of the evaluation of children with confirmed hypertension. Because up to 41% of children with hypertension have left ventricular hypertrophy, an echocardiogram, which can also assess for aortic coarctation, should also be considered as part of the evaluation.[17]

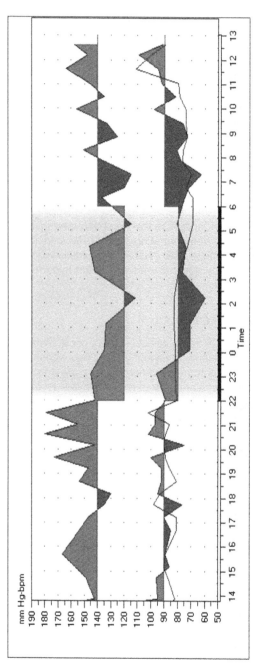

Fig. 1. Information reported from ABPM. Figure shows summary of a 24-hour ABPM session. The graph shows the sleep period as the shaded region from approximately 10:30 PM to 5:30 AM. The summary statistics provide overall average BP (145/86 mm Hg) as well as awake BP average (148/89 mm Hg), asleep BP (134/77 mm Hg), and percentage of asleep dipping (9.3% for systolic BP).

Diabetes Mellitus

Given that approximately 70% of diabetics have hypertension, and lowering high BP is important to reduce their CVD risk, the USPSTF recommends screening for type 2 diabetes in adults with sustained BP (either treated or untreated) greater than 135/80 mm Hg.[43] Compared with nondiabetics of the same age and sex, diabetics are at a 2 to 4-fold increased risk of cardiovascular events.[44] Among diabetics, aggressive BP control is more important than tight glucose control in reducing CVD events and slowing nephropathy.[45] The goal BP for diabetics is less than 130/80 mm Hg.[2] Aiming for tighter control (ie, <120 mm Hg systolic) does not improve outcomes and causes more adverse events.[46]

Given that patients with concomitant diabetes and hypertension are most at risk of cardiovascular events and nephropathy progressing to end-stage renal disease (ESRD), controlling BP is crucial, with the choice of pharmacologic therapy directed toward renoprotection and reducing microalbuminuria. Nephropathy occurs in up to 40% of patients with diabetes, and diabetic nephropathy is the single most important cause of ESRD. Annual urine albumin testing is recommended for all diabetics.[45] ACE inhibitors and ARBs delay the progression of nephropathy, and therefore one should be initiated (if not already in use) when microalbuminuria is detected.

Patients started on an ACE inhibitor or ARB should have their serum potassium and creatinine assessed within 2 weeks and then be periodically (eg, every 6 months) monitored for development of azotemia or hyperkalemia. In general, a rise of serum creatinine value of less than or equal to 30% and serum potassium value of less than or equal to 5.5 mmol/L are within acceptable limits.[45] Combining ACEs and ARBs has been shown to provide additional lowering of albuminuria but is not recommended because of causing worsening overall renal function.[47] Neither ACE inhibitors nor ARBs should be used during pregnancy, and they should probably be avoided in reproductive-aged women. If combination therapy is needed, which is likely, diuretics are recommended. If a third agent is needed, CCBs should be considered next.

African Americans

The prevalence of hypertension among African Americans is nearly 40%.[1] African Americans also tend to have earlier onset and more severe hypertension.[48] The Antihypertensive Lipid-Lowering Treatment to Prevent Heart Attack Trial (ALLHAT), examining the efficacy of several antihypertensive agents found that ACE inhibitor–induced angioedema and cough occurred more frequently among African American patients compared with other ethnicities. In addition, compared with lisinopril, chlorthalidone was more effective in reducing systolic BP in African Americans as the difference in systolic BP between the 2 drugs was twice as great (4 mm Hg) compared with non-Blacks. The rates of stroke and heart failure were higher among African Americans using lisinopril and amlodipine, respectively. Overall, diuretics and CCBs are preferred among African Americans, although beta-blocker, ACE inhibitor, or ARBs are indicated in the presence of compelling indications.[49]

Chronic Kidney Disease

CKD is defined by the presence of albuminuria (>300 mg/d or 200 mg albumin per gram of creatinine) or a glomerular filtration rate (GFR) less than 60 mL/min. Patients with CKD are at higher risk of morbidity and mortality from CVD and even higher with concomitant hypertension. In fact, hypertension itself is one of the leading causes of CKD, causing 25,000 new cases per year in the United States. Although most of the research has established that ACE inhibitors and ARBs reduce proteinuria and slow the progression of kidney damage among patients with diabetic nephropathy, similar results have been found among those with nondiabetic nephropathy.[50,51]

African Americans are 6 times more likely than Caucasians to develop hypertension-related kidney failure.[52,53] The African American Study of Kidney Disease and Hypertension (AASK) Trial demonstrated that ACE inhibitors are the most effective renoprotective drugs in African Americans; however, they are less effective as BP-lowering agents in this population.[52]

RESISTANT HYPERTENSION

RHTN is defined as BP above goal despite adherence to a combination of at least 3 optimally dosed antihypertensive medications of different classes, ideally one of which is a diuretic.[54] RHTN may affect up to 30% of hypertensive patients, with older age and obesity as major contributors.[54] Management of RHTN requires reevaluation for secondary causes, addressing potential lifestyle modifications, and optimization of multidrug regimens.

The initial approach to patients with possible RHTN is assessing their adherence to medication. Financial expense, multiple daily dosing, and side effects all contribute to poor adherence. It is therefore important to keep the medication regimen as simple as possible. Once-daily regimens and single-pill combinations improve patients' adherence to antihypertensive medications.[55,56] More importantly, single-pill combinations, many of which are available as generics, have been shown to achieve more rapid BP control (and thus improve cardiovascular outcomes) during the first year than initial monotherapy with add-on medications.[57] Asking about and addressing side effects may enhance patients' understanding and adherence. Antihypertensive side effects include sexual dysfunction (eg, from diuretics, beta-blockers), fatigue (eg, from beta-blockers), peripheral edema (eg, from CCBs), and cough and muscle pain (eg, from ACE inhibitors).[55]

When assessing possible RHTN, it is also important to ensure accuracy of BP measurement. Because there is some degree of measurement bias in methods using auscultation, automated BP cuffs are used in the office to standardize BP measurements. However, these devices cannot be used for patients with sustained arrhythmias (eg, atrial fibrillation) or severe atherosclerosis (because of poor compliance of arteries). Careful attention must be paid to technique (eg, feet on the floor, arm supported at heart level, no talking), and proper cuff size must be used. Too small a cuff will overestimate BP.[6]

Among patients with suspected RHTN, approximately one-third have normal BP on ABPM. Therefore, white coat effect must be excluded as an initial step.[54] If ABPM is not easily available, HBPM is used as first-line treatment. When the home BP measurements confirm elevated BP, treatment is intensified. In cases where office BP is elevated and home BP averages are normal, confirmation with ambulatory BP monitoring is advised.

Given that volume overload plays a role in RHTN, all patients (unless contraindicated) should be on one or more diuretics. One strategy is to increase the dose of diuretic or change to a more potent diuretic. Chlorthalidone has been shown to reduce BP more effectively and is longer acting compared with equivalent doses of hydrochlorothiazide.[58] In addition, compared with hydrochlorothiazide, it reduces progression to left ventricular hypertrophy and cardiovascular events to a greater degree.[59,60] The effectiveness of low-dose thiazides depends on adequate renal function.[55] In patients with a serum creatinine value greater than 1.8 mg/dL or GFR less than 30 mL/min, switch to a loop diuretic. Keep in mind that for BP control, short-acting loop diuretics (furosemide and bumetanide) must be dosed more than once daily. Torsemide is a longer-acting loop diuretic. Dietary sodium restriction is also important to control volume overload and therefore (along with the other lifestyle modifications) should be reiterated.

Other medications to consider include aldosterone antagonists (eg, spironolactone), an alpha-blocker (eg, terazosin), a combined alpha-beta blocker (labetalol or carvedilol), a vasodilator (eg, hydralazine), or centrally acting agents (eg, clonidine). Spironolactone can reduce systolic BP by approximately 20 mm Hg and diastolic BP by 10 mm Hg in patients with hypertension that is resistant to 3 or more drugs.[61] Hyperkalemia is a side effect and should be monitored carefully, especially in patients who are also taking an ACE inhibitor or an ARB. Other alternatives are eplerenone and amiloride. Aldosterone antagonists are contraindicated in patients with severe renal impairment. Consider concomitant beta-blockade for patients who develop reflex tachycardia with hydralazine. Clonidine is effective but should only be used in compliant patient as withdrawal causes severe rebound hypertension. Referral to a hypertension specialist is recommended when a patient's hypertension is not controlled satisfactorily despite adequate compliance with 4 agents.

REFERENCES

1. Centers for Disease Control (CDC). Vital signs: prevalence, treatment, and control of hypertension — United States, 1999–2002 and 2005—2008. MMWR Morb Mortal Wkly Rep 2011;60(4):103–8.
2. Chobanian AV, Bakris GL, Black HR, et al. The seventh report of the Joint National Committee on prevention, detection, evaluation, and treatment of high blood pressure: the JNC 7 report. JAMA 2003;289:2560–72.
3. Lewington S, Clarke R, Qizilbash N, et al. Age-specific relevance of usual blood pressure to vascular mortality: a meta-analysis of individual data for one million adults in 61 prospective studies. Lancet 2002;360:1903–13.
4. Singh V. Review: ACE-Is or ARBs reduce adverse CV outcomes regardless of baseline systolic blood pressure. Ann Intern Med 2012;157(2):JC1–8.
5. U.S. Preventive Services Task Force. Screening for high blood pressure: U.S. Preventive Services Task Force reaffirmation recommendation statement. AHRQ Publication No. 08-05105-EF-2, December 2007. Ann Intern Med 2007;147: 783–6.
6. Forrest B, Viera AJ. Hypertension. In: Sloane PD, Slatt LM, Ebell MH, et al, editors. Essentials of family medicine. 6th edition. Philadelphia: Wolters Kluwer/Lippincott Williams & Wilkins; 2011. p. 125–34.
7. Beckett NS, Peters R, Fletcher AE, et al. Treatment of hypertension in patients 80 years of age and older. N Engl J Med 2008;358:1887–98.
8. Khan N, Hemmelgarn B, Padwal R, et al. The 2007 Canadian Hypertension Education Program recommendations for the management of hypertension: part 2 – therapy. Can J Cardiol 2007;23:539–50.
9. Sacks FM, Svetkey LP, Volmer WM, et al. Effects on blood pressure of reduced dietary sodium and the Dietary Approaches to Stop Hypertension (DASH) diet. N Engl J Med 2001;135:1019–28.
10. Reid CM, Maher T, Jennings GL. Substituting lifestyle management for pharmacological control of blood pressure: a pilot study in Australian general practice. Blood Press 2000;9:267–74.
11. Qureshi AI, Sapkota BL. Blood pressure reduction in secondary stroke prevention. Continuum (Minneapolis Minn) 2011;17(6 2ndary Stroke Prevention):1233–41.

12. Goldstein L, Bushnell C, Adams R, et al. Guidelines for the primary prevention of stroke. Stroke 2011;42:517–84.
13. Law MR, Morris JK, Wald NJ. Use of blood pressure lowering drugs in the prevention of cardiovascular disease: meta-analysis of 147 randomised trials in the context of expectations from prospective epidemiological studies. BMJ 2009; 338:b1665.
14. Sierra C. Cerebral small vessel disease, cognitive impairment and vascular dementia. Panminerva Med 2012;54:179–88.
15. Grosso A, Veglio F, Porta M, et al. Hypertensive retinopathy revisited: some answers, more questions. Br J Ophthalmol 2005;89:1646–54.
16. Omura M, Saito J, Yamaguchi K, et al. Prospective study on the prevalence of secondary hypertension among hypertensive patients visiting a general outpatient clinic in Japan. Hypertens Res 2004;27:193–202.
17. U.S. Department of Health and Human Services, National Heart, Lung, and Blood Institute. The fourth report on the diagnosis, evaluation, and treatment of high blood pressure in children and adolescents. Revised May 2005. Available at: http://www.nhlbi.nih.gov/health/prof/heart/hbp/hbp_ped.pdf. Accessed August 27, 2012.
18. Viera AJ, Neutze DM. Secondary hypertension: an age-based approach. Am Fam Physician 2010;82:1471–8.
19. Eklof H, Ahlstrom H, Magnusson A, et al. A prospective comparison of duplex ultrasonagraphy, captopril renography, MRA, and CTA in assessing renal artery stenosis. Acta Radiol 2006;47:764–74.
20. Nadasdy T, Hebert LA. Infection-related glomerulonephritis: understanding mechanisms. Semin Nephrol 2011;31:369–75.
21. Tsai JD, Huang CT, Lin PY, et al. Screening high-grade vesicoureteral reflux in young infants with a febrile urinary tract infection. Pediatr Nephrol 2012;27: 955–63.
22. Mousa AY, Campbell JE, Stone PA, et al. Short- and long-term outcomes of percutaneous transluminal angioplasty/stenting of renal fibromuscular dysplasia over a ten-year period. J Vasc Surg 2012;55:421–7.
23. Olin JW, Sealove BA. Diagnosis, management, and future developments of fibromuscular dysplasia. J Vasc Surg 2011;53:826–36.
24. Hirsch AT, Jaskal ZJ, Hertzer NR, et al. ACC/AHA 2005 practice guidelines for the management of patients with peripheral arterial disease (lower extremity, renal, mesenteric, and abdominal aortic): executive summary. Circulation 2006; 113(11):1474–547.
25. Foy A, Ruggiero NJ 2nd, Filippone EJ. Revascularization in renal-artery stenosis. Cardiol Rev 2012;20:189–93.
26. Wheatley K, Ives N, Gray R, et al. Revascularization versus medical therapy for renal-artery stenosis. N Engl J Med 2009;361:1953–62.
27. Klein I, Danzi S. Thyroid disease and the heart. Circulation 2007;116:1725–35.
28. Acelajado MC, Calhoun DA. Aldosteronism and resistant hypertension. Int J Hypertens 2011;2011:837817.
29. Fogari R, Preti P, Zoppi A, et al. Prevalence of primary aldosteronism among unselected hypertensive patients: a prospective study based on the use of an aldosterone/renin ratio above 25 as a screening test. Hypertens Res 2007;30:111–7.
30. Armitage P, Rose GA. The variability of measurements of casual blood pressure: a laboratory study. Clin Sci 1966;30:325–35.
31. Pickering TG, Gerin W, Schwartz AR. What is the white-coat effect and how should it be measured? Blood Press Monit 2002;7:293–300.

32. Viera AJ, Hinderliter AL, Kshirsagar AV, et al. Reproducibility of masked hypertension in adults with untreated borderline office blood pressure: comparison of ambulatory and home monitoring. Am J Hypertens 2010;23:1190–7.
33. Shimbo D, Pickering TG, Spruill TM, et al. Relative utility of home, ambulatory, and office blood pressures in the prediction of end-organ damage. Am J Hypertens 2007;20:476–82.
34. Verberk WJ, Kroon AA, Kessels AG, et al. The optimal scheme of self blood pressure measurement as determined from ambulatory blood pressure recordings. J Hypertens 2006;24(8):1541–8.
35. Viera AJ, Cohen LW, Mitchell CM, et al. How and why do patients use home blood pressure monitors? Blood Press Monit 2008;13(3):133–7.
36. Cappuccio FP, Kerry SM, Forbes L, et al. Blood pressure control by home monitoring: meta-analysis of randomized trials. BMJ 2004;329:145–51.
37. Ohkubo T, Hozawa A, Yamaguchi J, et al. Prognostic significance of the nocturnal decline in blood pressure in individuals with and without high 24-hour blood pressure: the Ohasama study. J Hypertens 2002;20:2183–9.
38. Staessen JA, Thijs L, Fagard R, et al. Predicting cardiovascular risk using conventional vs ambulatory blood pressure in older patients with systolic hypertension. JAMA 1999;282:539–46.
39. Kario K, Pickering TG, Umeda Y, et al. Morning surge in blood pressure as a predictor of silent and clinical cerebrovascular disease in elderly hypertensives: a prospective study. Circulation 2003;107:1401–6.
40. Myers MG. Automated office blood pressure recorded at one minute intervals. J Hypertens 2011;29(e-supplement A):e426.
41. Myers MG, Godwin M, Dawes M, et al. Conventional versus automated measurement of blood pressure in the office (CAMBO) trial. Fam Pract 2012; 29:376–82.
42. Beckett L, Godwin M. The BpTRU automatic blood pressure monitor compared to 24-h ambulatory blood pressure monitoring in the assessment of blood pressure in patients with hypertension. BMC Cardiovasc Disord 2005;5:18.
43. U.S. Preventive Services Task Force. Screening for type 2 diabetes mellitus in adults, topic page. June 2008. Available at: http://www.uspreventiveservicestaskforce.org/uspstf/uspsdiab.htm. Accessed December 8, 2012.
44. Pignone M, Alberts MJ, Colwell JA, et al. Aspirin for primary prevention of cardiovascular events in people with diabetes. American Diabetes Association; American Heart Association; American College of Cardiology Foundation. J Am Coll Cardiol 2010;55:2878–86.
45. Buse JB, Ginsberg HN, Bakris GL, et al. Primary prevention of cardiovascular diseases in people with diabetes mellitus: a scientific statement from the American Heart Association and the American Diabetes Association. Circulation 2007;115:114–26.
46. ACCORD Study Group, Cushman WC, Evans GW, Byington RP, et al. Effects of intensive blood-pressure control in type 2 diabetes mellitus. N Engl J Med 2010;362:1575–85.
47. Mann JF, Schmieder RE, McQueen M, et al. Renal outcomes with telmisartan, ramipril, or both, in people at high vascular risk (the ONTARGET study): a multicenter, randomized, double-blind, controlled trial. Lancet 2008;372: 547–53.
48. Triplette MA, Rossi JS, Viera AJ, et al. The contribution of hypertension to black-white differences in likelihood of coronary artery disease detected during elective angiography. Am J Hypertens 2011;24:181–6.

49. Cushman WC, Davis BR, Pressel SL, et al. Mortality and morbidity during and after the Antihypertensive and Lipid-Lowering Treatment to Prevent Heart Attack Trial. J Clin Hypertens (Greenwich) 2012;14(1):20–31.
50. National Kidney Foundation Guideline. Clinical practice guidelines for chronic kidney disease: evaluation, classification, and stratification. Kidney Disease Outcome Quality Initiative. Am J Kidney Dis 2002;39:S1–246.
51. The GISEN Group (Gruppo Italiano di Studi Epidemiologici in Nefrologia). Randomised placebo-controlled trial of effect of ramipril on decline in glomerular filtration rate and risk of terminal renal failure in proteinuric, non-diabetic nephropathy. Lancet 1997;349:1857–63.
52. Wright JT, Bakris G, Greene T, et al, the African American Study of Kidney Disease and Hypertension (AASK) Study Group. Effect of blood pressure lowering and antihypertensive drug class on progression of hypertensive kidney disease: results of the AASK trial. JAMA 2002;288:2421–31.
53. United States Renal Data System. USRDS 2007 Annual data report. Bethesda (MD): National Institute of Diabetes and Digestive and Kidney Diseases, National Institutes of Health, U.S. Department of Health and Human Services; 2007.
54. Calhoun DA, Jones D, Textor S, et al. Resistant hypertension: diagnosis, evaluation, and treatment. A scientific statement from the American Heart Association Professional Education Committee of the Council for High Blood Pressure Research. Circulation 2008;117:e510–26.
55. Viera AJ, Hinderliter AL. Evaluation and management of the patient with difficult-to-control or resistant hypertension. Am Fam Physician 2009;79:863–9.
56. Bangalore S, Kamalakkannan G, Parkar S, et al. Fixed-dose combinations improve medication compliance: a meta-analysis. Am J Med 2007;120:713–9.
57. Egan BM, Bandyopadhyay D, Shaftman SR, et al. Initial monotherapy and combination therapy and hypertension control the first year. Hypertension 2012;59(6):1124–31.
58. Ernst ME, Carter BL, Goerdt CJ, et al. Comparative antihypertensive effects of hydrochlorothiazide and chlorthalidone on ambulatory and office blood pressure. Hypertension 2006;47:352–8.
59. Ernst ME, Neaton JD, Grimm RH, et al. Long-term effects of chlorthalidone versus hydrochlorothiazide on electrocardiographic left ventricular hypertrophy in the Multiple Risk Factor Intervention Trial. Hypertension 2011;58:1001–7.
60. Dorsch MP, Gillespie BW, Erickson SR, et al. Chlorthalidone reduces cardiovascular events compared with hydrochlorothiazide: a retrospective cohort analysis. Hypertension 2011;57:689–94.
61. Chapman N, Dobson J, Wilson S, et al. Effect of spironolactone on blood pressure in subjects with resistant hypertension. Hypertension 2007;49:839–45.

Hyperlipidemia as a Risk Factor for Cardiovascular Disease

Robert H. Nelson, MD

KEYWORDS

- Hypercholesterolemia • Hypertriglyceridemia • Dyslipidemia • Cardiometabolic risk
- CVD risk factors

KEY POINTS

- Elevated levels of blood lipids are well-documented risk factors for cardiovascular disease. Current classification schemes and treatment levels for hyperlipidemia are based on the National Cholesterol Education Panel's (NCEP) Adult Treatment Program-3 (ATP-III) guidelines.
- Statins are the preferred class of drugs to lower elevated low-density lipoprotein cholesterol (LDL-C). There are other classes to augment or substitute for statins, such as ezetimibe, fibrates, niacin, and dietary supplements.
- Extensive research over the past decade has raised the question of whether or not ATP-III guidelines are sufficiently aggressive. New guidelines from ATP-IV are expected to be released in the near future, but in the meantime physicians are faced with uncertainty about how low to target LDL-C, whether to pharmacologically treat high-density lipoprotein cholesterol (HDL-C) and triglyceride (TG) levels, and how best to achieve target goals.

INTRODUCTION

Modern primary care practitioners spend considerable time and effort on preventive medicine. Diagnosing and managing hyperlipidemia as a way to prevent cardiovascular disease (CVD) is a common activity for primary care physicians. According to the Centers for Disease Control and Prevention, data from a survey of 1492 physicians who provide ambulatory care in nongovernment settings, hyperlipidemia is second only to hypertension in the list of the 10 most common chronic conditions that were seen.[1] Hyperlipidemia is a strong risk factor for CVD. Hyperlipidemia refers to elevated cholesterol, elevated triglycerides (TGs) or both. The problem can be solely a result of hereditary factors, but more commonly it is an acquired condition. Physicians need to know the major categories of dyslipidemia and to have a well-reasoned action plan for

Funding Sources: NIDDK (DK82473), No industry funding.
Conflict of Interest: Nil.
Division of Endocrinology, Department of Family Medicine, Mayo College of Medicine, Mayo Clinic, 200 First Street Southwest, Rochester, MN 55905, USA
E-mail address: nelson.robert1@mayo.edu

dealing with each one, including knowing when to refer a case to a lipidology specialist. This article reviews the categories of hyperlipidemia, the current treatment recommendations, and the current controversies and unresolved questions. Some of the recent evidence-based data (~2000 to current year) and studies regarding hyperlipidemia are discussed.

DEFINITIONS OF HYPERLIPIDEMIA

For most primary care providers, hyperlipidemia is defined as elevations of fasting total cholesterol concentration that may or may not be associated with elevated TG concentration. Lipids are not soluble in plasma, however, but are instead transported in particles known as lipoproteins. Therefore, classifications of hyperlipidemia are also based on abnormalities of lipoproteins. See **Box 1**.

The National Cholesterol Education Panel (NCEP) created a standard using lipid levels in 2001 that is still the most commonly used clinical classification (**Table 1**).[2] The NCEP is currently revising its recommendations with an updated version of ATP-III guidelines expected to be released in the autumn of 2012.

SIGNIFICANCE OF HYPERLIPIDEMIA

Health care providers are concerned about hyperlipidemia because of the well-established association between lipid concentrations and the risk of CVD, the leading cause of death in the United States.[3] A landmark study that helped establish that therapeutic interventions to lower cholesterol levels result in reduced risk of cardiovascular morbidity or mortality was the Lipid Research Clinics Coronary Primary Prevention Trial, which was published in 2 parts (each using a different statistical analysis) in 1984.[4,5] Numerous other trials, both before and after 1984, also contributed to the evidence of a CVD-hyperlipidemia link; however, the scientific and medical communities took several decades to agree that this relationship truly exists. A complete history of the cholesterol controversy can be found in a multipart review (available online) that was published over a 3-year span in the *Journal of Lipid Research*.[6–10]

DIAGNOSIS

Most cases of hyperlipidemia are found because a lipid panel screen is done as part of a routine health care evaluation or because plasma lipids are checked after a cardiovascular event. The US Preventive Services Task Force has posted screening recommendations for lipid disorders on its Web site.[11] The group does not recommend universal screening. Its guidelines are summarized in **Box 2**.

Not all experts agree with these recommendations, primarily because they believe that the overall incidence of CVD in the United States is so high that screening should

---

Box 1
Classes of apolipoproteins

- Chylomicrons: Triglyceride (TG)-rich carrier of dietary fats.
- Very Low Density Lipoprotein (VLDL): TG-rich carrier of hepatic synthesized TGs.
- Intermediate-Density and Low-Density Lipoprotein (IDL and LDL): Cholesterol-rich remnant particles derived from lipolysis of triglycerides in VLDL.
- High-Density Lipoprotein (HDL): Cholesterol-rich particle that transports cholesterol to liver for disposal or recycling.

Table 1
Classification of hyperlipidemias as defined by the NCEP ATP-III

Low-density lipoprotein cholesterol

<100	Optimal
100–129	Near or above optimal
130–159	Borderline high
160–189	High
≥190	Very high

Total cholesterol

<200	Desirable
200–239	Borderline high
≥240	High

High-density lipoprotein cholesterol

<40	Low
≥60	High

Triglycerides

<150	Normal
150–199	Borderline high
200–499	High
≥500	Very high

All concentrations are expressed as mg/dL.

be more aggressive. For example, the American Heart Association states on its Web site[12] that "The American Heart Association urges all Americans to have their physicians determine their total and HDL blood cholesterol levels. This is very important for those people with a family history of heart disease, high blood pressure, or stroke." Screening refers to testing lipids in people who are without symptoms or associated disease. Any person who is diagnosed with diseases related to hyperlipidemia

Box 2
Recommendations of the US Preventive Services Task Force 2008

- Screen men aged 35 and older. (Grade A Recommendation)
- Screen men aged 20 to 35 if they are at increased risk for coronary heart disease.[a] (Grade B Recommendation)
- Screen women aged 45 and older if they are at increased risk for coronary heart disease. (Grade A Recommendation)
- Screen women aged 20 to 45 if they are at increased risk for coronary heart disease. (Grade B Recommendation)
- No recommendation for or against routine screening in men aged 20 to 35, or in women aged 20 and older who are not at increased risk for coronary heart disease. (Grade C Recommendation)

[a] Increased risk for CVD is defined by risk factors. These include men with diabetes, a family history of heart disease in a close male relative younger than 50 or a close female relative younger than 60, a family history of high cholesterol, or a personal history of multiple coronary disease risk factors (eg, smoking, high blood pressure).

(eg, hypothyroidism, diabetes, renal insufficiency) should have a lipid evaluation as a part of the diagnostic workup. This also holds true for anyone who presents with evidence of CVD (eg, angina, myocardial infarction, onset of claudication, discovery of a vessel bruit).

CLASSIFICATION OF HYPERLIPIDEMIA

Abnormal lipid profiles are generally a combination of abnormalities of the lipoprotein fractions noted in **Box 1**. The degree of increased risk of CVD depends on the exact pattern and the underlying cause. Primary care physicians do not necessarily need full knowledge of all hyperlipidemic syndromes, but all physicians should be fully aware of their own individual limitations and capabilities. It is vital to know common primary and secondary causes of elevated lipids and to recognize unusual patterns or physical findings that should trigger a referral to a lipidologist. Although rare in primary care practices, many genetic causes of hyperlipidemia carry an increased risk of premature CVD and/or other organ system disease. Some of these syndromes require treatment different from the usual primary care patient presenting with hyperlipidemia.

Hyperlipidemia can be broadly classified as an isolated elevation of cholesterol, isolated elevated TG, and elevations of both. The cause may be genetic, environmental, or both. **Table 2** is a list of genetic causes of hyperlipidemia with a brief clinical description including clues that should trigger consideration of a lipid specialty referral. In general, the clues to a genetic syndrome include very high cholesterol levels (>300 mg/dL), very high TG levels (>500 mg/dL), xanthomas, strong family history of hyperlipidemia or early CVD, or lack of expected response to maximal therapeutic doses of lipid-lowering agents.

Dyslipidemia has multiple secondary causes. These are listed in **Table 3**, which is divided into isolated cholesterol elevation, isolated TG elevation, and a mixed pattern.

An important secondary cause of high cholesterol is hypothyroidism. It is important to screen people with elevated cholesterol for hypothyroidism. This is because hypothyroidism causes elevations of cholesterol and reduced thyroid hormone concentrations increase the risk of statin-induced myopathy.[13] Other important contributors to secondary hyperlipidemia include diabetes, renal disease, and alcoholism. HIV is an important consideration, because both the infection and the use of protease inhibitors can contribute to lipid abnormalities.[14]

EVALUATION AND TREATMENT OF PATIENTS WITH HYPERLIPIDEMIA
CVD Risk Analysis

An important step in the interpretation of lipid-screening results is the performance of a cardiovascular risk assessment. This point is strongly emphasized in the report of ATP-III and in numerous peer-reviewed journal articles reviewing the topic of lipid management. The basic principle is that the higher a person's CVD risk, the greater the benefit in aggressively treating all modifiable risk factors, including hyperlipidemia. Any physician who is interpreting the results of a lipid panel needs to take the time to do a formal CVD risk analysis. One of the most commonly used validated instruments is the Framingham Risk Score; however, it has several limitations, such as underestimating the risk in a high-risk individual owing to the absence of some important risk factors in the scoring system.[15] Therefore, others have attempted to improve the scoring system to more precisely estimate the risk of a major cardiovascular event in differing groups.[16,17]

Table 2
Genetic causes of hyperlipidemia

Causes	Clinical Features
Isolated cholesterol elevation	
Genetic familial hypercholesterolemia	Relatively common (1 in 500 heterozygote); TC exceeds 300 mg/dL, family history of elevated TC common, associated with tendon xanthomas, premature (20–40 y old) CVD is common. Homozygotes are rare, but have TC >600 and if not treated usually die of MI before age 20.
Familial defective apolipoprotein B100	Increases LDL and has a phenotype that is indistinguishable from that of FH, including increased susceptibility to CHD.
Mutations associated with elevated LDL levels	Rare and isolated; suspect if elevated LDL unresponsive to treatment.
Elevated plasma lipoprotein(a)	Relationship to CVD unclear, studies contradictory.[48,49]
Polygenic hypercholesterolemia	No family history, no physical manifestations such as xanthomas, exact cause is unknown.
Lp(X)	Associated with obstructive hepatic disease, CVD risk unclear.
Sitosterolemia	Rare; plant sterols absorbed in large amounts, tendon xanthomas develop in childhood, LDL levels normal to high.
Cerebrotendinous Xanthomatosis	Rare; associated with neurologic disease, tendon xanthomas, and cataracts in young adults.
Elevated cholesterol and triglycerides	
Combined (familial) hyperlipidemia	May occur randomly or with strong family history of hyperlipidemia; type 2 diabetes and metabolic syndrome are associated and can make diagnosis more difficult.
Familial dysbetalipoproteinemia (type III hyperlipoproteinemia)	Severe hypertriglyceridemia and hypercholesterolemia (both often >300), associated with premature diffuse vascular disease, male predominance, palmar xanthomas are pathognomonic.
Hepatic lipase deficiency	Rare disorder with very high cholesterol and triglyceride concentrations, phenotypically similar to familial dysbetalipoproteinemia.
Isolated triglyceride elevations	
LPL deficiency	Results in elevated chylomicrons, which carry dietary fat; chylomicrons are generally not present after an overnight fast, so a creamy-looking plasma in a fasting specimen should be a clue to the diagnosis, especially if seen in young children; extremely high triglycerides can lead to pancreatitis.
ApoCII deficiency	This apolipoprotein is an activator of LPL; its absence causes a clinical picture identical to LPL deficiency.
Familial hypertriglyceridemia	Autosomal dominant inheritance; main defect is overproduction of VLDL triglycerides by the liver.

Abbreviations: CVD, cardiovascular disease; CHD, coronary heart disease; FH, familial hypercholesterolemia; LDL, low-density lipoprotein; LPL, Lipoprotein Lipase; TC, total cholesterol; VLDL, very low density lipoprotein.

Data from Semenkovich CF, Goldberg AC, Goldberg IJ. Disorders of lipid metabolism. In: Melmed S, Polonsky KS, Larsen PR, et al, editors. Williams textbook of endocrinology. 12th edition. Philadelphia: W.B. Saunders; 2011. p. 1633–56.

Table 3
Secondary causes of hyperlipidemia

Diet	Drugs	Disease and Disorders of Metabolism
Saturated & trans fats	Thiazide diuretics	Hypothyroidism
Excess calories	Beta-blockers	Obesity
Alcohol	Glucocorticoids	Type 2 diabetes
Red meat	Sex hormones	Metabolic syndrome
Whole milk	Retinoic acid derivations	Renal disease
High-sugar beverages and foods	Antipsychotics Antiretrovirals Immunosuppressive agents	HIV Polycystic ovarian syndrome

Novel Risk Factors

The emphasis on lowering LDL-C with statins has resulted in significant improvement in morbidity and mortality from CVD; however, despite the emphasis on control of LDL-C, a number of cardiac events occur in people without clinically abnormal LDL-C concentrations. This problem is often referred to as residual risk. One way of improving risk prediction and treatment has been to focus on non-HDL cholesterol levels rather than on just LDL-C. The reason for this is that other lipoprotein fractions contribute to the formation of atherosclerosis. These particles are intermediate or end products of triglyceride-rich lipoprotein (TGRL) catabolism, specifically very low density lipoprotein (VLDL) and chylomicrons. As TGs are removed from TGRLs by intravascular lipases, the particles become denser and have a greater portion of their composition as cholesterol. In the case of chylomicrons, which transport dietary fat, the end product of TG lipolysis is a small, dense Apo-B48–containing particle known as a chylomicron remnant. VLDL, which transports endogenously produced TGs, has a more complex catabolism. In a simplified version, the catabolic steps can be thought of as a conversion of VLDL to intermediate-density lipoproteins (IDLs), which are then converted to LDLs. The particles are defined by their different densities and TG:cholesterol ratios, but all of them contain apoB-100. These remnant particles are believed to be significant contributors to CVD because the particles not eliminated by the liver (the preferred disposal site) are taken up in arterial walls to eventually become lipid-laden macrophages, the well-known foam cells that are a hallmark of early atherosclerosis. In a meta-analysis of 38,153 statin-treated subjects in whom non–HDL-C, LDL-C, and Apo-B were compared, all 3 markers were predictive of CVD, with non–HDL-C showing a slightly greater association than the other two.[18] Even though statistically non–HDL-C was the best predictor, however, the 95% confidence intervals of the hazard ratio of CVD for each of the 3 markers overlapped sufficiently that this study cannot be considered conclusive.

Additional, markers for risk factor analysis are based on the contribution to CVD by inflammatory proteins and other cytokines. In 2011, a consensus panel of the National Lipid Association published a review of the clinical utility of various proposed markers. See **Box 3** for a partial list of markers that have been proposed.

In general, alternative risk factor markers have had mixed results in clinical trials. Even the most positive studies have not shown a dramatic improvement in prediction of future risk of CVD compared with traditional Framingham risk scoring. A major study, published in the *Journal of the American Medical Association* by the Emerging Risk Factors Collaboration, reviewed individual records from 37 prospective studies

---

Box 3
Summary of some novel or alternative risk factors with recommendations for their use based on different sources

- C-reactive protein: Recommended for routine measurement in intermediate risk subjects.

- Lp-PLA2: Consider for selected patients.

- Apo-B: Reasonable for many intermediate-risk patients.

- LDL-P: Reasonable for many intermediate-risk patients.

- Lp(a): Consider for selected patients.

- LDL Subfractions: Not recommended.

- HDL Subfractions: Not recommended.

Data from Davidson MH, Ballantyne CM, Jacobson TA, et al. Clinical utility of inflammatory markers and advanced lipoprotein testing: advice from an expert panel of lipid specialists. J Clin Lipidol 2011;5:338.

- Imaging (carotid intima thickening, coronary artery calcium by computed tomography): Primary value is asymptomatic individuals at intermediate cardiovascular risk. Further research is recommended.

Data from Peters SA, den Ruijter HM, Bots ML, et al. Improvements in risk stratification for the occurrence of cardiovascular disease by imaging subclinical atherosclerosis: a systematic review. Heart 2012;98:177–84.

- Fibrinogen: Not recommended (effective treatment not demonstrated).

Data from Wendland E, Farmer A, Glasziou P, et al. Effect of alpha linolenic acid on cardiovascular risk markers: a systematic review. Heart 2006;92:166.

- Homocysteine: Not recommended (effective treatment not demonstrated).

Data from Zhou YH, Tang JY, Wu MJ, et al. Effect of folic acid supplementation on cardiovascular outcomes: a systematic review and meta-analysis. PLoS One 2011;6:e25142.

---

containing 165,544 people without CVD at baseline.[19] The study compared traditional lipids to additional measures, including apolipoproteins B and A-I, lipoprotein(a), and lipoprotein-associated phospholipase A2 in individuals followed for a mean of 10 years. Those with CVD events during the study period were analyzed to determine if the alternative markers added significant predictive value. In an accompanying editorial, lipid expert Dr Scott Grundy concluded that "apolipoproteins are of limited value in reclassifying individuals among arbitrary risk categories, ie, low-risk, intermediate-risk, and high-risk."[20] Even when a particular test has been shown to add incremental improvement in predicting risk, there has not been sufficient evidence to use the test as a widespread screening tool. Most often, novel risk factors are useful for the patient who has intermediate risk and his or her physician desires additional information to make a decision regarding therapy. It should be considered that, for many novel risk markers, statin therapy does not reduce the marker levels[21] and evidence that treating the specific marker has any real impact on CVD is lacking. For example, it has been shown in multiple meta-analyses that folic acid reduces homocysteine, but does not reduce CVD hazard; moreover, the various tests available add cost, may add risk (eg, radiation for imaging), and many of the assays have not been widely standardized, thus resulting in difficulty interpreting the results. Based on current evidence, it is difficult to recommend these alternative risk markers for screening or for routine clinical use and they are probably most appropriate in carefully considered individual cases; however, this topic is an area of intense focus and ongoing research, so future studies may help elucidate a more clearly defined role for novel risk markers.

Treatment Goals

A portion of the current treatment goals, as outlined by the NCEP/ATP-III are listed in **Box 4**. The complete guidelines are available online from the National Institutes of Health as a quick reference guide.[22] These recommendations are generally accepted by some, but not all, medical specialty organizations. Others advocate for a more aggressive approach.

Regardless of the recommendations, it is useful to consider how successful the medical community has been in meeting guideline goals. A national survey conducted in 2003 (NEPTUNE II) showed 67% of the 4885 patients with elevated cholesterol achieved their LDL cholesterol treatment goal.[23] Data from the National Health and Nutrition Examination Surveys (NHANES) document a steady decline in total cholesterol over several decades, so that in 2002 no more than 17% of US adults had a total cholesterol level of 240 mg/dL or higher. More recent data from an identical survey in 2008 show that the Healthy People 2010 goal of an average cholesterol below 200 mg/dL in all adults ages 20 to 74 was met in both men and women by 2008.[24] The obvious problem in monitoring these trends is that the percentage of the population at or below goal varies considerably by demographic parameters. Therefore, it is useful for every practice to perform quality studies in its own population to determine how well current guidelines are met and to think innovatively about clinic initiatives that can address suboptimal treatment.

Lifestyle modification is the first step to reduce cholesterol levels. Changes in diet, weight loss, and increased exercise are all known to be effective. What is also well known is the difficulty in achieving these goals. There are major limitations in most weight-loss studies. For example, weight-loss programs show weight reduction reduces both cholesterol and TGs but long term almost half of the initial weight loss is regained after 1 year.[25] In a recent review of various weight-loss diets, the investigators concluded that the type of diet is less important than the its palatability and the ease of continuing it long term.[26] Given these drawbacks to lifestyle change, it may be prudent to achieve lipid-lowering goals by initiating medications sooner rather than later. If lifestyle change goals are achieved, the need for medication can be reassessed.

Pharmaceutical Options

Numerous studies have established that, for most patients, statins are the preferred medical treatment. Currently in the United States, the Food and Drug Administration has approved 6 drugs of this class (with some available in immediate-release or

---

Box 4
Comparison of LDL cholesterol and Non-HDL cholesterol goals for 3 risk categories based on ATP-III guidelines[a]

If CVD 10-year risk is:

- >20%, then LDL <100 and non-HDL <130

- ≤20% plus 2 or more risk factors, then LDL <130 and non-HDL <160

- 0–1 risk factors, then LDL <160 and non-HDL <190

[a] ATP-IV guidelines are expected this year and will probably significantly change these recommendations.

extended-release forms) (**Table 4**). Comparative data show that all of them reduce lipid levels to varying degrees, with atorvastatin and rosuvastatin considered to be the "strong" reducers of LDL. Although there are no trials comparing all of the available statins directly with each other, there are a few head-to-head comparisons of some of the statins. These are shown in **Table 5**.

Based on available evidence, there is no compelling reason to choose one statin over another for the usual primary care clinic patient; however, those patients with familial combined hyperlipidemia should probably be started on atorvastatin or rosu-vastatin.[27] Additionally, it has been shown that the presence of xanthomas in hetero-zygous familial hyperlipidemia confers additional CVD risk to these patients and specialty opinion should be sought.[28]

Alternatives to statins

Although statins have reached the status of preferred treatment for hyperlipidemia, there are reasons to consider other medications. Some physicians think that mono-therapy is preferable, whereas others believe that low to moderate doses of combina-tions of drugs produce better LDL-C reduction with fewer side effects. There are times when statin therapy is maximal, but the lipid goals have not been met. Finally, there are situations in which statins are either contraindicated or not tolerated. A full review of these options is beyond the scope of this article. A number of studies have looked at comparisons of drug combinations.[29] Some of the therapeutic options are listed in **Table 6**.

Use of complementary products (nutraceuticals, herbs, and so forth)

Many people prefer complementary and alternative medicines to pharmaceutical products. They want to use these products because they are less expensive to purchase, do not require a prescription, and are considered natural. Although there are no studies demonstrating that an alternative product is superior to statins in either lipid or CVD reduction, several reviews have shown modest reduction of plasma lipids with the use of substances such as garlic,[30] artichoke leaf extract,[31] nuts, plant stano-lols, psyllium, soluble fiber, orange juice, and red yeast rice.[32] Potential resources to help the interested reader learn more are found at the National Institutes of Health National Center for Complementary and Alternative Medicine official Web site (http://nccam.nih.gov/), which contains information that is organized both by product and by health condition. It also has links to systematic reviews and meta-analyses

Table 4
Current HMG-CoA-inhibitors

Drug	Trade Name	Dose Range	% LDL-C Decrease	% HDL-C Increase	% TG Decrease
Fluvastatin	Lescol	20–80 mg	22–35	3–11	17–21
Pravastatin	Pravachol	10–80 mg	22–37	2–12	15–24
Lovastatin	Altoprev/Mevacor	10–80 mg	21–42	2–8	6–21
Simvastatin	Zocor	5–80* mg	26–47	10–16	12–33
Atorvastatin	Lipitor	10–80 mg	39–60	5–9	19–37
Rosuvastatin	Crestor	5–40 mg	45–63	8–10	10–30
Pitavastatin	Livalo	1–4 mg	38–44	5–8	14–22

Abbreviations: HDL-C, high-density lipoprotein cholesterol; LDL-C, low-density lipoprotein choles-terol; TG, triglyceride.
* 80 mg dose only for those who have been taking it for more than 12 months and without evidence of myopathy.

Table 5
Studies of direct comparisons of 2 or more statins' efficacy in lipid lowering

Study Name	Number Participants	Drugs Compared	Conclusions
PATROL,[50,a]	302	Pitavastatin, atorvastatin, and rosuvastatin	The safety and efficacy of these 3 strong statins are equal
CIRCLE,[51,b]	743	Atorvastatin vs pitavastatin vs pravastatin	Pitavastatin or atorvastatin resulted in better reduction of LDL-C than pravastatin; pitavastatin significantly increased HDL-C compared with placebo, whereas the other two statins did not
SATURN,[52,a]	1039	Atorvastatin vs rosuvastatin	No difference in progression of arterial plaques by intravascular ultrasound despite statistically significant lower LDL with rosuvastatin

Abbreviations: HDL-C, high-density lipoprotein cholesterol; LDL-C, low-density lipoprotein cholesterol.
[a] Prospective randomized multicenter trial.
[b] Retrospective study.

conducted in the past 5 years about specific treatments. Another source is the Web site www.naturalstandard.com/. The Natural Standard Research Collaboration is a coalition of medical researchers that conducts and reviews research about natural remedies. They rate products using an evidence-based methodology and assign each review a grade (A–F) based on the available scientific evidence. Using traditional medical research sources (eg, PubMed), it is difficult to find systematic reviews of the evidence for the many natural remedies that have putative benefit in promoting a healthier lipid profile. Those that are available generally show only modest cholesterol lowering. A major deficiency in the study of alternative products is the lack of studies that use hard cardiovascular end points instead of a surrogate marker, such as changes in LDL-C. As was learned from the experience with products such as rosiglitazone[33,34] in people with type 2 diabetes, not all favorable changes in serum lipid characteristics translate into a reduction in CVD events. Thus, any study based solely on lipid lowering as an end point may be misleading.

UNANSWERED QUESTIONS AND CURRENT CONTROVERSIES

Despite the overall lowering of mean LDL-C and the overall incidence of CVD in the US population, CVD remains a significant health burden and a leading cause of mortality. There remain many unanswered questions and controversies regarding how best to further decrease these numbers. These questions are important because of the expected increase in CVD given the aging population and the obesity epidemic. These are addressed in this section in no particular order.

One of the potential reasons for continuing high rates of CVD is that the target LDL-C goals may be too modest. There are investigators and practitioners who advocate lowering LDL-C as low as can be achieved, possibly even to levels lower than 50 mg/dL. Others argue that the evidence to support this view has not been conclusively shown.

Table 6
Statin alternatives

Drug	Effects	Adverse Reactions
Bile acid sequestrants		
Cholestyramine (4–16 g) Colestipol (5–20 g) Colesevelam (2.6–3.8 g)	LDL: −15%–30% HDL: +3%–5% TG: No change or increase	Gastrointestinal distress Constipation Decreased absorption of other drugs
Nicotinic acid		
Immediate release (crystalline) nicotinic acid (1.5–3.0 g), extended release nicotinic acid (Niaspan) (1–2 g), sustained release nicotinic acid (1–2 g)	LDL: −5%–25% HDL: +15%–35% TG: −20%–50%	Flushing Hyperglycemia Hyperuricemia (or gout) Upper GI distress Hepatotoxicity
Fibric acids		
Gemfibrozil (600 mg BID) Fenofibrate (200 mg) Clofibrate (1000 mg BID)	LDL: −5%–20% (may be increased in patients with high TG) HDL: +10%–20% TG: −20%–50%	Dyspepsia Gallstones Myopathy
Ezetimibe		
Zetia (10 mg daily) As monotherapy, often combined with a statin	LDL-C: −18% HDL-C: +3% TG: −8%	Diarrhea Arthralgia Nasopharyngitis or sinusitis Controversial regarding reduction of CVD events
Omega 3 fatty acids		
Lovaza Fish oil Plant sources		Prescription fatty acid ester indicated only for treatment of TG >500 mg/dL to prevent pancreatitis. Fish oil has been shown to reduce elevated TG with subsequent mild reduction in LDL and non–HDL-C; however, a recent major study showed no benefit from fish oil capsules; consumption of fish is preferred. Plant sources of omega-3 FA have been subjected to few clinical trials with CVD end points.

Abbreviations: CVD, cardiovascular disease; FA, fatty acids; GI, gastrointestinal; HDL-C, high-density lipoprotein cholesterol; LDL-C, low-density lipoprotein cholesterol; TG, triglyceride.

A meta-analysis of trials with cardiovascular outcomes looked at 27,548 patients enrolled in 4 large studies. The investigators concluded that high-dose statins were significantly better than moderate-dose statins, primarily by reducing nonfatal cardiac events; however, they did not find a statistically significant difference between cardiovascular or all-cause mortality.[35] Another study that showed evidence of improved outcome from high-dose statins is the ASTEROID study.[36] The investigators used intravascular ultrasound to document atheroma regression after treatment with 40 mg daily of rosuvastatin. The average LDL-C achieved was ∼60 mg/dL. The study investigators concluded that lowering LDL-C below current recommended guidelines can cause regression of atherosclerosis in coronary disease patients. A third major study was the Treat to New Targets.[37] It found that lowering LDL-C to 80 mg/dL in the treatment group was superior in preventing CVD outcomes than lowering it to 100 mg/dL.

Another controversy regarding LDL-C target is the question of how best to achieve the desired goals. One side of the debate advocates high-dose statins, whereas the other prefers combination therapy in moderate doses. The question is based in part on a balance between benefit and risk. Statins are known to have beneficial effects in addition to lipid lowering. These pleiotropic effects include anti-inflammatory action and improvement in coagulability. The long-term risks of the statins are not fully known. There has been recent controversy over the question of whether statins cause type 2 diabetes.[38,39] In addition, there are questions about a possible link of statins to pancreatitis, although a recent review disputes this claim.[40] A number of the studies that have compared adjunctive therapy consisting of a statin plus another lipid-lowering drug with mono-statin treatment are reviewed in an exhaustive report from the Agency for Healthcare Research and Quality.[41] **Table 7** is a reproduction from the executive summary of the report. The main conclusion of the report is that there is insufficient evidence (especially morbidity/mortality data) to answer the question if high-dose monotherapy is different from combination therapy. Currently, there is no definitive answer to the question and each physician needs to make the decision based on incomplete data and a rational balance of risk versus benefit for each individual patient.

A significant unresolved problem in current medical practice is the issue of residual risk. Because a significant number of cases of CVD occur in people without traditional risk factors, some physicians have suggested using nontraditional biomarkers to identify those who are at increased risk for CVD despite normal lipid profiles. As previously discussed in the section on novel risk factors, there are no biomarkers that have been convincingly shown by large clinical trials or meta-analysis to be superior to current practice. Despite the scant evidence linking reduction of these markers to reduced incidence of CVD events, some believe cholesterol drugs should be used in healthy people with low probability of CVD.[42] This study is cited as an example of the type of analysis that leads some to argue for a more extensive use of statins because there was a significant decrease in CVD events. Others believe this liberal use of statins may constitute unacceptable risk in truly low-risk subjects. In the study cited previously, the number needed to treat to prevent a single death from any cause and to prevent a single nonfatal myocardial infarction was 239 and 153, respectively. Another approach to addressing residual risk is use of pharmacologic means to raise HDL-C. This idea has been challenged by recent trials that failed to show any lowering of CVD events despite raising HDL-C.[43,44] A recently published trial comparing genetic mutations that confer high HDL versus low HDL has called into question the well-established belief that HDL-C protects against CVD.[45] A third approach to addressing the problem of residual risk has been to focus on TGRLs as potential atherogenic agents. The idea is that lowering TG concentrations that are currently recognized as high, but not sufficiently so to treat pharmacologically (ie, 250–499 mg/dL), can have a major impact on CVD; however, recent trials in patients with type 2 diabetes treated with fibrates or niacin have created doubt about this hypothesis.[46,47] Current research is re-examining some of the long-held beliefs about the role of various lipid fractions in the etiology of CVD. This work includes both examination of the biochemical pathways to identify new potential drug targets and a detailed analysis of the negative studies to determine if the entire idea is wrong or just a portion.

To summarize, there is a solid link between elevated cholesterol (especially LDL-C) and CVD. It has been conclusively shown and become accepted practice to lower LDL-C in patients considered intermediate to high risk for CVD with a combination of therapeutic lifestyle change and medications. First-line drug therapy should be a statin, titrated to keep LDL-C at or below the target range recommended by the

Table 7
Summary of conclusions from evidence comparing use of a specific statin in combination with another lipid-modifying agent with use of a higher-dose statin in populations requiring intensive treatment and subgroups

Outcome	Strength of Evidence (GRADE)	Summary/Conclusions
Key Question 1. For patients who require intensive lipid-modifying therapy, what are the comparative long-term benefits and rates of serious adverse events of coadministration of different lipid-modifying agents (ie, a statin plus another lipid-modifying agent) compared with higher-dose statin monotherapy?		
All-cause mortality	Very low	Insufficient evidence was available regarding mortality. Based on small trials with few events, no difference in mortality was noted for any statin combination associated with ezetimibe or fibrates compared with higher-dose statin monotherapy. No evidence was available for other combinations.
Vascular death	—	No evidence was available for any statin combination vs higher-dose statin monotherapy.
SAEs[a]	Very low	Up to a maximum follow-up of 24 wk, no intervention was significantly safer when statin-ezetimibe combination was compared with higher-dose statin monotherapy. No evidence was available for other combinations.
Key Question 2. Do these regimens differ in reaching LDL targets (or other surrogate markers), short-term side effects, tolerability, and/or adherence?		
Attainment of ATP-III LDL-C goals	Very low	Ezetimibe plus simvastatin therapy is more likely to result in attainment of LDL-C target than higher-dose simvastatin, based on 2 small trials. Results for statin-fibrate combination (1 trial) were indeterminate. No evidence was available for other combinations.
Key Question 3. Compared with higher-dose statins and with one another, do combination regimens differ in benefits and harms within subgroups of patients?		
All-cause mortality, vascular death, and attainment of ATP-III LDL-C goals	Very low	There is insufficient evidence to draw any meaningful conclusions in subgroups for any combination.
SAEs	—	Because absent to scant subgroup evidence was anticipated, SAEs were examined across all trial populations (see above).
Intercombination, indirect comparison of syntheses		We are unable to confirm a difference in benefits or harms between combinations due to the lack of evidence.

Abbreviations: ATP-III, Adult Treatment Panel III (of the National Cholesterol Education Program); GRADE, Grading of Recommendations Assessment, Development and Evaluation; LDL-C, low-density lipoprotein cholesterol; SAE, serious adverse events.

[a] Because of scant evidence for those in need of intensive lipid lowering, SAEs were examined across all trial populations.

ATP-III guidelines. Multiple alternatives are available for those who are either statin intolerant or who fail to achieve therapeutic goals. Although these statements are relatively simple, it took decades for them to become standard medical practice. Considerable work is ongoing to identify what factors are most important to residual risk. This work plus ongoing effectiveness research in clinical practice networks should lead to significant changes in how practitioners approach dyslipidemia over the next 1 to 2 decades.

REFERENCES

1. National Ambulatory Medical Care Survey: 2009 Summary Tables. In: National Ambulatory Medical Care Survey: 2009 Summary Tables, The Ambulatory and Hospital Care Statistics Branch of the Centers for Disease Control and Prevention's National Center for Health Statistics, 2009, p. Table 16. Presence of selected chronic conditions at office visits, by patient age and sex: United States 2009. Available at: http://www.cdc.gov/nchs/data/ahcd/namcs_summary/2009_namcs_web_tables.pdf. Accessed September 5, 2012.
2. National Cholesterol Education Program (NCEP) Expert Panel on Detection, Evaluation, and Treatment of High Blood Cholesterol in Adults (Adult Treatment Panel III). Third Report of the National Cholesterol Education Program (NCEP) Expert Panel on detection, evaluation, and treatment of high blood cholesterol in adults (Adult Treatment Panel III) final report. Circulation 2002;106:3143–421.
3. Murphy SL, Xu JQ, Kochanek KD. Deaths: preliminary data for 2010. National vital statistics reports, Table B. Hyattsville (MD): National Center for Health Statistics; 2012.
4. The Lipid Research Clinics Coronary Primary Prevention Trial results. I. Reduction in incidence of coronary heart disease. JAMA 1984;251:351–64.
5. The Lipid Research Clinics Coronary Primary Prevention Trial results. II. The relationship of reduction in incidence of coronary heart disease to cholesterol lowering. JAMA 1984;251:365–74.
6. Steinberg D. Thematic review series: the pathogenesis of atherosclerosis. An interpretive history of the cholesterol controversy: part I. J Lipid Res 2004;45:1583–93.
7. Steinberg D. Thematic review series: the pathogenesis of atherosclerosis. An interpretive history of the cholesterol controversy: part II: the early evidence linking hypercholesterolemia to coronary disease in humans. J Lipid Res 2005;46:179–90.
8. Steinberg D. Thematic review series: the pathogenesis of atherosclerosis: an interpretive history of the cholesterol controversy, part III: mechanistically defining the role of hyperlipidemia. J Lipid Res 2005;46:2037–51.
9. Steinberg D. The pathogenesis of atherosclerosis. An interpretive history of the cholesterol controversy, part IV: the 1984 coronary primary prevention trial ends it—almost. J Lipid Res 2006;47:1–14.
10. Steinberg D. Thematic review series: the pathogenesis of atherosclerosis. An interpretive history of the cholesterol controversy, part V: the discovery of the statins and the end of the controversy. J Lipid Res 2006;47:1339–51.
11. US Preventive Services Task Force. Screening for lipid disorders in adults. 2008. Available at: http://www.uspreventiveservicestaskforce.org/uspstf/uspschol.htm. Accessed August 29, 2012.
12. American Heart Association. Public cholesterol screening. 2011. Available at: http://www.heart.org/HEARTORG/Conditions/Cholesterol/SymptomsDiagnosisMonitoringofHighCholesterol/Public-Cholesterol-Screening-Adults-and-Children_UCM_305617_Article.jsp. Accessed September 5, 2012.

13. Semenkovich CF, Goldberg AC, Goldberg IJ. Disorders of lipid metabolism. In: Melmed S, Polonsky KS, Larsen PR, et al, editors. Williams textbook of endocrinology. 12th edition. Philadelphia: W.B. Saunders; 2011. p. 1655.
14. Aberg JA. Lipid management in patients who have HIV and are receiving HIV therapy. Endocrinol Metab Clin North Am 2009;38:207–22.
15. Chapter 3.3 Assessment of cardiovascular risk. In: Cooper A, Nherera L, Calvert N, et al, editors. Clinical guidelines and evidence review for lipid modification: cardiovascular risk assessment and the primary and secondary prevention of cardiovascular disease. London: National Collaborating Centre for Primary Care and Royal College of General Practitioners; 2008. p. 49–54.
16. Peters SA, den Ruijter HM, Bots ML, et al. Improvements in risk stratification for the occurrence of cardiovascular disease by imaging subclinical atherosclerosis: a systematic review. Heart 2012;98:177–84.
17. Yeboah J, McClelland RL, Polonsky TS, et al. Comparison of novel risk markers for improvement in cardiovascular risk assessment in intermediate-risk individuals. JAMA 2012;308:788–95.
18. Boekholdt SM, Arsenault BJ, Mora S, et al. Association of LDL cholesterol, non-HDL cholesterol, and apolipoprotein B levels with risk of cardiovascular events among patients treated with statins: a meta-analysis. JAMA 2012;307:1302–9.
19. Di Angelantonio E, Gao P, Pennells L, et al. Lipid-related markers and cardiovascular disease prediction. JAMA 2012;307:2499–506.
20. Grundy SM. Use of emerging lipoprotein risk factors in assessment of cardiovascular risk. JAMA 2012;307:2540–2.
21. Balk EM, Lau J, Goudas LC, et al. Effects of statins on nonlipid serum markers associated with cardiovascular disease: a systematic review. Ann Intern Med 2003;139:670–82.
22. ATP-III at-a-glance: quick desk reference 2001. Available at: http://www.nhlbi.nih.gov/guidelines/cholesterol/dskref.htm. Accessed September 5, 2012.
23. Davidson MH, Maki KC, Pearson TA, et al. Results of the National Cholesterol Education (NCEP) Program Evaluation ProjecT Utilizing Novel E-Technology (NEPTUNE) II survey and implications for treatment under the recent NCEP Writing Group recommendations. Am J Cardiol 2005;96:556–63.
24. Centers for Disease Control and Prevention. QuickStats: average total cholesterol level among men and women. Atlanta (GA): Department of Health and Human Services; 2009. p. 1045.
25. Curioni CC, Lourenco PM. Long-term weight loss after diet and exercise: a systematic review. Int J Obes (Lond) 2005;29:1168–74.
26. Makris A, Foster GD. Dietary approaches to the treatment of obesity. Psychiatr Clin North Am 2011;34:813–27.
27. Hemphill LC. Familial hypercholesterolemia: current treatment options and patient selection for low-density lipoprotein apheresis. J Clin Lipidol 2010;4:346–9.
28. Oosterveer DM, Versmissen J, Yazdanpanah M, et al. Differences in characteristics and risk of cardiovascular disease in familial hypercholesterolemia patients with and without tendon xanthomas: a systematic review and meta-analysis. Atherosclerosis 2009;207:311–7.
29. Sharma M, Ansari MT, Abou-Setta AM, et al. Systematic review: comparative effectiveness and harms of combination therapy and monotherapy for dyslipidemia. Ann Intern Med 2009;151:622–30.
30. Stevinson C, Pittler MH, Ernst E. Garlic for treating hypercholesterolemia. A meta-analysis of randomized clinical trials. Ann Intern Med 2000;133:420–9.

31. Wider B, Pittler MH, Thompson-Coon J, et al. Artichoke leaf extract for treating hypercholesterolaemia. Cochrane Database Syst Rev 2009;(4):CD003335.
32. Nies LK, Cymbala AA, Kasten SL, et al. Complementary and alternative therapies for the management of dyslipidemia. Ann Pharmacother 2006;40:1984–92.
33. Nissen SE, Wolski K. Effect of rosiglitazone on the risk of myocardial infarction and death from cardiovascular causes. N Engl J Med 2007;356:2457–71.
34. Jonas D, Van Scoyoc E, Gerrald K, et al. Drug class review: newer diabetes medications, TZDs, and combinations: final original report [Internet]. Portland (OR): Oregon Health & Science University; 2011. Available at:. http://www.ncbi.nlm.nih.gov/books/NBK54209/. Accessed August 31, 2012.
35. Cannon CP, Steinberg BA, Murphy SA, et al. Meta-analysis of cardiovascular outcomes trials comparing intensive versus moderate statin therapy. J Am Coll Cardiol 2006;48:438–45.
36. Nissen SE, Nicholls SJ, Sipahi I, et al. Effect of very high-intensity statin therapy on regression of coronary atherosclerosis: the ASTEROID trial. JAMA 2006;295: 1556–65.
37. LaRosa JC, Grundy SM, Waters DD, et al. Intensive lipid lowering with atorvastatin in patients with stable coronary disease. N Engl J Med 2005;352:1425–35.
38. Sattar N, Preiss D, Murray HM, et al. Statins and risk of incident diabetes: a collaborative meta-analysis of randomised statin trials. Lancet 2010;375:735–42.
39. Preiss D, Seshasai SR, Welsh P, et al. Risk of incident diabetes with intensivedose compared with moderate-dose statin therapy: a meta-analysis. JAMA 2011;305:2556–64.
40. Preiss D, Tikkanen MJ, Welsh P, et al. Lipid-modifying therapies and risk of pancreatitis: a meta-analysis. JAMA 2012;308:804–11.
41. Sharma M, Ansari MT, Soares-Weiser K, et al. Comparative effectiveness of lipid-modifying agents. Prepared by the University of Ottawa Evidence-based Practice Center under contract No. 290-02-0021. In: Comparative effectiveness review. Rockville (MD): Agency for Healthcare Research and Quality; 2009. p. ES1–14. Available at: www.effectivehealthcare.ahrq.gov/reports/final.cfm. Accessed September 5, 2012.
42. Conly J, Clement F, Tonelli M, et al. Cost-effectiveness of the use of low- and high-potency statins in people at low cardiovascular risk. CMAJ 2011;183:E1180–8.
43. Boden WE, Probstfield JL, Anderson T, et al. Niacin in patients with low HDL cholesterol levels receiving intensive statin therapy. N Engl J Med 2011;365: 2255–67.
44. Ghosh RK, Ghosh SM. Current status of CETP inhibitors in the treatment of hyperlipidemia: an update. Curr Clin Pharmacol 2012;7:102–10.
45. Voight BF, Peloso GM, Orho-Melander M, et al. Plasma HDL cholesterol and risk of myocardial infarction: a mendelian randomisation study. Lancet 2012;380: 572–80.
46. Ginsberg HN, Elam MB, Lovato LC, et al. Effects of combination lipid therapy in type 2 diabetes mellitus. N Engl J Med 2010;362:1563–74.
47. Keech A, Simes RJ, Barter P, et al. Effects of long-term fenofibrate therapy on cardiovascular events in 9795 people with type 2 diabetes mellitus (the FIELD study): randomised controlled trial. Lancet 2005;366:1849–61.
48. Gregson J, Stirnadel-Farrant HA, Doobaree IU, et al. Variation of lipoprotein associated phospholipase A2 across demographic characteristics and cardiovascular risk factors: a systematic review of the literature. Atherosclerosis 2012; 225:11–21.

49. Nordestgaard BG, Chapman MJ, Ray K, et al. Lipoprotein(a) as a cardiovascular risk factor: current status. Eur Heart J 2010;31:2844–53.
50. Teramoto T. The clinical impact of pitavastatin: comparative studies with other statins on LDL-C and HDL-C. Expert Opin Pharmacother 2012;13:859–65.
51. Maruyama T, Takada M, Nishibori Y, et al. Comparison of preventive effect on cardiovascular events with different statins. The CIRCLE study. Circ J 2011;75: 1951–9.
52. Nicholls SJ, Ballantyne CM, Barter PJ, et al. Effect of two intensive statin regimens on progression of coronary disease. N Engl J Med 2011;365:2078–87.

Pericarditis, Myocarditis, and Other Cardiomyopathies

Nicolas W. Shammas, MD, EJD, MS[a,b,]*, Rafat F. Padaria, MD[b],
Edmund P. Coyne, MD[b]

KEYWORDS

- Pericarditis • Cardiomyopathy • Acute myocarditis • Pericardial effusion
- Therapeutics • Etiology

KEY POINTS

- Acute pericarditis requires at least 2 of the following 4 criteria for diagnosis: (1) chest pain characteristics of pericarditis, (2) pericardial rub, (3) characteristic electrocardiographic (ECG) changes, and (4) new or worsening pericardial effusion.
- Pericardial effusion in the setting of neoplasm does not always indicate neoplastic infiltration to the pericardial sac.
- Pharmacologic treatment of dilated cardiomyopathy (DCM) includes β-blockers and angiotensin-converting enzyme inhibitors (ACEI).
- Acute myocarditis may present with mild symptoms to severe heart failure (HF) requiring mechanical support or fulminant myocarditis that leads to death.

PERICARDITIS

Pericardium is the thin covering of the heart that separates it from the rest of the mediastinum. It consists of 2 layers: the outer fibrous pericardium and the inner double-layer serous pericardium. Layers of the serous pericardium are the visceral epicardium (covers the heart and great vessels) and the parietal pericardium (covers the fibrous pericardium). The pericardial cavity is enclosed between the visceral and parietal pericardium and normally contains from 15 to 50 mL of clear fluid, which is an ultrafiltrate of plasma. The pericardium is not essential to heart function but can have significant clinical consequences. Pericardial disease can present itself as pericaridtis (acute or

Disclosure: None as it relates to this manuscript from any of the authors. Full corresponding author disclosure at http://mcrfmd.com/?page=235.
Funding: Supported by the Nicolas and Gail Research Fund at the Midwest Cardiovascular Research Foundation, Davenport, IA.
[a] Midwest Cardiovascular Research Foundation, 1622 East Lombard Street, Davenport, IA 52803, USA; [b] Cardiovascular Medicine, PC, 1236 East Rusholme, Suite 300, Davenport, IA 52803, USA
* Corresponding author.
E-mail address: shammas@mchsi.com

http://dx.doi.org/10.1016/j.pop.2012.11.009
0095-4543/13/$ – see front matter © 2013 Elsevier Inc. All rights reserved.

chronic recurrent), pericardial effusion (with or without hemodynamic consequences), or constrictive pericardial disease.[1]

Acute Pericarditis

Acute pericarditis is an inflammatory process involving the pericardium that occurs in 0.1% of hospitalized patients and up to 5% of noncoronary patients seen in the emergency room with chest pain.[2] **Box 1** illustrates the common causes of acute pericarditis.

Diagnosis

Pericarditis is primarily a clinical diagnosis, made by a proper history, physical examination, and the ECG. It is generally agreed upon that at least 2 of the following 4 criteria need to be met for the diagnosis of acute pericarditis[1]: (1) chest pain characteristics of pericarditis, (2) pericardial rub, (3) characteristic ECG changes, and (4) new or worsening pericardial effusion.

Chest pain is the most common symptom in patients with pericarditis. It is generally sharp, worsens with deep breath or on lying backward, and improves with leaning forward, and it may radiate to the trapezius muscle.

A pericardial friction rub may be heard in patients with pericarditis. It is best heard with the patient leaning forward, during inspiration, at the left lower sternal border. The rub is scratchy in character and may have 3 components: atrial systole, ventricular systole, and early ventricular diastole. However, 1 or 2 components may also be present.

Diffuse concave ST segment elevation with PR segment depression is seen. ST elevation is seen on the 12-lead ECG in patients with new-onset acute pericarditis (**Fig. 1**). There are 4 consecutive stages of pericarditis seen on the ECG (**Fig. 2**):

- Stage I: ST elevation in both arms and precordial leads.
- Stage II: pseudonormalization of ST elevation

Box 1
Causes of acute pericarditis

Idiopathic

Infectious—bacterial, viral, fungal, parasitic, human immunodeficiency virus

Systemic diseases—immune mediated

Myocardial infarction

Radiation

Postoperatively after open heart surgery

Aortic dissection

Chest wall trauma

Malignancy

    Primary—mesothelioma, angiosarcoma

    Metastatic—lung, breast, bone, lymphoma, melanoma

Metabolic—uremia, hypothyroidism

Pharmacologic

    Penicillin, phenytoin, procainamide, hydralazine, minoxidil, cromolyn sodium, methysergide, doxorubicin

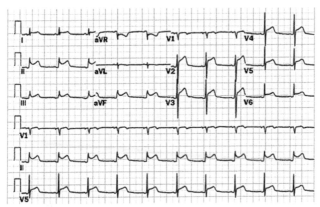

Fig. 1. Electrocardiogram in acute pericarditis. Note the diffuse ST elevation across the precordial and arm leads.

- Stage III: inverted T waves
- Stage IV: normalization of T waves

All these stages are seen in about 60% of patients.[3] Stage I is seen in 80% of patients.[4] These changes need to be placed in their clinical context because ischemia cannot be ruled out particularly if the pain is anginal in nature and the levels of cardiac enzymes are elevated.

Chest radiograph may show cardiomegaly when a minimum of 200 mL of pericardial effusion is present.[2] When acute pericarditis is suspected, the presence of a pericardial effusion and/or bright thickened pericardium will further confirm the diagnosis. However, echocardiography (**Fig. 3**) may be most cost effective when no improvement in symptoms is seen within 1 to 2 weeks of the diagnosis or if there is hemodynamic instability or recent cardiac surgery. Also, in acute pericarditis, cardiac computed tomography (CT) may show thickening of the pericardium, but this finding is nonspecific. In addition, cardiac magnetic resonance (CMR) is sensitive in acute pericarditis, showing a delayed enhanced gadolinium uptake in the inflamed pericardium.[1] Finally, serology in the case of acute pericarditis is of low yield and markers for autoimmune diseases are not necessary to obtain unless there is a clinical suspicion of their occurrence. Antiviral titers are also not useful and will not change the management of the patient with acute viral pericarditis.[5,6]

Treatment
It is important to focus initially on triaging patients who are hemodynamically unstable or imminently likely to become unstable. In patients with hemodynamic instability,

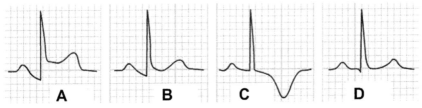

Fig. 2. Stages of electrocardiographic changes in acute pericarditis. (*A*) stage I, ST elevation in both arms and precordial leads. (*B*) Stage II: pseudonormalization of ST elevation. (*C*) stage III: inverted T waves. (*D*) Stage IV: normalization of T waves.

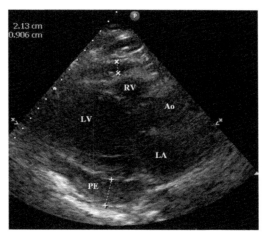

Fig. 3. Pericardial effusion seen on echocardiography. Ao, aorta; LA, left atrium; LV, left ventricle; PE, pericardial effusion; RV, right ventricle.

elevated jugular venous pressure with pulsus paradoxus and Kussmaul sign are present. Patients will likely have sinus tachycardia, low voltage, and signs of acute pericarditis on the ECG. Electrical alternans, a specific and less-sensitive sign of cardiac tamponade, indicates swinging of the heart in the pericardial fluid and is identified with alteration of the QRS amplitude or axis in between beats. Cardiac tamponade needs to be considered in patients with hypotension, cardiac shock, or pulseless electrical activity. An echocardiogram will confirm the diagnosis and allow immediate treatment to be initiated with volume expansion and pericardiocentesis or surgical removal of the pericardial fluid. Typical findings on the echocardiogram are late diastolic collapse of the right atrium, early diastolic collapse of the right ventricle (RV), and significant mitral inflow variability. Also, the echocardiogram may be helpful in identifying aortic dissection or cardiac free wall rupture as causes of tamponade. Right heart catheterization is rarely needed to confirm the diagnosis. Typical findings on the right atrial pressure tracing is a prominent a wave with a blunted y descent. This pattern is associated with a drop in aortic pressure with inspiration compared with expiration (pulsus paradoxus).

When hemodynamic stability is present, outpatient treatment is appropriate with close follow-up. When acute pericarditis is suspected, a few tests can be performed including a chest radiograph, ECG, erythrocyte sedimentation rate, and C-reactive protein. Viral serology is unlikely to be helpful. However, if human immunodeficiency virus infection or tuberculosis is suspected, appropriate testing needs to be performed to confirm the diagnosis. If the clinical picture suggests an autoimmune disorder, then antinuclear antibody test can be performed. Specific testing is also needed if malignancy is suspected. Irrespective of such testing, if a patient is likely to develop tamponade, hospitalization is warranted. Several features are likely to predict a worse prognosis and need for in-hospital management.[7] These features include a large pericardial effusion, high fever with leukocytosis, elevated troponin levels, failure of nonsteroidal antiinflammatory drugs (NSAIDs), trauma, and reduced immunity. If a patient has a large pericardial effusion (>20 mm on echocardiogram), it is recommended that this be electively drained because nearly one-third of these patients develop tamponade unexpectedly, particularly if the effusion persists for more than 1 month or early right atrial collapse is seen.[1]

Key Points

Acute pericarditis requires at least 2 of the following 4 criteria for diagnosis: (1) chest pain characteristics of pericarditis, (2) pericardial rub, (3) characteristic ECG changes, and (4) new or worsening pericardial effusion.

Echocardiography is most cost effective when no improvement in symptoms is seen within 1 to 2 weeks of the diagnosis or if there is hemodynamic instability or recent cardiac surgery.

The initial focus should be on triaging patients who are hemodynamically unstable or imminently likely to become unstable.

The mainstay of treatment is NSAIDs, colchicine, and in autoimmune pericarditis, steroids. In general, steroids are to be avoided because they increase the rate of recurrent pericarditis.

The mainstay of treatment is NSAIDs.[8] Ibuprofen, high-dose aspirin, and indomethacin have been used successfully.[3] Treatment duration is typically 3 weeks (1 week high dose of NSAIDs and then taper to lower dose). Gastroprotection with proton pump inhibitors is recommended. Aspirin is preferred in patients with acute coronary syndrome and history of coronary artery disease. Coronary blood flow is reduced with indomethacin, and therefore it is best to avoid this drug in patients with coronary artery disease.[9] If response to NSAIDs is poor after 1 week of therapy, colchicine[10] is recommended for 4–6 weeks. Colchicine should be avoided in patients with severe hepatic or renal impairment. High-dose steroids with a 3-week taper is a very effective treatment for suppressing the inflammatory response in acute pericariditis, but its use should be limited to cases in which NSAIDs and colchicine have failed. Treatment with steroids is associated with a higher incidence of relapse of pericarditis.[10] Steroids for acute pericarditis may be considered as first-line treatment in cases of autoimmune disease or uremic pericarditis.[8]

Recurrent pericarditis is challenging to treat. It can be incessant with recurrence within the first 6 weeks of stopping treatment or relapsing with recurrence after 6 weeks.[11] This condition is thought to be autoimmune in origin and does respond well to steroids or immunosuppressants. The diagnosis of recurrent pericarditis is similar to diagnosing acute pericarditis as described earlier. The typical time for recurrence is within 18 to 20 months after the initial attack.[12] Colchicine is also very effective in reducing recurrent pericarditis. Because steroids are associated with higher recurrences of pericariditis, it is recommended to be reserved to those patients who fail NSAIDs and colchicine or in patients with autoimmune pericarditis.[1]

Pericardiectomy is rarely needed and is reserved for patients with recurrent pericarditis and constrictive pericarditis despite aggressive medical treatment. Pericardiectomy may not always suppress the symptoms of recurrent pericarditis.

Constrictive Pericarditis

Constrictive pericarditis is a chronic form of pericarditis in which a fibrotic, thickened, and adherent pericardium restricts diastolic filling and cardiac output. Constrictive pericarditis results in right-sided HF. This condition is often underdiagnosed. Confirming the diagnosis remains a challenge. **Box 2** illustrates the common causes of constrictive pericarditis.

Diagnosis

Constrictive pericarditis presents with diastolic failure because of the inability of the myocardium to expand once it reaches the thickened and stiffened pericardium. The compliance of the ventricle and the systolic function are generally preserved.

Box 2
Causes of constrictive pericarditis

Idiopathic

Infectious: tuberculosis, viral, purulent

Traumatic

Postcardiac surgery

Postmediastinal radiation

Chronic inflammatory disease: systemic lupus erythematosus, rheumatoid arthritis

Uremia

Neoplastic disease

Asbestosis

Sarcoidosis

Patients present with lower-extremity edema, elevated jugular venous distention, anasarca, enlarged liver, postprandial discomfort, and third spacing with abdominal and pleural effusions. In addition to a picture of right-sided heart failure, patients can also present with a low cardiac output syndrome with dyspnea and fatigue. Constrictive pericarditis can be of insidious or acute onset. When constrictive pericarditis presents acutely, patients also have agitation, tachycardia, or the Beck triad of elevated venous pressure, systemic hypotension, and a small quiet heart. A history of cardiac surgery or systemic inflammatory disease should raise the suspicion of constrictive pericarditis.

On examination, the jugular vein has a deep y descent. During inspiration, there is a paradoxic rise in venous pressure with more distension of the jugular vein (Kussmaul sign). On auscultation, there is a diastolic knock, a loud third heart sound that occurs because of abrupt cessation of flow at the end of the rapidly filling phase of the ventricles. Pulsus paradoxus is uncommon in constrictive pericarditis.

Diagnostic tests
The ECG features are nonspecific for constrictive pericarditis. Nonspecific ST and T abnormalities are typically seen. Low QRS voltage and atrial fibrillation are present in some patients. Approximately 25% of patients have pericardial calcification on a plain chest radiograph.[13] Echocardiographic findings are shown in **Box 3**. In constrictive pericarditis, mitral annular velocity is preserved because the main mechanism of cardiac diastolic filling is the longitudinal motion of the heart. This feature is in contrast to restrictive cardiomyopathy (RCM) in which myocardial relaxation is reduced and so is the mitral annular velocity.[1]

Thickening of pericardium (>4 mm) and calcification[13] may be apparent on CT and CMR imaging (**Fig. 4**). Angiographic assessment of constrictive pericardial disease can be challenging and may be difficult to distinguish from RCM. Equalization of diastolic pressures and a dip and plateau pattern or square root sign are seen when simultaneous RV and left ventricular (LV) pressure is obtained and is seen in both constrictive and restrictive cardiomyopathies. In constrictive pericarditis, there is increased ventricular interdependence not seen in RCM.[14] With inspiration, less LV filling occurs allowing more RV filling. Therefore, with inspiration, the LV pressure is decreased and RV pressure is increased. This discordance of pressure is a highly specific sign of constrictive pericarditis that is not seen with RCM.

> **Box 3**
> **Echocardiographic findings in patients with constrictive pericarditis**
>
> 2D echo
>
> Pericardial thickening
>
> Normal left ventricular size and systolic function
>
> Abnormal ventricular septal motion
>
> Biatrial enlargement
>
> Flattened diastolic wall motion
>
> Dilated inferior vena cava and hepatic veins
>
> Doppler findings
>
> Restrictive mitral inflow velocities with respiration
>
> Restrictive tricuspid inflow velocities with respiration
>
> Preserved medial mitral annulus early diastolic velocity
>
> Hepatic vein: decreased diastolic forward flow with expiration and increase in diastolic flow reversal

Treatment

In acute constrictive pericarditis, medical therapy is the first-line therapy. Complete pericardiectomy is the standard treatment for patients with chronic constrictive pericarditis. Pericardiectomy is associated with a high mortality of more than 6% that is more likely to occur in elderly patients with advanced HF, pulmonary hypertension, and chronic renal insufficiency.[15,16]

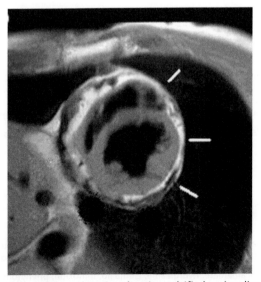

Fig. 4. Cardiac magnetic resonance imaging showing calcified pericardium in a patient with constrictive pericarditis (*white lines*).

Key Points

The main presentation of constrictive pericarditis is right-sided heart failure and symptoms of dyspnea and fatigue.

Thickening of the pericardium may be seen on computed tomography and cardiac magnetic resonance imaging.

Echocardiographic findings can assist in the diagnosis of constrictive pericarditis.

Medical therapy is the first-line therapy. Pericardiectomy is reserved for patients with chronic constrictive pericarditis.

Pericardial Effusion

Pericardial effusion is defined as an increased amount of pericardial fluid. **Box 4** shows the common causes of pericardial effusion. Sometimes the cause of

---

Box 4
Causes of pericardial effusion

Idiopathic

Infectious

    Viral

    Pyogenic: pneumococci, streptococci, staphylococci, *Neisseria*, *Legionella* species

    Tuberculous

    Fungal: histoplasmosis, coccidioidomycosis, *Candida*

    Syphilitic

    Protozoal

    Parasitic

Neoplastic

Postcardiac surgery

Uremia

Myxedema

Severe pulmonary hypertension

Radiation therapy

Acute myocardial infarction—including the complication of free wall rupture

Aortic dissection—leading to hemorrhagic effusion from leakage into the pericardial sac

Trauma

Hyperlipidemia

Chylopericardium

Familial Mediterranean fever

Whipple disease

Hypersensitivity or autoimmune related: systemic lupus erythematosus, rheumatoid arthritis, ankylosing spondylitis, rheumatic fever, scleroderma, Wegener granulomatosis

Drug associated: procainamide, hydralazine, isoniazid, minoxidil, phenytoin, anticoagulants, methysergide

a pericardial effusion may be obvious to the physician in the setting of a known disease such as end-stage renal disease, neoplasm, postcardiac surgery, and myocardial infarction.[17,18] Neoplastic disease can involve the pericardium through several mechanisms such as direct extension from mediastinal structures or the cardiac chamber, retrograde extension from the lymphatic system, and hematologic seeding. Pericardial effusion in the setting of neoplasm does not always indicate neoplastic infiltration to the pericardial sac. In one study, a malignant pericardial effusion was found in only 58% of patients with cancer.[19] In a large study of 322 patients with moderate to large pericardial effusions,[20] the most common diagnosis was acute idiopathic pericarditis (20%), followed by iatrogenic effusion (16%), neoplasm (13%), and chronic idiopathic pericardial effusion (9%). In 2 published series and when tamponade was present (clinically or hemodynamically on echocardiogram), neoplastic pericardial effusions were most prevalent.[21,22]

Diagnosis

Patients may present with chest pain, pressure, or discomfort that is characteristically relieved by sitting up and leaning forward and is intensified by lying supine. They may also have light headedness, syncope, palpitations, cough, dyspnea, or hoarseness.

A large effusion causing hemodynamic compromise may present with one or all the components of the Beck triad of hypotension, muffled heart sounds, and jugular venous distention. Pulsus paradoxus, an exaggeration of physiologic respiratory variation in systemic blood pressure, defined as a decrease in systolic blood pressure of more than 10 mm Hg with inspiration signaling falling cardiac output during inspiration may also be detected. Other physical signs that may be present include a pericardial friction rub, Kussmaul sign, tachycardia, tachypnea, and decreased breath sounds.

The presence of a pericardial effusion can easily be identified with echocardiography, CT, or magnetic resonance imaging (MRI). The most cost-effective and readily available test is the echocardiogram. Echocardiography can identify patients with hemodynamic compromise before it becomes clinically overt. The presence of both right atrial and RV collapse has a positive predictive value of 74% for clinical tamponade.[23] Respiratory variation in RV and LV diastolic filling of more than 25% also suggests the presence of hemodynamically significant effusion.

Treatment

Pharmacotherapy for pericardial effusion includes the use of the one of the following agents, depending on cause: aspirin or other NSAIDs, colchicine, steroids, or antibiotics. In patients with acute inflammatory signs such as fever, pericardial rub, or chest pain, aspirin or other NSAIDs are the first line of therapy. Colchicine is effective in

---

Key Points

Pericardial effusion in the setting of neoplasm does not always indicate neoplastic infiltration to the pericardial sac.

The presence of a pericardial effusion can easily be identified with echocardiography, computed tomography, or magnetic resonance imaging.

Hypotension, jugular venous distention, pulsus paradoxus, tachycardia, tachypnea, and decreased breath sounds indicate hemodynamic compromise.

Purulent pericarditis and recurrent neoplastic effusion should be drained with subxiphoid pericardiotomy.

relapsing pericarditis and may be used as first line in first episode of pericarditis.[8,10] Corticosteroids and NSAIDs are helpful in patients with autoimmune conditions, but steroids should be avoided otherwise because they increase the chance of relapse.[8] Antineoplastic therapy (systemic chemotherapy, radiation) in conjunction with pericardiocentesis has been shown to be effective in reducing recurrences of malignant effusions. Purulent pericarditis and recurrent neoplastic effusion should be drained with subxiphoid pericardiotomy.

CARDIOMYOPATHIES

HF is estimated to affect 2% of the American population and accounts for approximately 277,000 deaths annually. HF is the leading cause of hospitalization for patients older than 65 years and accounts for nearly 2% of hospital admissions.[24] The disorder leads to 12 million to 15 million office visits per year. In 2010, the estimated total cost of HF in the United States was $39.2 billion.[25] Primary care physicians, cardiologists, and intensivists encounter patients with HF and the corresponding clinical challenges on a daily basis. Several proposed reforms in the US health care delivery system are anticipated to put intense focus on chronic disease management, and HF is often cited as the condition that will receive much attention.

HF is a complex clinical syndrome that results from the heart's failure to adequately provide circulation to satisfy the body's metabolic needs at rest or with activity. This failure may relate to the LV's failure to adequately fill in diastole or eject blood in systole. Although fluid retention with subsequent edema and pulmonary congestion are the expected hallmarks of HF, some patients do not present with volume excess but instead describe dyspnea and fatigue with diminished exercise capacity. The development of pulmonary congestion may be related to the rapidity of the development of volume overload, but it is not a universally consistent finding in patients with volume excess. Because pulmonary congestion may often be absent in the patient with chronic HF, the term "heart failure" is preferred over the older but still widely used term "congestive heart failure."

HF may be related to several cardiac conditions, including disease of the myocardium, the pericardium, or the cardiac valves. In certain individuals, arrhythmia may lead to HF. High-output HF usually relates to noncardiac conditions, which lead to increased arterial to venous shunting (eg, thiamine deficiency, thyrotoxicosis, Paget disease of the bone, severe anemia) and typically occurs in patients with underlying structural heart disease.

Cardiomyopathy is a common cause of HF. It should be clarified, however, that the cardiomyopathy is, in and of itself, not HF. Any of the cardiomyopathies, whether ischemic or nonischemic (dilated, restrictive, or hypertrophic) may lead to HF, but HF remains a clinical diagnosis made evident by symptoms of fatigue/dyspnea, with or without the finding of volume overload and pulmonary congestion. Cardiomyopathy, in the absence of these symptoms or findings, is treated with measures very similar to those used to treat HF, but the patient without circulatory compromise at rest or with activity is not considered to have HF.

Unless otherwise stated, the remainder of this review focuses on the evaluation and management of patients with cardiomyopathy, a common cause of HF. Cardiomyopathy can be classified as ischemic or nonischemic. Ischemic heart disease, with underlying coronary artery disease, is thought to be responsible for two-thirds of the cases of HF with low ejection fraction (EF). The prevalence of ischemic disease in the HF population, however, depends largely on the population being studied. Nonischemic cardiomyopathy can be classified as DCM, hypertrophic cardiomyopathy (HCM), and RCM.

Dilated Cardiomyopathy (DCM)

The LV myocardium may be injured for any number of reasons. At present, neurohormonal responses to LV injury are thought to lead to a progressive decline in LV systolic function and enlargement of LV cavity size, a process known as remodeling. Compounds that circulate in greater concentration (or are expressed in greater tissue concentrations) after myocardial injury and lead to a further decline in myocardial function include norepinephrine, angiotensin II, aldosterone, tumor necrosis factor, endothelin, vasopressin, and cytokines. These agents, alone or in combination, may lead to sodium retention and arterial vasoconstriction. In addition, these compounds may have direct toxic effects on myocardial cells (norepinephrine)[26] or may stimulate the development of increased fibrosis within the myocardial interstitium (angiotensin II, aldosterone). Finally, increased degradation of nitric oxide, reduced synthesis and release of NO, and formation of reactive oxygen species occur and contribute to vasoconstriction.[27–29]

Viral cardiomyopathy may be the most common cause of nonischemic cardiomyopathy. Viral DNA has been found within the genome of myocardial cells of 67.4% of consecutive patients with idiopathic DCM studied with myocardial biopsy and polymerase chain reaction analysis of the genome.[30] A variety of viral DNAs were discovered within the myocardial genome, and the evidence for a causative role could only be postulated. However, the high prevalence of evidence of prior viral infection in this population was very suggestive.

Familial DCM is not recognized clinically with high frequency, but it is estimated that 30% of patients with idiopathic DCM have a genetic cause. Familial DCM is an inherited autosomal dominant condition. Symptoms and age of onset are variable among families. A complete review of family history is important in patients with familial cardiomyopathy including cases of unexplained sudden cardiac death or syncope. Echocardiography is the tool of choice to diagnose this entity.[31]

Alcoholic cardiomyopathy[32] was previously thought to be related to various nutritional deficiencies, but more recent evidence indicates a direct toxic effect of alcohol on cardiomyocytes. Some studies suggest that a genetic vulnerability to the toxic effects of alcohol must exist for damage to occur. Alcoholic cardiomyopathy can be asymptomatic or symptomatic. Alcohol consumption of approximately 7 to 8 standard drinks per day for more than 5 years may lead to alcoholic cardiomyopathy with subsequent dilation and thinning of the ventricle. Abstinence from alcohol and treatment with HF drugs are essential to improve heart function.

Peripartum cardiomyopathy is a rare disorder that is usually apparent in the otherwise healthy woman who develops HF with depressed LV function in the peripartum period. This condition occurs in the last trimester of pregnancy or in the first 5 months after delivery. Peripartum cardiomyopathy is a rare condition that occurs in 1 in every 2289 live births in the United States.[33] Although the acute HF may be severe, the cardiomyopathy is usually reversible. There is evidence that women with peripartum cardiomyopathy are at increased risk for recurrent disease with subsequent pregnancies. A high index of suspicion is needed when a pregnant woman develops signs of HF. Providers need to avoid using ACEI or angiotensin receptor blockers (ARB) because of harmful effects to the fetus.[34]

Tachycardia-induced cardiomyopathy is defined as atrial or ventricular dysfunction seen in patients with prolonged rapid heart rate, and it resolves on controlling the arrhythmia. This condition is frequently seen in long-standing unrecognized atrial fibrillation with a poorly controlled ventricular rate. Other tachycardias may also play a role in this context.[35–37] The function of the LV usually improves significantly when the ventricular rate is ultimately controlled.

Cardiomyopathy mediated by premature ventricular beats is caused by very frequent premature ventricular beats that cause dyssynchrony of the LV contraction and may lead to a maladaptive response similar to that seen with other myocardial injuries. One recent study[38] revealed that a premature ventricular complex (PVC) burden of over 24% best separated the patient populations with decreased EF from those with normal EF (sensitivity 79%, specificity 78%). This cardiomyopathy often improves with treatment of the ventricular ectopy.[37]

Takotsubo cardiomyopathy or apical ballooning syndrome may be responsible for 1% to 2% of patients presenting with acute coronary syndrome. These patients are typically women older than 50 years and with a recent history of severe emotional or physiologic stress with evidence of acute ischemia and severe depression of LV function (especially involving the LV apex) and normal coronary arteries. HF develops in 20% to 45% of patients. In over 90% of patients, LV function normalizes. The symptoms of Takotsubo cardiomyopathy can be similar to those of heart attack and is often difficult to distinguish. Patients present with chest pain, shortness of breath, ECG, and enzymatic abnormalities similar to myocardial infarction. Angiography is the best way to distinguish between these 2 entities with the classical ballooning of the LV and the lack of significant coronary artery disease. Traditional risks of myocardial infarction do not apply to patients with Takotsubo cardiomyopathy, and strictly speaking, these patients are not labeled as patients with heart attack. The long-term prognosis is good, and no further deterioration of heart muscle is seen in these patients.[39]

Drug-induced cardiomyopathy: certain antineoplastic drugs, including the anthracyclines (doxorubicin), high-dose cyclophosphamide, trastuzumab (Herceptin), and tyrosine kinase inhibitors (sunitinib) have widely recognized relationships to either temporary (Herceptin) or permanent (anthracyclines such as doxorubicin) myocardial depression. Doxorubicin (Adriamycin) cardiomyopathy is dose dependent with higher doses likely to cause the cardiomyopathy (400 mg/m^2 of body surface area, 5%; 500 mg/m^2, 16%; 550 mg/m^2, 26%; and 700 mg/m^2, 48%).[40] Doxorubicin-induced myopathy could occur from 1 month to several years after the treatment and is likely to occur more frequently in patients who receive other antineoplastic agents.[41,42] Trastuzumab is a recombinant IgG monoclonal antibody that binds to the human epidermal growth factor receptor 2 protein (HER2) and has been shown to cause HF and cardiomyopathy.[43] It is used to treat breast cancers that overexpress HER2. Cocaine was also reported as a rare cause of DCM.[44] Patients are typically young males with tachycardia, signs of adrenergic excess, heart failure, and frequent arrhythmias including atrial fibrillation and with no prior prodromal syndrome.[45] Other drugs that lead to cardiomyopathy include Ecstasy (3, 4-methylenedioxymethamphetamine),[46] Ma Huang (*Ephedra*),[47] and amphetamine.[48]

Valvular cardiomyopathy is secondary to severe valvular insufficiency (mitral or aortic) or severe valvular stenosis (aortic). A close follow-up of these patients with echocardiography is indicated to monitor for cardiac cavity size, thickness, and ejection fraction. The American College of Cardiology/American Heart Association (ACC/AHA) 2006 guidelines recommend transthoracic echocardiography for reevaluation of asymptomatic patients on a yearly basis for severe aortic stenosis and every 1–2 years for moderate aortic stenosis. Moderate to severe mitral valve insufficiency needs to be monitored on a semiannual basis. An early reduction in ejection fraction (<60% for mitral insufficiency and <50% for aortic valve insufficiency) or an enlargement of the cavity size (LV end-systolic dimension >55 mm for aortic valve insufficiency or >40 mm for mitral valve insufficiency) are indications for surgical intervention. Patients may become symptomatic with dyspnea, HF, chest pain, or syncope before cardiac remodeling occurs, and surgery is also indicated for these patients to relieve symptoms and alter prognosis. Aortic valve replacement is indicated in patients with severe aortic valve stenosis if they are symptomatic, undergoing concomitant bypass surgery, or undergoing surgery of the aorta and other valves, or in asymptomatic patients with ejection fraction of 50% or less. At present, patients who are at excessively high risk for aortic valve replacement for severe aortic stenosis can be considered for transcatheter aortic valve replacement.[49]

Idiopathic cardiomyopathy indicates a DCM with no identifiable cause.

Several *systemic conditions* may lead to LV dysfunction, and these diagnoses may become apparent as a complete history and physical examination is completed. Some of these include hypertension, hyperthyroidism, hemochromatosis, and amyloidosis.

Treatment

Patients with DCM are treated in a way similar to those with the syndrome of HF. Treatment targets improvement in heart function, prevention of sudden cardiac death, and reduction of the chance of developing HF and recurrent hospitalizations. The following paragraphs provide a brief summary of pharmacologic and mechanical approaches in the treatment of patients with DCM.

Pharmacologic treatment

Diuretics Diuretic therapy is reserved for patients who have fluid overload or patients with symptoms of HF. Thiazide diuretics increase the fractional excretion of sodium by 5% to 10%. The ability of thiazides to cause natriuresis declines with declining creatinine clearance. Loop diuretics, including furosemide, torsemide, and bumetanide, increase the fractional excretion of sodium by 20% to 25% and maintain natriuretic properties even at relatively low Glomerular filtration rates (GFRs). Loop diuretics have evolved as the mainstay of diuretic therapy for patients with HF. Non-loop diuretics, most commonly metolazone, can be added to a loop diuretic to enhance diuresis in resistant cases of fluid overload and HF.

β-Blockers In over 20 published trials, enrolling over 20,000 patients with HF, the β-blockers carvedilol, metoprolol succinate, and bisoprolol have been shown to have significant clinical benefit. These β-blockers reduce the risk of death, reduce the combined end point of death and hospitalization, enhance well-being, and lessen symptoms in patients with HF. Trial data do not exist for the use of β-blockers in patients with asymptomatic LV dysfunction. Despite the lack of data from a randomized controlled trial, the use of β-blockers in this population is a Class I recommendation in the most recent ACC/AHA Guidelines on the management of HF.[50] Unless otherwise contraindicated, all patients with HF due to depressed LV systolic function should be treated with one of the 3 β-blockers that have been proved to have the greatest clinical benefit. These drugs should be started as soon as LV dysfunction is diagnosed and normovolemia is accomplished.[51–53]

Angiotensin-converting enzyme inhibitors (ACEI) or angiotensin receptor blockers (ARB) ACEI have been studied in over 30 trials enrolling more than 7000 patients with HF. These trials have consistently shown that ACEI can improve mortality and the combined risk of death and hospitalization.[54,55] In addition, these agents improve symptomatic status and improve the sense of well-being of the patient with HF. Benefits have been demonstrated in patients with mild, moderate, or severe symptoms. Asymptomatic patients have been proved to have a mortality benefit from long-term ACEI therapy.[56] In the absence of contraindication, all patients with LV systolic dysfunction, whether symptomatic or asymptomatic, should be treated with ACEI. When patients are unable to tolerate ACEI, the use of ARB is an acceptable alternative.[57]

Digoxin The benefit of digoxin is limited to improving symptoms in patients with advanced systolic HF and atrial fibrillation. Digoxin has not been shown to alter prognosis of patients with severe HF.[58]

Aldosterone antagonists Aldosterone antagonists can improve survival and reduce hospitalization in patients with advanced HF symptoms (Class III and IV NYHC [New York Heart Class]). The role of these antagonists in less-symptomatic patients with DCM is not established.[59]

Anticoagulation Chronic HF is associated with an increased risk of cerebral embolus, presumably related to LV thrombi, which may form as a consequence of a localized hypercoagulable state. The value of chronic anticoagulation in patients with atrial fibrillation has been well documented. The value of chronic anticoagulation in patients with depressed LV systolic function in sinus rhythm was recently studied in the warfarin versus aspirin in reduced cardiac ejection fraction (WARCEF) trial.[60] In this study, the risk of ischemic stroke was reduced from 4.7% in patients treated with aspirin to 2.5% in patients treated with warfarin to a target international normalized ratio (INR) of 2.0 to 3.5. The primary outcome of the trial, however, was a composite of death, ischemic stroke, or intracerebral hemorrhage, and there was no significant difference between the 2 groups with regard to the primary outcome. The reduction in embolic stroke risk by chronic anticoagulation therapy was offset by an increased risk of major bleeding in the WARCEF trial. At this time, there seems to be no trial evidence that would support the use of warfarin in patients with HF in sinus rhythm.

Mechanical treatment

Cardiac resynchronization therapy (biventricular pacing) Prolonged QRS on the ECG in patients who develop HF has been associated with cardiac dyssynchrony that has deleterious effects on ventricular function and HF symptoms. This association has been identified as a predictor of sudden death, worsening HF, and total mortality. Biventricular pacing has been developed as a treatment of the dyssynchrony seen in patients with HF with a wide QRS. In this procedure, pacing leads are placed in the RV and LV. Clinical trials studying patients with moderate to severe HF and wide QRS complexes on the ECG have demonstrated a 30% reduction in hospitalization and a 24% to 36% reduction in mortality.[61–63] Most patients studied in cardiac resynchronization trials (CRT) have had an left bundle branch block (LBBB). Uncertainty persists in the magnitude of benefit of biventricular pacing in patients with wide QRS due to right bundle branch block. CRT in patients with less-symptomatic HF was studied in the multicenter automatic defibrillator implantation trial (MADIT)-CRT trial.[64] Relatively asymptomatic patients were randomized to implantable cardiac defibrillator (ICD) therapy with CRT versus ICD therapy alone. All patients had an EF less than 30% and a QRS greater than 130 ms. Survival free of HF was significantly improved in patients randomized to CRT, and these patients were also found to have a 11% increase in their left ventricular ejection fraction (LVEF). Based on these results and other studies, biventricular pacing is now often performed in patients without severe HF symptoms with an EF less than 30% and a wide complex QRS.

Implantable defibrillators for prevention of sudden cardiac death Patients with depressed LV systolic function and prior history of ventricular fibrillation or sustained ventricular tachycardia have a high risk of recurrent life-threatening arrhythmia. Implantation of a defibrillator is associated with improved mortality outcomes in these patients, and, in the absence of contraindications to defibrillator therapy (eg, concomitant illness that would limit lifespan independent of arrhythmia therapy), such therapy is indicated.[65–67]

Key Points

Pharmacologic treatment of dilated cardiomyopathy includes β-blockers and angiotensin-converting enzyme inhibitors.

In patients with decompensated dilated cardiomyopathy, aldosterone blockers and digoxin may be added.

Alcohol should be avoided in patients with dilated cardiomyopathy.

Biventricular pacing in patients with reduced EF and wide QRS complex on electrocardiogram can improve EF, reduce hospitalization, and reduce mortality.

Implantable defibrillators reduce the occurrence of sudden death in patients with an EF of <35%.

In patients with dilated cardiomyopathy and normal sinus rhythm, warfarin is not indicated.

Takotsubo cardiomyopathy is stress mediated and generally reversible with good prognosis.

The role of defibrillator therapy for patients with depressed LV systolic function but without prior life threatening arrhythmia has been the subject of randomized clinical investigation. In the MADIT II trial, mortality rates were reduced from 19.8% to 14.2% in patients with prior myocardial infarction and an EF of 30% or less. In 2005, Bardy and colleagues[68] reported in the Sudden Cardiac Death in Heart Failure Trial (SCD-HeFT) that the risk of death was reduced from 29% to 22% by the use of defibrillator therapy in patients with an EF of 35% or less, regardless of the cause of the LV dysfunction. Patients with nonischemic as well as ischemic cardiomyopathy benefited in the improvement of mortality with ICD therapy. Although antiarrhythmic therapy may be used in patients with recurring ventricular arrhythmias, in the hope of minimizing discharges of a defibrillator, empirical antiarrhythmic therapy for primary prevention of life-threatening arrhythmia has not been associated with a mortality benefit. The most efficacious antiarrhythmic with the least proarrhythmic potential (amiodarone) was studied in SCD-HeFT, and the overall mortality was not improved with drug therapy. ICDs are now advised for patients with an EF of 35% or less at least 40 days from a myocardial infarction and on optimal medical therapy. As a significant number of patients will have an improvement in their EF with a period of optimal medical therapy, a time interval from the time of HF diagnosis to implantation of an ICD is advised.

Restrictive Cardiomyopathy

RCM is defined as a heart muscle disease that impairs ventricular filling because of muscle stiffness characterized by diastolic dysfunction and diastolic heart failure. Typically, either or both ventricles have normal or decreased diastolic filling with normal systolic ventricular function at least in the early phases of the disease.[69]

RCM may be idiopathic, infiltrative, treatment-induced, or due to malignancy. RCM may be seen in systemic diseases such as amyloidosis (**Fig. 5**) (most common cause in the United States), sarcoidosis, hemochromatosis, hypereosinophilic syndromes in its 2 forms Loeffler endocarditis and endomyocardial fibrosis (the latter seen in tropical areas and also known as Davie disease), carcinoid heart disease, progressive systemic sclerosis, and glycogen storage of the heart, and it may be iatrogenically induced by radiation and chemotherapy (anthracycline toxicity).[70,71] RCM accounts for about 5% of all primary heart muscle disease. RCM needs to be distinguished from constrictive pericarditis because the latter may present clinically and hemodynamically in a similar way but its treatment is very different.

Both patients with RCM and constrictive pericarditis may present with dyspnea on exertion or nocturnal dyspnea, poor exercise tolerance, lower extremity edema,

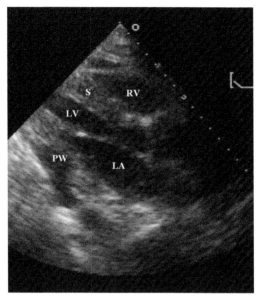

Fig. 5. Echocardiographic appearance of amyloid-induced hypertrophic cardiomyopathy showing the thickened septum (S) and posterior wall (PW). LA, left atrium; LV, left ventricle; RV, right ventricle.

cough, and overall malaise and fatigue. On examination, the jugular vein is elevated with deep x and y descents. Kussmaul sign is also present. Peripheral edema, ascites, and hepatomegaly may be present. In RCM an S3 is present. Extracardiac manifestations of a systemic disorder may provide a clue to the cause of RCM. When pleural effusions are present, diminished breath sounds are noted on pulmonary examination.

Echocardiographic findings of RCM show restrictive mitral inflow velocities with respiration. Also, hepatic vein systolic flow reversals are more noticeable with inspiration. These findings can help distinguish RCM from constrictive pericardial disease.

The following paragraphs briefly discuss specific entities of RCM.

Idiopathic RCM has no known cause and presents itself with restrictive hemodynamics. It is equally present in males and females. A familial pattern is present in some cases. Both right-sided and left-sided HF are typically present, and one-third of the patients may have thromboembolic complications. Patients do not need to have significant left ventricular hypertrophy (LVH) or distinct pathologic findings. Generally, interstitial fibrosis is present to various degrees, minimal to extensive.

Amyloidosis-induced RCM is secondary to amyloid protein deposit in the cardiac cells. Depending on the amyloid protein composition, amyloidosis is classified into 4 different types:

- Primary amyloidosis or myeloma related: because of myeloma protein fibrils are diffusely deposited throughout the myocardium in all 4 cardiac chambers.
- Secondary amyloidosis
- Senile amyloidosis: common in elderly patients
- Familial amyloidosis

Echocardiography shows (see **Fig. 5**) a granular sparkling appearance. This is not, however, diagnostic of amyloidosis. Biventricular thickening and biatrial enlargement

---

Key Points

Restrictive cardiomyopathy needs to be distinguished from constrictive pericarditis because both present very similarly.

Echocardiography helps in distinguishing restrictive myocardial disease from constrictive pericarditis.

Treatment targets the cause of restrictive cardiomyopathy when it is known.

Amyloidosis in the most common cause of restrictive cardiomyopathy in the United States.

---

are seen. The ejection fraction is typically normal. Doppler echo shows a restrictive filling pattern. Results of a cardiac biopsy can confirm the diagnosis.

Hypereosinophilic-syndrome-induced RCM can be due to Loeffler endocarditis and endomyocardial fibrosis (Davie disease). Eosinophilic cardiomyopathy or Loeffler endocarditis occurs because of prolonged eosinophilia infiltrating the myocardium and causing heart injury. Endomyocardial fibrosis occurs as a result, along with thickening of the myocardium, obliteration of the ventricular cavity, and thrombus formation. Endomyocardial fibrosis, seen in tropical areas, does not exhibit eosinophilia but is pathologically similar to Loeffler endocarditis. Generally, patients have poor prognosis with diffuse involvement of the heart.

Treatment

Treatment targets the cause of RCM when it is known. Generally, prognosis is poor and therapy is mostly to improve quality of life. The main categories of medications used are anticoagulants, diuretics, antiarrhythmics, steroids, and chemotherapy. These medications are tailored to each individual case. Heart transplant may be considered in severely symptomatic cases.

Hypertrophic Cardiomyopathy (HCM)

HCM affects 0.2% of the general population.[72,73] HCM is defined as an unexplained degree of LVH with a normal LV cavity size. The hallmark of HCM is LVH with a maximal LV wall thickness of greater than or equal to 15 mm. Although it is a genetic disease, phenotypic expression may range from no hypertrophy to maximal hypertrophy with a pattern of diffuse or segmental hypertrophy.[74–76] The disease is caused by autosomal dominant mutations in genes encoding protein components of the sarcomere and its myofilaments.[77,78]

The clinical presentation of HCM is variable ranging from normal life expectancy with no symptoms to serious complications including sudden cardiac death.[79–81] Progression of HCM to complications can be the result of ventricular arrhythmias, HF, and/or atrial fibrillation with secondary thrombotic complications.[82] Obstructive HCM is dynamic and changes with contractility and preload/afterload changes of the ventricles. Obstructive HCM is present when the peak instantaneous LV outflow gradient is more than 30 mm Hg at rest or with provocative measures.[83,84] In symptomatic patients with gradients greater than or equal to 50 mm Hg (at rest or with provocation), septal reduction therapy is indicated. Familial inheritance and genetic counseling is recommended in patients with HCM. Patients at high risk of sudden cardiac death are those with a prior history of ventricular arrhythmias, family history of sudden death, unexplained syncope, nonsustained ventricular tachycardia on Holter monitoring, and wall thickness that is equal to or exceeds 30 mm.

Echocardiography is commonly used to diagnose HCM. CMR imaging is increasingly being used to diagnose HCM particularly in patients in whom echocardiography

---

Key Points

The hallmark of HCM is LVH with a maximal left ventricular wall thickness greater than or equal to 15 mm.

Obstructive HCM is present when the peak instantaneous LV outflow gradient is more than 30 mm Hg at rest or with provocative measures.

Echocardiography and cardiac magnetic resonance are used to diagnose hypertrophic cardiomyopathy.

High-dose diuretics and vasodilators should be avoided because they worsen the degree of LV outflow obstruction.

β-Blockers (first-line therapy) or cardioselective calcium channel blockers (verapamil) are the mainstay of pharmacology therapy.

Surgical septal myectomy and alcohol septal ablation should be reserved to patients with severe symptoms and should be avoided in asymptomatic patients.

---

is inconclusive. CMR provides a sharp contrast between blood and the myocardium and can define well the presence and pattern of hypertrophy. Patients with HCM should be screened for risk factors for atherosclerosis. Myocardial perfusion imaging is less reliable in patients with HCM because it can lead to reversible or fixed defects even in the absence of obstructive coronary disease.

Multiple therapeutic interventions have been implemented to treat patients with HCM. Patients with HCM should avoid strenuous activity or competitive sports.[85] High-dose diuretics and vasodilators should be avoided because they worsen the degree of LV outflow obstruction. β-Blockers (first-line therapy) or cardioselective calcium channel blocker (verapamil) are the mainstay of pharmacology therapy. Disopyramide can be combined with β-blockers or verapamil in symptomatic patients who do not respond to these medications alone. In the setting of acute hypotension in patients with left ventricular outflow tract (LVOT) obstruction, intravenous phenylephrine or another selective vasoconstrictor is needed. ICD to prevent sudden cardiac death (in severely symptomatic patients with EF ≤50% on maximal medical therapy) and various pharmacologic therapies to treat HF symptoms and atrial fibrillation have been used. In patients refractory to medical treatment, permanent pacing may be considered. Surgical septal myectomy and alcohol septal ablation should be reserved to patients with severe symptoms and should be avoided in asymptomatic patients.

MYOCARDITIS

Myocarditis is an acute injury to the myocardium with secondary activated autoimmune response leading to severe inflammatory reaction and subsequent myocardial damage and HF.[86] The most common cause is a viral infection. **Box 5** outlines the causes of myocaditis.

Diagnosis

Adults with acute myocarditis may present with chest pain, shortness of breath, fainting spells, reduced functional capacity, fatigue and malaise, and new-onset atrial or ventricular arrhythmias. Pericarditis symptoms also could be present because the pericardium may be involved (myopericarditis). Symptoms may range from mild to severe HF requiring mechanical support or fulminant myocarditis that leads to death. A history of viral prodromal syndrome may precede the onset of the myocarditis by several days to weeks.[87]

Box 5
Causes of acute myocarditis

Infection: viral, bacterial, protozoal, spirochetal, fungal, rickettsial

Autoimmune disease: giant cell myocarditis, lupus

Systemic diseases: sarcoidosis, celiac disease, hypereosinophilic syndrome

Drug reactions: anthracyclines, cocaine

Environmental: lead, carbon monoxide

Radiation therapy

The ECG in acute myocarditis shows mostly nonspecific T-wave abnormalities. Occasionally, ST elevation is seen and can mimic ST elevation myocardial infarction. Supraventricular or ventricular arrhythmias are also seen in more than half of the patients. A new LBBB is generally associated with a higher rate of adverse events.[88,89]

Cardiac MRI is being used more frequently in the diagnosis of acute myocarditis. Cardiac MRI can identify areas of cardiac edema, hyperemia, and necrosis. MRI-guided endomyocardial biopsy increases the yield of diagnosing myocarditis.[86] Echocardiography provides nonspecific findings of cardiac dilatation, reduced LV function, pericardial effusion, and diastolic dysfunction. The LV is mostly affected, but RV dysfunction is a poor prognostic indicator in acute myocarditis.[90] Endomyocardial biopsy is generally not needed except in 2 situations: recent unexplained HF in the setting of fulminant myocarditis with normal or dilated LV and suspected giant cell myocarditis.[86]

Treatment

Most patients recover with pharmacologic therapy alone with a good prognosis. Patients with HF are treated the same way as those with HF with systolic dysfunction. β-Blockers, angiotensin blockers, and aldosterone inhibitors should be administered. NSAIDs should be avoided because they worsen prognosis.[91] Mechanical hemodynamic support in the acute phase is generally needed for severe cases with hemodynamic compromise. Immunosuppressive therapy is beneficial in chronic virus-negative DCM. Avoidance of aerobic exercise for 6 months is important because it may increase mortality.

Prognosis

Most patients with acute myocarditis recover well with no long-term poor prognosis. If, however, they have HF and reduced EF on presentation, they have 56% mortality

---

Key Points

Acute myocarditis may present with mild symptoms to severe heart failure requiring mechanical support or fulminant myocarditis that leads to death.

Cardiac magnetic resonance imaging (MRI) is being used more frequently in the diagnosis of acute myocarditis.

The left ventricle is mostly affected, but right ventricular dysfunction is a poor prognostic indicator in acute myocarditis.

Patients who survive the acute phase have excellent long-term prognosis except those with giant cell myocarditis.

within 4 years.[92] Patients who survive the acute phase have excellent long-term prognosis except those with giant cell myocarditis in whom transplantation may be necessary.

REFERENCES

1. Khandaker MH, Espinosa RE, Nishimura RA, et al. Pericardial disease: diagnosis and management. Mayo Clin Proc 2010;85:572–93.
2. Spodick DH. Acute cardiac tamponade. N Engl J Med 2003;349:684–90.
3. Imazio M, Demichelis B, Parrini I, et al. Day-hospital treatment of acute pericarditis: a management program for outpatient therapy. J Am Coll Cardiol 2004; 43:1042–6.
4. Bruce MA, Spodick DH. Atypical electrocardiogram in acute pericarditis: characteristics and prevalence. J Electrocardiol 1980;13:61–6.
5. Zayas R, Anguita M, Torres F, et al. Incidence of specific etiology and role of methods for specific etiologic diagnosis of primary acute pericarditis. Am J Cardiol 1995;75:378–82.
6. Permanyer-Miralda G. Acute pericardial disease: approach to the aetiologic diagnosis. Heart 2004;90:252–4.
7. Imazio M, Cecchi E, Demichelis B, et al. Indicators of poor prognosis of acute pericarditis. Circulation 2007;115:2739–44.
8. Maisch B, Seferovic PM, Ristic AD, et al. Guidelines on the diagnosis and management of pericardial diseases executive summary: the task force on the diagnosis and management of pericardial diseases of the European Society of Cardiology. Eur Heart J 2004;25:587–610.
9. Schifferdecker B, Spodick DH. Nonsteroidal anti-inflammatory drugs in the treatment of pericarditis. Cardiol Rev 2003;11:211–7.
10. Imazio M, Bobbio M, Cecchi E, et al. Colchicine in addition to conventional therapy for acute pericarditis: results of the COlchicine for acute PEricarditis (COPE) trial. Circulation 2005;112:2012–6.
11. Soler-Soler J, Sagrista-Sauleda J, Permanyer-Miralda G. Relapsing pericarditis. Heart 2004;90:1364–8.
12. Imazio M, Demichelis B, Parrini I, et al. Management, risk factors, and outcomes in recurrent pericarditis. Am J Cardiol 2005;96:736–9.
13. Ling LH, Oh JK, Breen JF, et al. Calcific constrictive pericarditis: is it still with us? Ann Intern Med 2000;132:444–50.
14. Talreja DR, Nishimura RA, Oh JK, et al. Constrictive pericarditis in the modern era: novel criteria for diagnosis in the cardiac catheterization laboratory. J Am Coll Cardiol 2008;51:315–9.
15. Bertog SC, Thambidorai SK, Parakh K, et al. Constrictive pericarditis: etiology and cause-specific survival after pericardiectomy. J Am Coll Cardiol 2004;43:1445–52.
16. DeValeria PA, Baumgartner WA, Casale AS, et al. Current indications, risks, and outcome after pericardiectomy. Ann Thorac Surg 1991;52:219–24.
17. Sagristà-Sauleda J, Sarrias Mercé A, Soler-Soler J. Diagnosis and management of pericardial effusion. World J Cardiol 2011;3:135–43.
18. Galve E, Garcia-Del-Castillo H, Evangelista A, et al. Pericardial effusion in the course of myocardial infarction: incidence, natural history, and clinical relevance. Circulation 1986;73:294–9.
19. Posner MR, Cohen GI, Skarin AT. Pericardial disease in patients with cancer. The differentiation of malignant from idiopathic and radiation-induced pericarditis. Am J Med 1981;71:407–13.

20. Sagristà-Sauleda J, Mercé J, Permanyer-Miralda G, et al. Clinical clues to the causes of large pericardial effusions. Am J Med 2000;109:95–101.
21. Levine MJ, Lorell BH, Diver DJ, et al. Implications of echocardiographically assisted diagnosis of pericardial tamponade in contemporary medical patients: detection before hemodynamic embarrassment. J Am Coll Cardiol 1991;17:59–65.
22. Guberman BA, Fowler NO, Engel PJ, et al. Cardiac tamponade in medical patients. Circulation 1981;64:633–40.
23. Mercé J, Sagristà-Sauleda J, Permanyer-Miralda G, et al. Correlation between clinical and Doppler echocardiographic findings in patients with moderate and large pericardial effusion: implications for the diagnosis of cardiac tamponade. Am Heart J 1999;138:759–64.
24. Haney S, Sur D, Xu Z. A review and primary care perspective. J Am Board Fam Pract 2005;18:189–98.
25. Roger VL, Go AS, Lloyd-Jones DM, et al. Heart disease and stroke statistics–2011 update: a report from the American Heart Association. Circulation 2011; 123:e18–209.
26. Mann DL, Kent RL, Parsons B, et al. Adrenergic effects on the biology of the adult mammalian cardiocyte. Circulation 1992;85:790–804.
27. Opie LH. The neuroendocrinology of congestive heart failure. Cardiovasc J S Afr 2002;13:171–8.
28. Bauersachs J, Schafer A. Endothelial dysfunction in heart failure: mechanisms and therapeutic approaches. Curr Vasc Pharmacol 2004;2:115–24.
29. Tousoulis D, Charakida M, Stefanadis C. Inflammation and endothelial dysfunction as therapeutic targets in patients with heart failure. Int J Cardiol 2005;100:347–53.
30. Kuhl U, Pauschinger M, Noutsiast M, et al. High prevalence of viral genomes and multiple viral infections in the myocardium of adults with 'idiopathic' left ventricular dysfunction. Circulation 2005;111:887–93.
31. Schmidt MA, Michels VV, Edwards WD, et al. Familial dilated cardiomyopathy. Am J Med Genet 1988;31:135–43.
32. Piano MR. Alcoholic cardiomyopathy: incidence, clinical characteristics, and pathophysiology. Chest 2002;121:1638–50.
33. Mielniczuk LM, Williams K, Davis DR, et al. Frequency of peripartum cardiomyopathy. Am J Cardiol 2006;97:1765–8.
34. Ramaraj R, Sorrell VL. Peripartum cardiomyopathy: causes, diagnosis, and treatment. Cleve Clin J Med 2009;76:289–96.
35. Aguinaga L, Primo J, Anguera I, et al. Long term follow up in patients with PJRT treated with radiofrequency ablation. Pacing Clin Electrophysiol 1998;21:2073–8.
36. Cruz FE, Cheriex EC, Smeets JL, et al. Reversibility of tachycardia induced cardiomyopathy after cure of incessant SVT. J Am Coll Cardiol 1990;16:739–44.
37. Grimm W, Menz V, Hoffmann J, et al. Reversal of tachycardia induced cardiomyopathy following ablation of repetitive monomorphic RV outflow tract tachycardia. Pacing Clin Electrophysiol 2001;24:166–71.
38. Baman TS, Lange DC, Ilg KJ, et al. Relationship between burden of premature ventricular complexes and left ventricular function. Heart Rhythm 2010;7:865–9.
39. Sharkey SW, Lesser JR, Maron BJ. Takotsubo (stress) cardiomyopathy. Circulation 2011;124:e460–2.
40. Swain SM, Whaley FS, Ewer MS. Congestive heart failure in patients treated with doxorubicin: a retrospective analysis of three trials. Cancer 2003;97(11):2869–79.
41. Lipshultz SE, Lipsitz SR, Mone SM, et al. Female sex and drug dose as risk factors for late cardiotoxic effects of doxorubicin therapy for childhood cancer. N Engl J Med 1995;332:1738–43.

42. Steinherz LJ, Steinherz PG, Tan CT, et al. Cardiac toxicity 4 to 20 years after completing anthracycline therapy. JAMA 1991;266:1672–7.
43. Jones LW, Haykowsky MJ, Swartz JJ, et al. Early breast cancer therapy and cardiovascular injury. J Am Coll Cardiol 2007;50:1435–41.
44. Felker GM, Hu W, Hare JM, et al. The spectrum of dilated cardiomyopathy. The Johns Hopkins experience with 1,278 patients. Medicine (Baltimore) 1999; 78(4):270–83.
45. Maraj S, Figueredo VM, Lynn Morris D. Cocaine and the heart. Clin Cardiol 2010; 33:264–9.
46. Mizia-Stec K, Gasior Z, Wojnicz R, et al. Severe dilated cardiomyopathy as a consequence of Ecstasy intake. Cardiovasc Pathol 2008;17:250–3.
47. Samenuk D, Link MS, Homoud MK, et al. Adverse cardiovascular events temporally associated with ma huang, an herbal source of ephedrine. Mayo Clin Proc 2002;77:12–6.
48. Crean AM, Pohl JE. 'Ally McBeal heart?'– drug induced cardiomyopathy in a young woman. Br J Clin Pharmacol 2004;58(5):558–9.
49. Bonow RO, Carabello BA, Chatterjee K, et al. ACC/AHA 2006 guidelines for the management of patients with valvular heart disease: a report of the American College of Cardiology/American Heart Association Task Force on Practice Guidelines (Writing Committee to Develop Guidelines for the Management of Patients With Valvular Heart Disease). J Am Coll Cardiol 2006;48:e1–148.
50. Hunt SA, Baker DW, Chin MH, et al. ACC/AHA guidelines for the evaluation and management of chronic heart failure in the adult: executive summary. Circulation 2001;104:2996–3007.
51. CIBIS-II Investigators. The cardiac insufficiency bisoprolol study II (CIBIS-II): a randomised trial. Lancet 1999;353:9–13.
52. Hjalmarson A, Goldstein S, Fagerberg B, et al. Effects of controlled-release metoprolol on total mortality, hospitalizations, and well-being in patients with heart failure: the Metoprolol CR/XL Randomized Intervention Trial in congestive heart failure (MERIT-HF). MERIT-HF Study Group. JAMA 2000;283:1295–302.
53. Packer M, Bristow MR, Cohn JN, et al. The effect of carvedilol on morbidity and mortality in patients with chronic heart failure. U.S. Carvedilol Heart Failure Study Group. N Engl J Med 1996;334:1349–55.
54. Effect of enalapril on survival in patients with reduced left ventricular ejection fractions and congestive heart failure. The SOLVD Investigators. N Engl J Med 1991; 325:293–302.
55. Effects of enalapril on mortality in severe congestive heart failure. Results of the Cooperative North Scandinavian Enalapril Survival Study (CONSENSUS). CONSENSUS Trial Study Group. N Engl J Med 1987;316:1429–35.
56. Effect of enalapril on mortality and the development of heart failure in asymptomatic patients with reduced left ventricular ejection fractions. The SOLVD Investigators. N Engl J Med 1992;327:685–91.
57. Eisenberg MJ, Gioia LC. Angiotensin II receptor blockers in congestive heart failure. Cardiol Rev 2006;14:26–34.
58. The effect of digoxin on mortality and morbidity in patients with heart failure. The Digitalis Investigation Group. N Engl J Med 1997;336:525–33.
59. Pitt B, Zannad F, Remme WJ, et al. The effect of spironolactone on morbidity and mortality in patients with severe heart failure. Randomized Aldactone Evaluation Study Investigators. N Engl J Med 1999;341:709–17.
60. Homma S, Thompson JL, Pullicino PM, et al, WARCEF Investigators. Warfarin and aspirin in patients with heart failure and sinus rhythm. N Engl J Med 2012;366:1859–69.

61. Bristow MR, Saxon LA, Boehmer J, et al. Comparison of medical therapy, pacing, and defibrillation in heart failure (COMPANION) Investigators. Cardiac-resynchronization therapy with or without an implantable defibrillator in advanced chronic heart failure. N Engl J Med 2004;350:2140–50.

62. Leon AR, Abraham WT, Brozena S, et al, InSync III Clinical Study Investigators. Cardiac resynchronization with sequential biventricular pacing for the treatment of moderate-to-severe heart failure. J Am Coll Cardiol 2005;46:2298–304.

63. Leon AR, Abraham WT, Curtis AB, et al, MIRACLE Study Program. Safety of transvenous cardiac resynchronization system implantation in patients with chronic heart failure: combined results of over 2,000 patients from a multicenter study program. J Am Coll Cardiol 2005;46:2348–56.

64. Moss AJ, Hall WJ, Cannom DS, et al, MADIT-CRT Trial Investigators. Cardiac-resynchronization therapy for the prevention of heart-failure events. N Engl J Med 2009;361:1329–38.

65. Moss AJ. MADIT-I and MADIT-II. J Cardiovasc Electrophysiol 2003;14(Suppl 9):S96–8.

66. Moss AJ, Greenberg H, Case RB, et al, Multicenter Automatic Defibrillator Implantation Trial-II (MADIT-II) Research Group. Long-term clinical course of patients after termination of ventricular tachyarrhythmia by an implanted defibrillator. Circulation 2004;110:3760–5.

67. Moss AJ, Zareba W, Hall WJ, et al, Multicenter Automatic Defibrillator Implantation Trial II Investigators. Prophylactic implantation of a defibrillator in patients with myocardial infarction and reduced ejection fraction. N Engl J Med 2002; 346:877–83.

68. Bardy GH, Lee KL, Mark DB, et al, Sudden Cardiac Death in Heart Failure Trial (SCD-HeFT) Investigators. Amiodarone or an implantable cardioverter–defibrillator for congestive heart failure. N Engl J Med 2005;352:225–37.

69. Kushwaha SS, Fallon JT, Fuster V. Restrictive cardiomyopathy. N Engl J Med 1997;336:267–76.

70. Nihoyannopoulos P, Dawson D. Restrictive cardiomyopathies. Eur J Echocardiogr 2009;10:iii23–33.

71. Wald DS, Gray HH. Restrictive cardiomyopathy in systemic amyloidosis. QJM 2003;96:380–2.

72. Zou Y, Song L, Wang Z, et al. Prevalence of idiopathic hypertrophic cardiomyopathy in China: a population-based echocardiographic analysis of 8080 adults. Am J Med 2004;116:14–8.

73. Maron BJ, Gardin JM, Flack JM, et al. Prevalence of hypertrophic cardiomyopathy in a general population of young adults: echocardiographic analysis of 4111 subjects in the CARDIA Study Coronary Artery Risk Development in (Young) Adults. Circulation 1995;92:785–9.

74. Maron BJ, Yeates L, Semsarian C. Clinical challenges of genotype positive (+)-phenotype negative (-) family members in hypertrophic cardiomyopathy. Am J Cardiol 2011;107:604–8.

75. Klues HG, Schiffers A, Maron BJ. Phenotypic spectrum and patterns of left ventricular hypertrophy in hypertrophic cardiomyopathy: morphologic observations and significance as assessed by two-dimensional echocardiography in 600 patients. J Am Coll Cardiol 1995;26:1699–708.

76. Maron MS, Maron BJ, Harrigan C, et al. Hypertrophic cardiomyopathy phenotype revisited after 50 years with cardiovascular magnetic resonance. J Am Coll Cardiol 2009;54:220–8.

77. Seidman JG, Seidman C. The genetic basis for cardiomyopathy: from mutation identification to mechanistic paradigms. Cell 2001;104:557–67.

78. Alcalai R, Seidman JG, Seidman CE. Genetic basis of hypertrophic cardiomyopathy: from bench to the clinics. J Cardiovasc Electrophysiol 2008;19:104–10.
79. Cannan CR, Reeder GS, Bailey KR, et al. Natural history of hypertrophic cardiomyopathy: a population-based study, 1976 through 1990. Circulation 1995;92: 2488–95.
80. Maron BJ. Hypertrophic cardiomyopathy: a systematic review. JAMA 2002;287: 1308–20.
81. Elliott PM, Poloniecki J, Dickie S, et al. Sudden death in hypertrophic cardiomyopathy: identification of high risk patients. J Am Coll Cardiol 2000;36:2212–8.
82. Gersh BJ, Maron BJ, Bonow RO, et al. 2011 ACCF/AHA guideline for the diagnosis and treatment of hypertrophic cardiomyopathy: executive summary: a report of the American College of Cardiology Foundation/American Heart Association Task Force on Practice Guidelines. J Am Coll Cardiol 2011;58:2703–38.
83. Panza JA, Petrone RK, Fananapazir L, et al. Utility of continuous wave Doppler echocardiography in the noninvasive assessment of left ventricular outflow tract pressure gradient in patients with hypertrophic cardiomyopathy. J Am Coll Cardiol 1992;19:91–9.
84. Sasson Z, Yock PG, Hatle LK, et al. Doppler echocardiographic determination of the pressure gradient in hypertrophic cardiomyopathy. J Am Coll Cardiol 1988; 11:752–6.
85. Spirito P, Seidman CE, McKenna WJ, et al. The management of hypertrophic cardiomyopathy. N Engl J Med 1997;336:775–85.
86. Blauwet LA, Cooper LT. Myocarditis. Prog Cardiovasc Dis 2010;52:274–88.
87. Hufnagel G, Pankuweit S, Richter A, et al. The European Study of Epidemiology and Treatment of Cardiac Inflammatory Diseases (ESETCID). First epidemiological results. Herz 2000;25:279–85.
88. Dec GW Jr, Waldman H, Southern J, et al. Viral myocarditis mimicking acute myocardial infarction. J Am Coll Cardiol 1992;20:85–9.
89. Morgera T, Di Lenarda A, Dreas L, et al. Electrocardiography of myocarditis revisited: clinical and prognostic significance of electrocardiographic changes. Am Heart J 1992;124:455–67.
90. Mendes LA, Dec GW, Picard MH, et al. Right ventricular dysfunction: an independent predictor of adverse outcome in patients with myocarditis. Am Heart J 1994; 128:301–7.
91. Khatib R, Reyes MP, Smith FE. Enhancement of Coxsackievirus B3 replication in Vero cells by indomethacin. J Infect Dis 1990;162:997–8.
92. Mason JW, O'Connell JB, Herskowitz A, et al. A clinical trial of immunosuppressive therapy for myocarditis. The Myocarditis Treatment Trial Investigators. N Engl J Med 1995;333:269–75.

Index

Note: Page numbers of article titles are in **boldface** type.

Prim Care Clin Office Pract 40 (2013) 237–252
http://dx.doi.org/10.1016/S0095-4543(13)00009-2
0095-4543/13/$ – see front matter © 2013 Elsevier Inc. All rights reserved.

primarycare.theclinics.com

Moving?

Make sure your subscription moves with you!

To notify us of your new address, find your **Clinics Account Number** (located on your mailing label above your name), and contact customer service at:

Email: journalscustomerservice-usa@elsevier.com

800-654-2452 (subscribers in the U.S. & Canada)
314-447-8871 (subscribers outside of the U.S. & Canada)

Fax number: 314-447-8029

Elsevier Health Sciences Division
Subscription Customer Service
3251 Riverport Lane
Maryland Heights, MO 63043

*To ensure uninterrupted delivery of your subscription, please notify us at least 4 weeks in advance of move.